RHINOLOGY AND SINUSOLOGY
Diagnosis • Medical Management • Surgical Approaches

Series Editor

Howard L. Levine, M.D., F.A.C.S.
Director, The Mt. Sinai Nasal-Sinus Center
Chief, Section of Nasal-Sinus Surgery
The Mt. Sinai Medical Center
Cleveland, Ohio

Trauma of the Nose and Paranasal Sinuses

Robert H. Mathog, M.D.
Professor and Chairman
Department of Otolaryngology–Head and Neck Surgery
Wayne State University School of Medicine
Detroit, Michigan

Richard L. Arden, M.D.
Assistant Professor
Department of Otolaryngology–Head and Neck Surgery
Wayne State University School of Medicine
Detroit, Michigan

Steven C. Marks, M.D.
Assistant Professor
Department of Otolaryngology–Head and Neck Surgery
Wayne State University School of Medicine
Detroit, Michigan

Illustrated by William Loechel

1995
THIEME MEDICAL PUBLISHERS, INC. New York
GEORG THIEME VERLAG Stuttgart • New York

Thieme Medical Publishers, Inc.
381 Park Avenue South
New York, New York 10016

TRAUMA OF THE NOSE AND PARANASAL SINUSES
Robert H. Mathog
Richard L. Arden
Steven C. Marks

Library of Congress Cataloging-in-Publication Data
Mathog, Robert H., 1939–
Trauma of the nose and paranasal sinuses / Robert H. Mathog, Richard L. Arden, Steven C. Marks ; illustrated by William Loechel.
p. cm.—(Rhinology and sinusology)
Includes bibliographical references and index.
ISBN 0-86577-526-5 (Thieme Medical Publishers).—ISBN 3-13-100141-0 (G. Thieme Verlag)
1. Nose—Wounds and injuries. 2. Paranasal sinuses—Wounds and injuries. I. Arden, Richard L. II. Marks, Steven C. III. Title. IV. Series.
[DNLM: 1. Paranasal Sinuses—injuries. 2. Paranasal Sinuses—surgery. 3. Nasal Bone—injuries. 4. Nasal Bone—surgery. 5. Surgery, Plastic. WV 340 M432t 1995]
RF437.M38 1995
617.5′23044—dc20
DNLM/DLC
for Library of Congress 95-26571
CIP

Important note: Medicine is an ever-changing science. Research and clinical experience are continually broadening our knowledge, in particular our knowledge of proper treatment and drug therapy. Insofar as this book mentions any dosage or applications, readers may rest assured that the authors, editors, and publishers have made every effort to ensure that such references are strictly in accordance with the state of knowledge at the time of production of the book. Nevertheless, every user is requested to carefully examine the manufacturers' leaflets accompanying each drug to check on his own responsibility whether the dosage schedules recommended therein or the contraindications stated by the manufacturers differ from the statements made in the present book. Such examination is particularly important with drugs that are either rarely used or have been newly released on the market.

Printed in the United States of America.

5 4 3 2 1

TMP ISBN 0-86577-526-5
GTV ISBN 3-13-100141-0

Contents

Contributors

Richard L. Arden, M.D.
Assistant Professor
Department of Otolaryngology–Head and Neck Surgery
Wayne State University School of Medicine
Detroit, Michigan

Don L. Burgio, M.S., M.D.
Assistant Professor
Department of Otolaryngology–Head and Neck Surgery
Wayne State University School of Medicine
Detroit, Michigan

Gary B. Coleman, M.D.
Resident
Department of Otolaryngology–Head and Neck Surgery
Wayne State University School of Medicine
Detroit, Michigan

James K. Dziadziola, Jr., M.D.
Resident
Department of Otolaryngology–Head and Neck Surgery
Wayne State University School of Medicine
Detroit, Michigan

Ben Goldwyn, M.D.
Resident
Department of Otolaryngology–Head and Neck Surgery
Wayne State University School of Medicine
Detroit, Michigan

Jorge D. Latoni, M.D.
Resident
Department of Otolaryngology–Head and Neck Surgery
Wayne State University School of Medicine
Detroit, Michigan

Jeffrey S. Leider, M.D.
Clinical Assistant Professor
Department of Otolaryngology–Head and Neck Surgery
Wayne State University School of Medicine
Detroit, Michigan

Steven C. Marks, M.D.
Assistant Professor
Department of Otolaryngology–Head and Neck Surgery
Wayne State University School of Medicine
Detroit, Michigan

Robert H. Mathog, M.D.
Professor and Chairman
Department of Otolaryngology–Head and Neck Surgery
Wayne State University School of Medicine
Detroit, Michigan

Robert J. Meleca, M.D.
Resident
Department of Otolaryngology–Head and Neck Surgery
Wayne State University School of Medicine
Detroit, Michigan

Kevin L. Robinson, M.D.
Department of Otolaryngology
Harper Hospital
Detroit, Michigan

Terry Shibuya, M.D.
Resident
Department of Otolaryngology–Head and Neck Surgery

Wayne State University School of Medicine
Detroit, Michigan

Duane Smith, M.D.
Resident
Department of Otolaryngology–Head and Neck Surgery
Wayne State University School of Medicine
Detroit, Michigan

Foreword

Trauma to the Nose and Paranasal Sinuses is another volume in the ongoing textbook series *Rhinology and Sinusology*. Each of the volumes attempts to present to the health professional accurate and current information on a specific topic of importance in the area of nasal and sinus disorders.

Most of our lives today are fast paced and activity filled. We are all susceptible to nasal and sinus trauma caused by such things as automobile accidents, sports, and violence.

Injuries to the nose and paranasal sinuses often result in some combination of aesthetic and functional problems that may alter a patient's lifestyle. Patients experiencing trauma can be devastated by the alteration in their appearance with its concomitant psychosocial implications. Functional disturbances can affect breathing, olfaction, eating and chewing, and vision. Because of the ramifications of these injuries, proper diagnosis and management of trauma to this area are of the utmost importance.

The authors attempt to provide a complete guide to the sophisticated practitioner managing trauma to the nose and paranasal sinuses. The book deals with both soft tissue and bony injuries. It discusses management of nasal trauma as well as trauma to each of the sinuses. It describes the management of complex injuries, complications from trauma, and long-term sequelae.

Trauma to the Nose and Paranasal Sinuses should serve as a valuable guide and compendium for up-to-date information on the management of injuries in this complex area.

Howard L. Levine, M.D.
Director, The Mt. Sinai Nasal Sinus Center
Cleveland Ear, Nose, Throat and Facial Surgery
Chief, Nasal Sinus Surgery
Division of Otolaryngology, Department of Surgery
The Mt. Sinai Medical Center
Cleveland, Ohio

Preface

Given the complexity of the craniofacial skeleton, and its intimate association with overlying and underlying soft tissue structures, isolated injury of a paranasal sinus or sinuses is uncommon. Rather, concomitant soft tissue trauma, and the immediate and delayed sequela of the injury, frequently eventuate in both functional and aesthetic compromises for the patient. The proximity of the cranial, orbital, and oral cavities to the nasal and paranasal sinuses provides both the mechanism and the means by which complex injury patterns may arise from seemingly "minor" sinus trauma. A thorough understanding of these anatomical relations, related pathophysiology, and essential steps in diagnosis and management are essential for proper care of the patient.

Trauma of the Nose and Paranasal Sinuses is intended to provide a basic conceptual framework for residents and practicing surgeons who deal with trauma in these regions. Its purpose is to supplement, not surplant, more comprehensive, broader scope texts that deal with facial injury. An emphasis has been placed on diagnosis and management with numerous references cited from many overlapping multispecialty fields. The text is organized into chapters individually addressing trauma to a given sinus subsite, as well as related chapters associated with complications of certain injuries (ie, CSF fistula, mucoceles, nasal obstruction). An attempt has been made to incorporate and review standard surgical techniques gleaned from the literature and, whenever possible, to provide the author's personal approach in the management of certain injuries and pathologic states. The numerous illustrations utilized represent original drawings by William Loechel, a noted medical illustrator. We hope readers of this text will find this to be a useful basic reference for understanding nasal and paranasal sinus trauma, and that it stimulates further reading and enhanced clinical practice in this area.

Robert H. Mathog, M.D.
Richard L. Arden, M.D.
Steven C. Marks, M.D.

1

Soft Tissue Trauma

JORGE D. LATONI, M.D.
TERRY SHIBUYA, M.D.
RICHARD L. ARDEN, M.D.

The face delineates one's physical characteristics, hereditary features, and emotional feelings. It is the primary vehicle through which expressive and nonexpressive language is communicated. It is therefore very important for the surgeon who manages soft tissue trauma of the head and neck region to be well acquainted with the basic concepts of soft tissue repair. It is incumbent on the managing physician to see that the best possible result is attained after facial trauma.

The public has become increasingly aware of the health care professionals who specialize in soft tissue trauma to the face. With this knowledge, and the ever-growing medicolegal climate surrounding aesthetic injuries, specialists are often requested to evaluate injuries in the emergency room. When the patient's injuries are severe, a team approach of specialists may be necessary to provide the best comprehensive treatment for an injury to the head and neck region.

MECHANISM OF INJURY

The majority of injuries to the facial region are the result of motor vehicle accidents (Table 1–1). The type of injury sustained is directly related to the position of the victim within the car at the time of the collision. The front-seat passenger is the most vulnerable. Collision studies have shown that the front-seat passenger sustains injuries when thrown forward with the initial collision, then sustains a second crash when being thrown back from the windshield into the front seat.[1]

Advances in windshield construction, airbag systems, and mandatory seat belt laws have prevented more deaths. Survivors though may have more soft tissue injuries of the head and neck. Quite often, injury to the forehead and face show numerous small superficial lacerations, small avulsion flaps, abrasions, hematomas, and soft tissue swelling (Fig. 1–1).

Injuries sustained at home occur more frequently than expected. They may be the result of a slip, fall, or projectile object. They can range in severity from minor to major.

Table 1–1. Causes of Major Facial Injuries from 1042 Consecutive Cases Treated over a 10-Year Period

CAUSE	NO. OF PATIENTS	(%)
Automobile accident	565	(54)
Home accident	171	(17)
Athletic injury	118	(11)
Animal bite	60	(6)
Other	55	(5)
Intended injury	46	(4)
Work injury	27	(3)
Total	1042	(100)

From Schultz.[1]

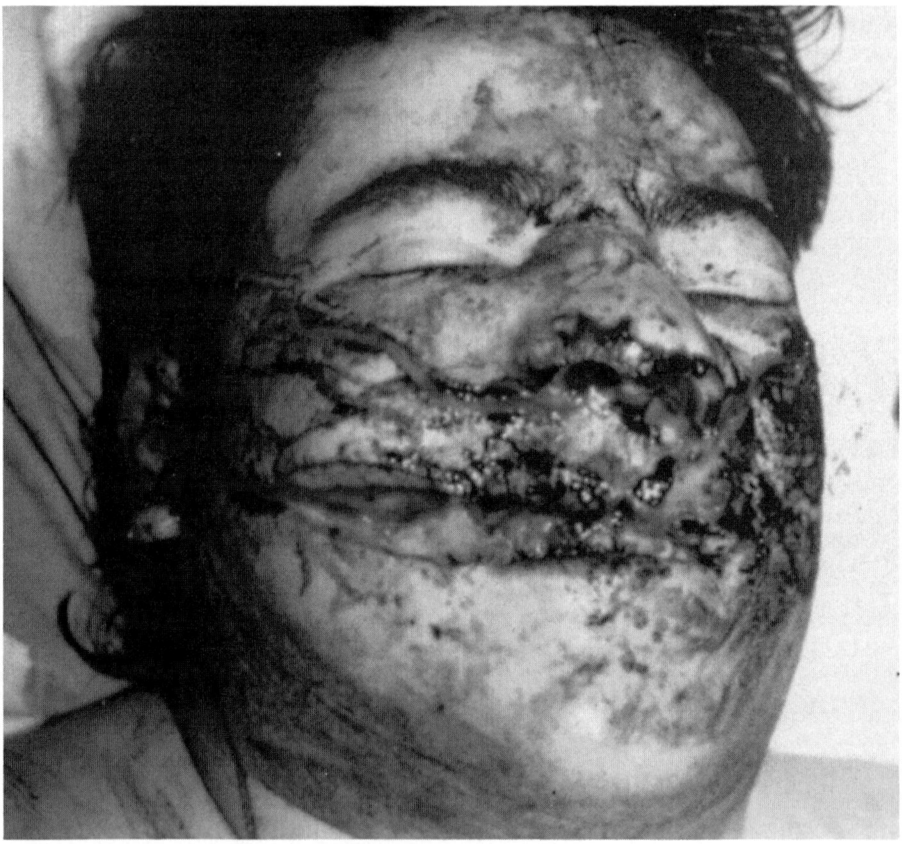

Figure 1–1. Individual who had an explosion in his face resulting in multiple soft tissue and bony injuries of the face.

Animal and human bites create a special problem. Quite often these wounds are contaminated with bacteria and saliva. Facial injuries due to dog bites are the most common in this category and are usually sustained by young children.[2] These wounds are often tearing or avulsive in nature. Careful cosmetic repair of such injuries is very important as it can impact on the child's later psychosocial development.

Athletic injuries account for only a small percentage of injuries to the head and neck region. Most injuries are minor in nature consisting of abrasions, contusions, and lacerations. The injuries should be managed in a timely fashion with appropriate treatment. Injuries may include split lips, avulsed nasal tissue, eyelid lacerations, and auricular hematomas.

Work or industrial accidents are not as common. These accidents may cause severe facial injury. Massive crush injuries, explosions, fires, penetrating objects, and burns to the face may occur. Management of such injuries may be challenging and one should not overlook the possibility of intracranial damage.[1]

Soft tissue injuries resulting from assaults are not as common in suburban or rural environments. Surgeons practicing in an inner city or urban setting are often exposed to patients who have sustained penetrating knife or gunshot injuries to the head and neck. These wounds may not show extensive soft tissue trauma, but may result in more severe internal bony and visceral damage. Thorough investigation of underlying injuries is always warranted.

ANATOMY

The microscopic anatomy of the facial and scalp skin is composed of three main layers: epidermis, dermis, and subcutaneous connective tissue.

The thinnest skin of the head and face is located in the eyelids whereas the thickest skin is found in the hair-bearing areas of the scalp and beard. Epidermal thickness ranges from 0.02 to 1.4 mm, whereas dermal thickness varies from 0.40 to 2.4 mm.[3]

The epidermis is composed of four layers (Fig. 1–2). Cells proliferate from the basal layer to the outer keratotic layer. The stratum basale is a single layer of cells resting on the basal lamina and underlying dermis. Cells in this layer are cuboidal or low columnar and form the germinal layer for proliferating epithelial cells. The next most superficial layer is the stratum spinosum, composed of basophilic cells that have spinous processes. This layer comprises cells distinguished by their development of lamellated granules or membrane-coated granules and tonofibrils. Overlying this layer is the stratum granulosum, which consists of three to five layers of flattened cells that possess irregularly shaped coarse keratohyalin granules that stain intensely with basic dyes and hematoxylin. The stratum corneum, the most superficial layer, is characterized by many layers of flat, cornified cells that lack a nucleus and have a cytoplasm filled with filaments of keratin. This layer loosens and desquamates over time. The entire cytomorphosis takes 15 to 30 days to occur depending on the region of the body. Palmar and plantar skin exhibit a unique layer of stratum lucidum between the stratum granulosum and the stratum corneum.[4]

The dermis underlies the epidermis and provides support and nutrition for the epidermis (Fig. 1–3). The superficial portion of the dermis, known as the papillary dermis, has widely separated collagen and elastic fibers ensheathed by a dermal capillary plexus. The

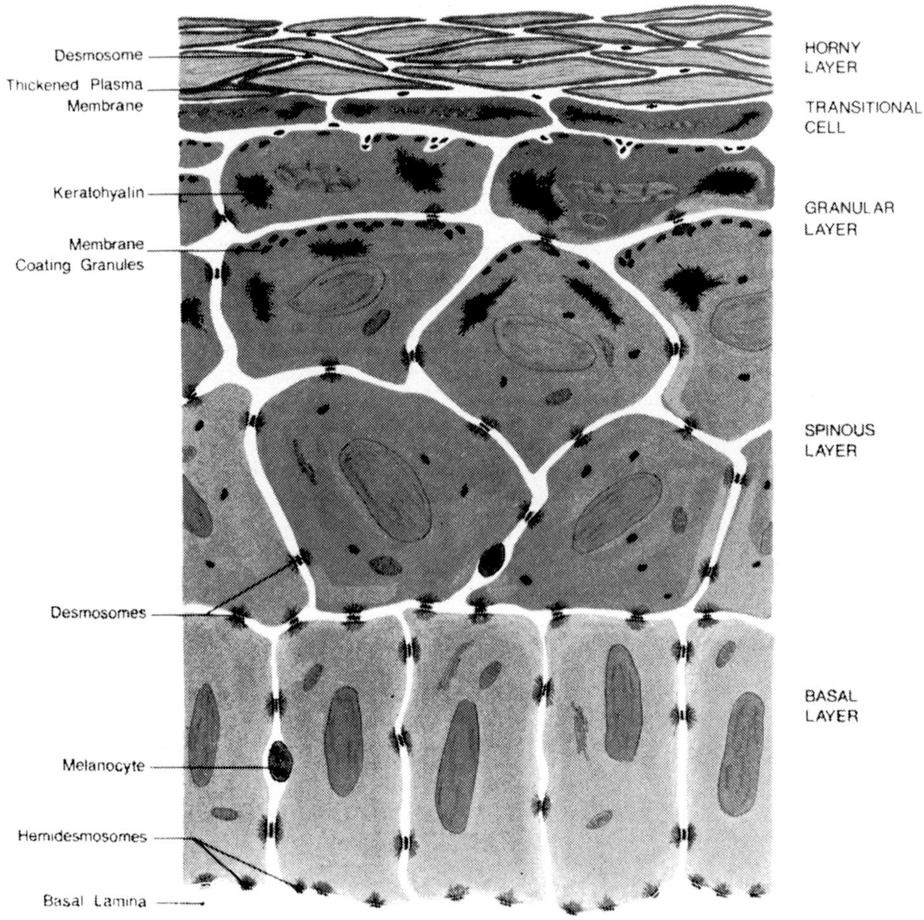

Figure 1–2. Epidermal layers. (Reprinted with permission from Simpson.[3])

deeper layer of dermis is the reticular layer, which has a much more dense connective tissue network. Collagen and elastic fibers running within it are abundant and are oriented parallel to the epidermal surface. The muscles of facial expression terminate in the reticular layer.[4]

The epidermal-dermal junction consists of interdigitating epidermal rete pegs and vascularized dermal papillae. At this junction, neural fibers are found. After soft tissue injury, optimal cutaneous repair is dependent on early reestablishment of a healthy epidermal and dermal relationship. If a laceration penetrates below the depth of the dermal subpapillary plexus of vessels, the blueprint for duplicating skin is lost and scar tissue develops.[3]

The subcutaneous layer is hypodermal in position. This layer has collagen and elastic fibers that are continuous with the overlying dermis. Varying number of fat cells develop in this layer that also contains large blood vessels and nerve trunks.[4]

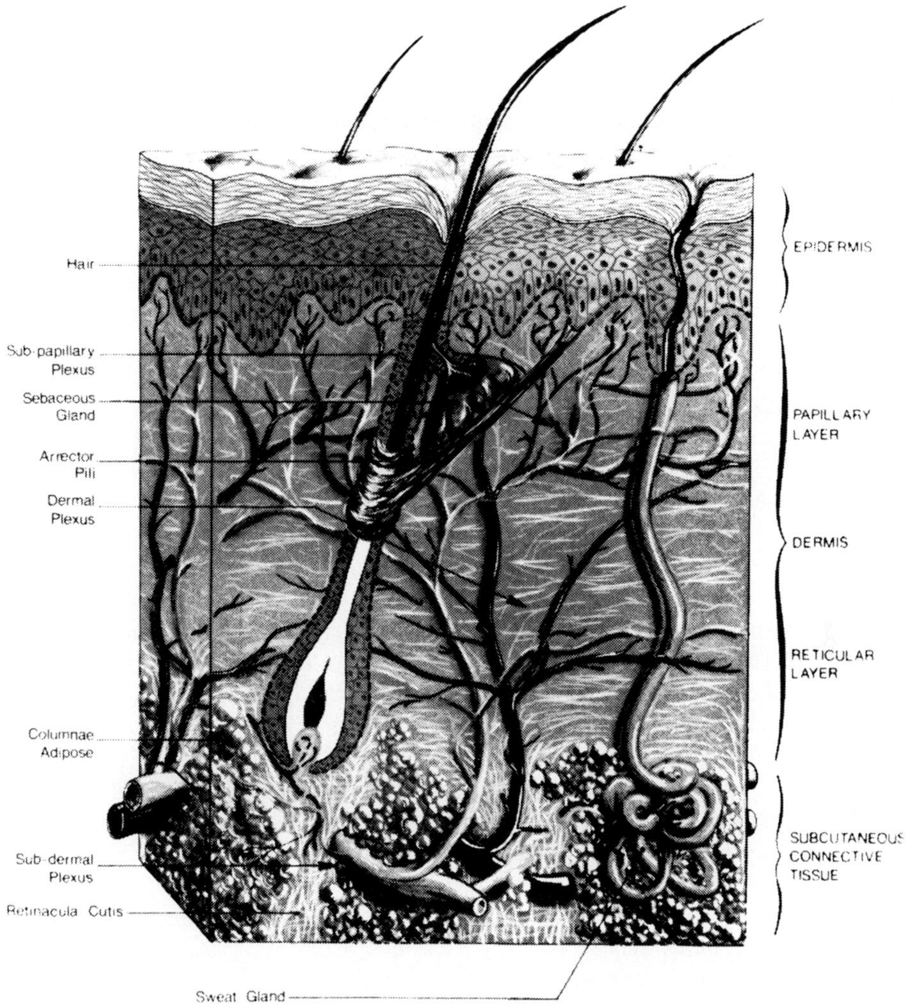

Figure 1–3. Normal skin structures. (Reprinted with permission from Simpson.[3])

INITIAL EVALUATION

When asked to evaluate a patient in the emergency room for a soft tissue injury there are some important questions that should be asked. First, is the patient in stable condition? Has the patient been evaluated adequately by the emergency room service, and have the ABCs of life support been implemented? Oftentimes, in a crowded and busy emergency room injuries can be overlooked, and the consulting physician should not omit a complete physical examination. It is important to make sure the patient's airway is secure. With facial trauma the patient may suffer an injury that can compromise the airway. If necessary, the patient may need to be intubated or have a tracheotomy for adequate airway control. If the patient is bleeding, it is wise to apply a direct pressure dressing to the wound rather than blindly clamp inside an open wound. Clamping blindly may cause more harm by injuring exposed neurovascular structures. Once adequate lighting and instrumentation are available the wound may then be properly examined.

Next, has the patient been cleared from a neurological standpoint regarding intracranial or spinal injuries? If these questions have not been addressed it is important that they be adequately answered before any manipulation of the patient. If the patient is not in stable condition, and other life-threatening injuries need to be treated first, the soft tissue injuries may be covered and managed once the patient is stable.

When treating a soft tissue injury it is important to consider the mechanism and timing of the injury. This will help determine whether the wound is clean and can be closed primarily, or whether the wound is contaminated and should be closed secondarily. The mode of injury will also provide clues about what underlying injuries may exist. High velocity injuries quite often have underlying fractures, whereas sharp penetrating injuries may have underlying vascular or visceral damage.

The patient's tetanus immunization history should also be reviewed. If the patient has not been vaccinated, active and passive immunization should be administered. If no booster has been given in the last 5 years, one should be given. For particularly dirty wounds a booster may be considered even if the patient has received one within the last 5 years.

At the time of initial evaluation a comprehensive physical examination should be performed and a decision should be made as to whether the patient will be better served by closing the soft tissue injury in the operating room or in the emergency room. The presence of a foreign body, facial fracture, injury to the facial nerve, laceration of the parotid duct, or injury to the lacrimal drainage system almost always requires a trip to the operating room. Other indications for repairing injuries in the operating room include an uncooperative patient (ie, children), extensive lacerations with loss of tissue, extensive time needed for repair, or inadequate lighting or instrumentation available for repair.

Additional questions regarding the patient's past medical history should be asked. If the patient is unconscious or unable to answer, a family member may be of assistance. A history of diabetes mellitus, chronic obstructive pulmonary disease, smoking, or peripheral vascular disease may impede the wound-healing process. Consent should be obtained from the patient or family member with the understanding that further scar revision or reconstructive procedures may be necessary and no guarantees of esthetic results can be made. Photographic documentation of selected injuries are also valuable adjuncts in today's medicolegal climate.

TREATMENT

Cleansing and Debridement

Proper cleansing of the wound is vital to provide the optimal healing environment while minimizing the chance of infection and scarring. Sharp debridement with scalpels and mechanical abrasion with scrub brushes are the mainstays of management for cleansing the grossly contaminated wound. Dirt and foreign bodies may be removed using mild soap, normal saline, or diluted povidone-iodine solution. Irrigation is an important adjunct to sharp debridement. Irrigation should be performed with a pulsating jet lavage system as this has been shown to remove significantly more bacteria and results in fewer wound infections than more conventional low pressure irrigation.[5] In the emergency room or operating room a 19-gauge needle attached to a syringe may be used as a modification of the pulsating jet lavage. If grease or oil is present, it may be removed with ether, acetone, or xylol. The use of hydrogen peroxide for cleansing wounds is discouraged as it creates an exothermic reaction that is toxic to the tissues and hinders the wound healing process.

Foreign particles due to asphalt or other material imbedded in the dermal layer should be removed as soon as possible. They will become fixed in the tissue in approximately 12 to 24 hours. This is best done with the patient under general anesthesia. Scrubbing the involved area with a sterile scrub brush and mild soap may be adequate. If the foreign particles are already fixed in the tissue it may be necessary to use a dermabrader to clean the area. Isolated foreign bodies may be individually removed using a no. 11 blade scalpel. When using the scrub brush or dermabrader it is very important for the surgeon not to remove the papillary dermal layer or permanent damage and scarring may result.[6]

Extensive debridement of facial soft tissues is generally not advisable, particularly in the nasal alae, eyelid, and lip regions. Because the face has an excellent blood supply, tissue injured in these regions almost always survives, and extensive debridement may lead to poor aesthetic and functional results.

Lacerations that have minimal tissue injury, but have jagged edges, typically benefit from freshening of the wound edges. Excision of 2 to 3 mm of tissue around the edges is performed to provide precise tissue alignment and reduced scarring.

ANESTHESIA

Local anesthesia utilizing injectable xylocaine with epinephrine is usually adequate for the management of minor injuries. An accurate assessment for possible sensory or motor nerve injuries should precede local infiltration with the anesthetic solution. When feasible, regional nerve blocks are preferred as they require less anesthetic and result in less tissue distortion. If a procedure requires a longer length of time, the use of a longer acting local anesthetic such as Marcaine or bupivacaine should be considered. When using a local agent with epinephrine, it is important to wait at least 15 minutes to allow maximal vasoconstrictor effect to occur. If a large amount of local anesthetic is required, always check the maximal dose of medication that may be administered calculated for weight and age of the patient. Procedures requiring extensive work, or involving an uncooperative patient, typically benefit from a general anesthetic.

TIMING OF CLOSURE

Once the patient has been cleared from a medical standpoint to have the wound closed the surgeon must determine whether the wound should be closed primarily or secondarily. All soft tissue injuries are contaminated to some degree. If a wound is contaminated with greater than 10^5 bacteria per gram of tissue, or is culture positive for β-hemolytic streptococci, this is a contraindication for wound closure.[7] Unfortunately, quantitative wound cultures take approximately 18 to 36 hours for results and are not the most cost-effective means of determining contamination. An accurate history of the wounding event is generally the most helpful information in determining the extent to which a wound is contaminated. Wounds that have been exposed to dirt, gravel, grease, animal bites, human bites, saliva, or dirty objects are considered contaminated and may benefit from a delayed closure. Wounds that have been caused by clean objects, and wounds that are immediately cleaned and protected from contaminating foreign bodies, may be considered clean and closed primarily. If the extent of contamination is questionable, a representative specimen may be removed from the wound, weighed, diluted, and homogenized. A 0.02-mL aliquot of the suspension is then placed on a glass slide and gram stained. If a single organism is seen on the slide, the bacterial count in the original biopsy will be greater than 10^5 organisms per gram of tissue. If no organisms are seen, the count will be less than 10^5 organisms per gram of tissue.[8] This procedure usually takes approximately 15 minutes.

The majority of injuries may be closed primarily. Robson et al[9] reported that in 80 wounds (upper extremity, 30; lower extremity, 33; scalp, 9; face, 8) presenting to an urban emergency room department, approximately 20% yielded at least 10^5 organisms per gram of tissue. In this study, 75% of the wounds were limited to the skin and subcutaneous tissue whereas 25% of the wounds involved deeper structures.

Animal bites are contaminated wounds that are usually caused by dogs. Studies have shown that dogs that are fed meal compared with meat have lower bacterial levels in their saliva. Dogs fed meal had 10^4 to 10^5 bacteria per milliliter of saliva whereas dogs fed meat had 10^7 to 10^8 bacteria per milliliter of saliva. This may be of use when trying to determine whether to close a bite wound primarily or secondarily.[5]

In addition, human saliva contains high bacterial counts (10^7 to 10^8 bacteria per milliliter of saliva) and is the justification for delayed primary closures in this setting.[5]

Elapsed time from wounding is another factor that needs to be taken into account prior to closure. Studies have shown patients with less than 10^2 bacteria per gram of wound tissue presented for treatment an average of 2.2 hours after their injury. Patients with 10^2 to 10^5 bacteria per gram of wound tissue presented for treatment an average of 3 hours after their injury, and those with greater than 10^5 organisms per gram presented for treatment an average of 5.17 hours after their injury.[9] The facial region is fortunate to have an excellent blood supply that enables it to handle a bacterial inoculum for a longer period of time by comparison with other regions of the body. With these factors in mind, maximal time for primary closure involving injuries to the head and neck should generally be restricted to 6 to 8 hours. If the wound cannot be closed in this time period because of an unstable medical condition, or delays in seeking medical attention, secondary closure should be considered. Quantitative cultures showing less than 10^5 bacteria per gram of tissue, and qualitative cultures showing no β-hemolytic streptococci growth, will give optimal conditions for secondary closure.[5] Krizek et al[10] have shown that in a series of 50 skin grafts, if the recipient granulation bed had less than 10^5 bacteria per gram of tissue on the day of grafting, there was a 93% success rate. By contrast, if the recipient granulation bed had greater than 10^5 bacteria per gram of tissue on the day of grafting, there was only a 19% success rate.

TECHNIQUE

Undermining

The purpose of undermining wound edges before their approximation is to increase tissue mobilization for better distribution of skin tension during closure. This may also aid skin eversion by facilitating the accurate placement of subcutaneous sutures.

If a wound is initially closed under excessive tension it is likely that scar widening will occur. In soft tissue trauma it is sometimes not a good idea to perform wide undermining for fear that further tissue anoxia may occur; however, judicious undermining in some cases is necessary to assist in the approximation of tissue layers under minimal tension. In general, the greater the tissue loss, the greater the resultant tension on the wound edges will be when primary closure is attempted. This increased tension will necessitate wider undermining of the wound edges to improve skin edge mobilization and thus reduce the skin tension. Increased tension at the skin edges is also seen in wounds that lie perpendicular to the relaxed skin tension lines and in wounds overlying highly mobile areas. Older patients, with increased skin laxity, may require less undermining than a child for example, to close a similar size wound edge gap under minimal tension.

Some authors suggest using skin hooks for atraumatic eversion of skin edges to facilitate undermining and suture placement. Alternatively, fine noncrushing forceps can be effectively utilized as well. Undermining is accomplished in the upper subcutaneous tissue layer with the help of a pair of fine scissors (eg, Iris) or with the belly of a no. 15 blade (Fig. 1–4). The middle finger of the hand holding the skin hook, or forceps, is kept over the skin surface of the wound edge being undermined to help assess the depth of the undermining process. The desired depth is just below the dermis at the dermal–subcutaneous tissue junction.

Undermining is generally performed over the entire length of the wound and on both sides of the wound. The width of the undermining generally depends on the presence or absence of tissue loss, the orientation of the wound, the anatomic site, and to a lesser degree, on the age of the patient. It should not produce distortion of adjacent facial features such as the angle of the mouth, palpebral fissure, or nasal ala. Undermining may also be more extensive on one side of the wound than the other to avoid damage to vessels, nerves, and other important structures.

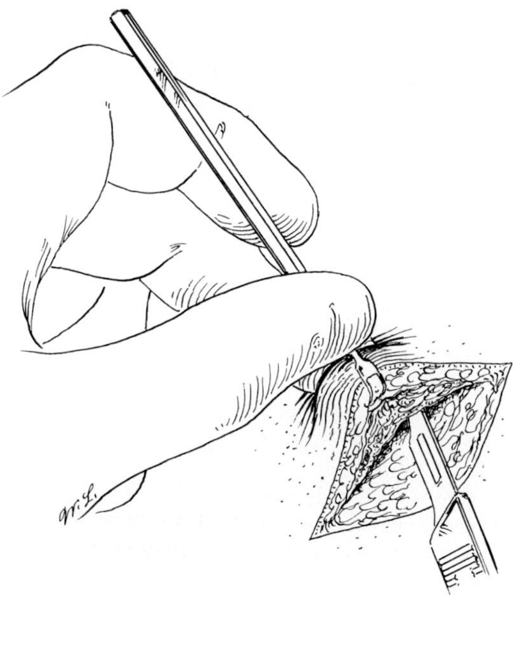

Figure 1–4. Undermining with no. 15 scalpel blade.

It must be remembered that as a scar matures it contracts in a three-dimensional manner, with the resultant tissue forces imparting depression and widening of the final scar. For this reason, it is important to intentionally evert the skin edges during subcutaneous closure, and to minimize skin tension at the wound edges with proper undermining and subcutaneous closure techniques.

One must remember to undermine with a precise even-thickness, particularly near the skin margins, to prevent inaccurate approximation of the skin layers. Some authors suggest creating a beveled, or slightly undercut skin margin, to help create the desired skin eversion during approximation. This eversion, as mentioned earlier, generally flattens with time.

Overzealous undermining increases wound trauma, enhances the possibility of hematoma formation, and may compromise the blood supply to the wound edge. These conditions may contribute to an unacceptable final scar.

In the "trap-door" deformity, a curvilinear laceration produces an avulsed flap of tissue with a pedicle attaching it to the remaining skin (Fig. 1–5). In the usual situation, the skin and the underlying soft tissues are injured in such a way that the laceration produces a slanting or oblique wound of varying thickness. Sometimes the skin laceration lies in an

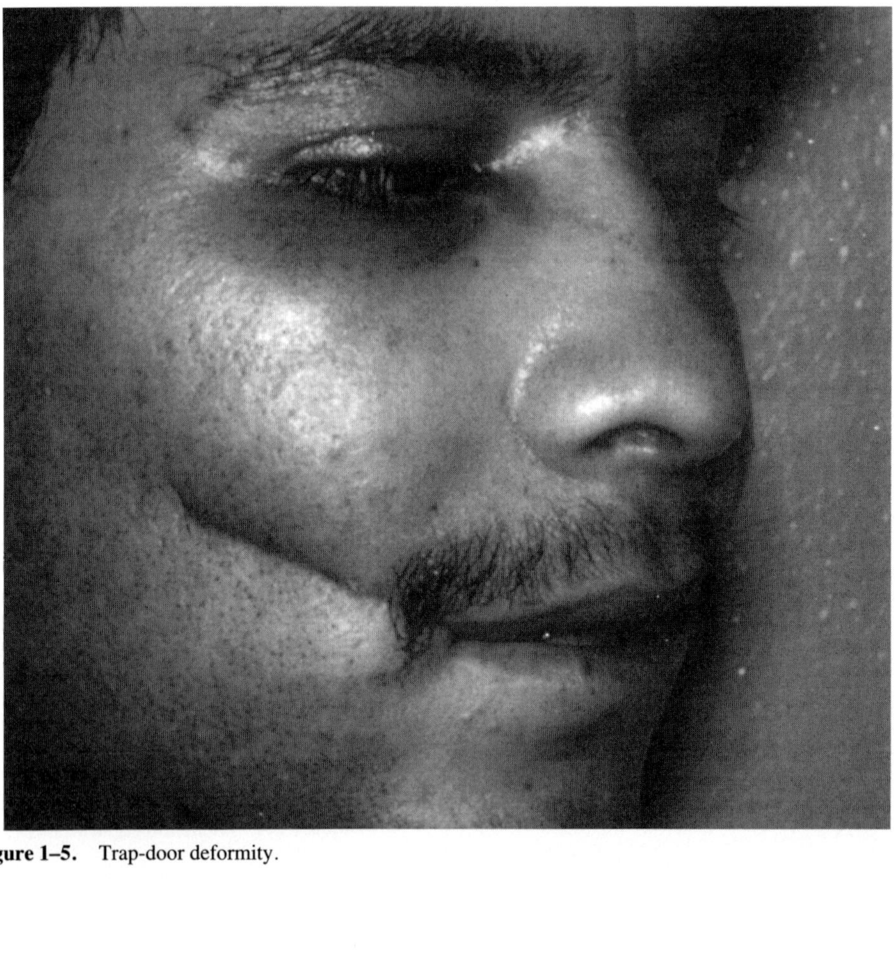

Figure 1–5. Trap-door deformity.

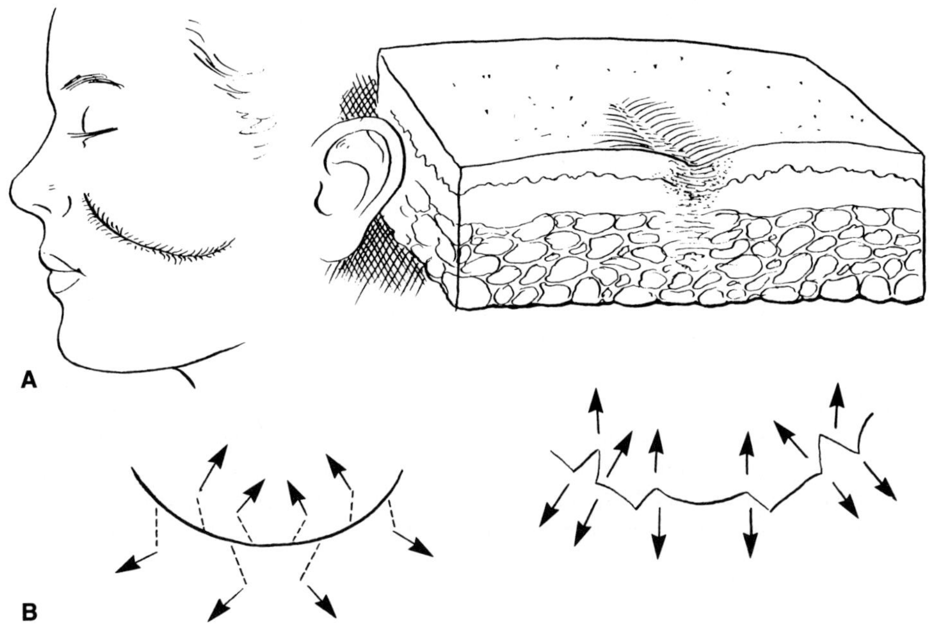

Figure 1–6. (A) Profile of a trap-door deformity and cross-sectional view. (B) Multiple Z-plasty correction of trap-door injury.

inferior or dependent position, leaving the pedicle carrying the blood supply in an antigravity relation, potentially interfering with venous return from the flap.[11]

If these wounds are not closed properly, edema of the avulsed segment (particularly if based superiorly) and contracture of the nonlinear scar can lead to the raised trap-door deformity. The inside skin margin of the scar may contract thus creating a depressed scar that can alternate with areas of scar hypertrophy (Fig. 1–6).[11]

According to the "convergence of forces" theory,[11] when a curvilinear or V-shaped scar is formed, the vector forces are not equally distributed and will result in a divergence of forces outside and a convergence of forces within the central scar area (Fig. 1–7). These convergent forces result in alteration of the soft tissue bulk within the scar confines, leading to the elevation and bunching up of the tissues characteristically seen in a trap-

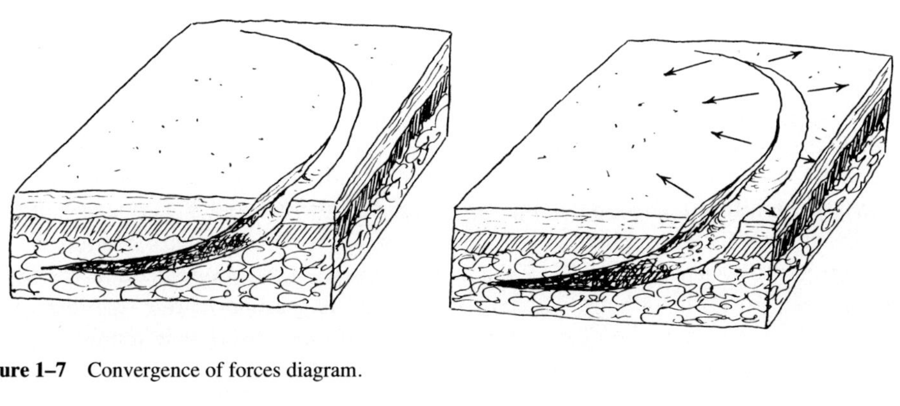

Figure 1–7 Convergence of forces diagram.

door deformity.[11] This untoward result can be minimized by trimming some of the thin oblique edges of the flap such that the wound can be approximated in a vertical plane. Also, by undermining the skin edges opposite the flap for approximately the same distance as the lacerated flap, the tissue layers can be more carefully approximated and the tension better distributed in a layer by layer basis.[11,12] Two-layer undermining (one between the dermis and the subcutaneous tissue, another beneath the subcutaneous tissue) is sometimes necessary in this circumstance for a more precise approximation of tissue layers.

The Z-plasty technique, in conjunction with undermining and soft tissue debulking, can later be useful in improving the appearance of the trap-door deformity during scar revision. Multiple Z-plasties along the curvilinear scar produce a reorientation of the contraction vectors, thereby reducing the effect of the convergence of forces thought to contribute to its characteristic appearance (Fig. 1–6B).[11]

A beveled laceration, even when properly sutured, may still show vascular compromise on the beveled side, particularly when the wound edges are approximated under tension. In these situations the beveled edge should be excised for a short distance, including the opposite side if necessary, to achieve accurate approximation of the wound edges in a vertical plane. It should be remembered that it is not necessary to excise the beveled edge all the way back to the beginning of the beveling.[13]

Subcutaneous Closure

The purpose of the subcutaneous closure is to reduce the dead space (thus reducing the probability of fluid accumulation), to reduce skin wound tension, and to assist in alignment, approximation, and eversion of appropriately undermined skin edges.

Wound management requires meticulous approximation of wound layers. The most common cause of residual scarring is due to a single layer closure with large sutures, which allows separation and depression of the scar, particularly after the removal of the epidermal sutures. Approximation of mucosa, perichondrium with cartilage, and the muscles of facial expression should be performed, when indicated, prior to subcutaneous closure. In most cases, at least a dermal and epidermal approximation are necessary, with the dermal layer being the most important step of wound closure.[14]

Accumulation of fluid within the wound is likely to cause an inflammatory reaction that can result in wound breakdown, secondary infection (and necessitate drainage), or eventuate in organization and fibrosis. Alone or in combination all of these factors will lead to suboptimal scar formation.

If a wound is believed to be contaminated, or if hemostasis or fluid accumulation is a concern, a drain should be placed prior to wound closure and left in place for at least 24 hours. Large neck wounds can be drained effectively by utilizing continuous suction through soft perforated tubes (eg, Jackson-Pratt drains), for which wound closure must be airtight. Smaller wounds can be passively drained using a 1/4-in. Penrose drain, a sterile rubber band, no. 90 polyethylene tubing, or a size 0 sterile silk suture.[15]

Unless significant tension on the skin edges is present, an absorbable suture is generally utilized for approximation of the deeper layers. When approximating fat and muscle layers, silk and chromic gut are the most commonly used suture materials.[16] Silk is composed of natural fibers held together by an adhesive gum derivative that disappears after several years and is therefore thought of as a slowly absorbable suture.[16] It also possesses good handling characteristics and tensile strength.

Catgut is an animal protein that is commercially available in chromate-coated form to lengthen its absorption time and to reduce tissue reaction. Its tensile strength retention is lost by 2 to 3 weeks[17] (rate varying with individual patient characteristics); however, one of its disadvantages is that it can be unequally degraded enzymatically anywhere along the stitch, which may result in premature breakage. Catgut is absorbed faster in inflamed wounds and, for that reason, it can be used safely in most subepidermal wound closures except for those that are infected, inflamed, or under tension. Additionally, hypersensitivity to chromate salts is infrequent but should ideally be investigated prior to usage.

In infected wounds, a multifilamentous suture is preferably avoided. Bacteria and debris may be trapped within the suture material interstices and serve as a nidus for infection. In this situation, Prolene (polypropylene) provides a nonabsorbable, synthetic, monofilamentous material that retains its in vivo tensile strength for years and is generally unweakened by tissue enzymes. Prolene is available blue or clear (undyed), possesses low tissue drag, elicits a minimal inflammatory reaction, and is the least thrombogenic of all suture materials. As an elastic suture with high memory, knot security is low, and necessitates multiple throws to safeguard against slippage.

For the dermal closure, chromic gut, Vicryl (polyglactin 910), and Dexon (polyglycolic acid) are generally used. Vicryl and Dexon are stronger than gut, possess tying characteristics similar to those of silk, induce less tissue reaction (absorbed by hydrolysis rather than enzymatically), and retain their tensile strength (50% at 2 to 3 weeks) longer than chromic gut.[17] These advantages render Vicryl and Dexon the suture of choice by some surgeons for dermal closure in facial wounds and in other areas associated with mobility or tension.

Polydioxanone (PDS) is a synthetic monofilament absorbable material, made available in recent years, that possesses good tensile strength for prolonged periods of time (50% at 4 weeks, 25% at 6 weeks). The PDS polymer contains an oxygen ether group that provides the soft and pliable characteristic of this suture. However, according to the experience of some surgeons, PDS eventually "spits" through the tissues. For this reason, it is recommended that it be used only in deeper tissues that are at least 2 mm beneath the skin surface.[17]

Monocryl (poliglecaprone 25) is another synthetic absorbable monofilament suture that is very pliable and easy to handle. Monocryl is an excellent choice for suture when wound closure requires high initial strength with a short strength retention profile (50% at 1 week, 25% at 2 weeks).

When prolonged wound support is desired, and as a first line alternative to PDS, polyester sutures may be employed. Available in undyed or green, these nonabsorbable synthetic sutures possess good handling characteristics owing to their multifilamentous and braided construct. As a group, they retain extremely high tensile strength properties, second only to stainless steel. The uncoated varieties (Mersilene, Dacron) are associated with increased tissue drag but evoke a minimal tissue reaction. Conversely, the coated forms (Tevdek, Tri-Cron, Ethibond) slide through tissue more easily but are associated with greater inflammatory tissue reactions.

Similar to undermining, a skin hook or fine forceps is used to reflect the skin edges and facilitate the placement of dermal stitches. The dermal suture is first passed from below through the upper subcutaneous layer of the undermined skin edge (Fig. 1–8). Then, following the curve of the needle, the suture is passed through the dermis in a manner such that the suture lies closest to the epidermis at the point farthest away from the skin edge to

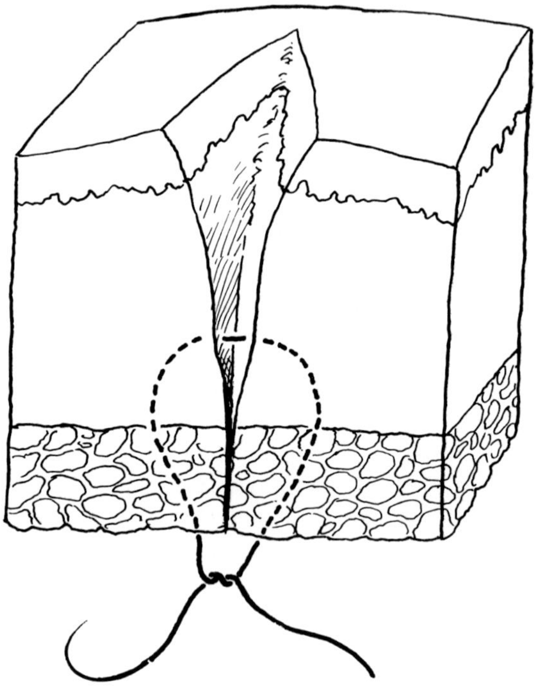

Figure 1–8. Subcutaneous closure.

assist in skin eversion. The suture then exits through the dermis, and the same is repeated on the opposite wound edge, entering at the same dermal depth. When the knot is tied it should lie buried underneath the dermis, and as the wound edges are approximated, skin eversion must be accomplished. Subcutaneous sutures should be placed approximately every 5 mm.[18]

With an absorbable suture, a slight dimpling of the skin surface where the suture lies closest to the epidermis is acceptable. With a nonabsorbable suture, however, permanent dimpling may result if the suture is not replaced.

Epidermal Closure

Cutaneous scarring may be decreased by the accurate approximation of skin margins closed under minimal tension. The purpose of the epidermal sutures is not to pull the skin edges together, but to ensure that the properly everted skin edges are more accurately approximated and are held tightly in this position during healing. When tissue is missing, and simple undermining will not effect an adequate tension-free closure, the surface should then be covered by a flap or graft.

Stitch marks, also called crosshatch scars, may be punctate or linear and are usually created as a result of strangulation of the skin edge along the suture line (Fig. 1–9). This may be secondary to stitches that were tied too tightly or left in too long. The aesthetic results worsen if there is a tendency for keloid formation, if stitch abscesses develop, or in thick-skinned regions.

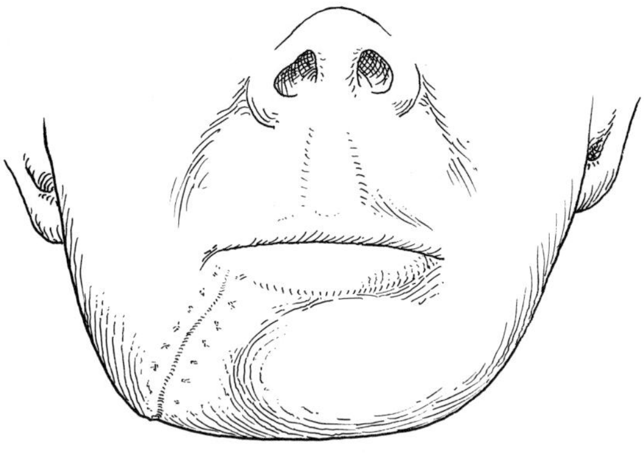

Figure 1–9. Crosshatch mark deformity.

Sutures that are tied too tightly may result in wound margin ischemia or in the suture actually cutting into the underlying skin.[13] Additionally, if a skin defect is closed with undue tension, the stitches will probably need to be tied tight and left in for a longer period of time to help prevent wound dehiscence. The use of thick suture material will add to the amount of foreign body and tissue reaction in the wound and can be deleterious to optimal wound healing.[19] To obviate the likelihood of suture marks, it is necessary to place epidermal sutures that are small in caliber, relatively inert, allow for a tension-free closure, and remove them relatively early.

Needle holders designed by Webster, Castroviejo, or Gillies are designed for small needles. Small skin hooks and tissue forceps can hold the tissue atraumatically as the stitches are being placed. Iris scissors can be used for trimming contused or macerated skin edges.

In general, monofilamentous nonabsorbable sutures are preferred for epidermal closure because they are associated with less epidermal and bacterial ingrowth into the suture tract, which helps minimize tissue reaction. 5-0 and 6-0 sutures are the most commonly used suture sizes to approximate the epidermis of facial wounds.

Nylon is the most common facial skin suture used today mainly because of its minimal tissue reactivity and the way it glides through the tissues. Like other synthetic material, nylon has "strand memory" and is prone to unravel so it is better tied with a surgeon's knot first followed by several square knots. When used as a buried permanent suture, nylon loses about 20% of its initial tensile strength in 1 year and is generally degraded within 1 to 2 years. Similar to silk, it behaves like a semipermanent suture.

Owing to its low tissue reactivity and long-lasting tensile strength, Prolene has also become a popular choice among some surgeons as an alternative to nylon for epidermal closure.

Small cutting needles are fairly atraumatic especially when the sutures are swaged to them. Swaged needles prevent the need to pass a needle eye or double suture strand through the suture tract, thus avoiding further tissue trauma. Several needle sizes and curvatures are available, enabling needles to be selected based on the manipulation required to obtain adequate closure. Generally, a half-circle needle for deeper layer closure within the wound edge, and a one-fourth or three-eighths needle for epithelial closure, will help minimize the amount of manipulation and surgical motion required.

Facial sutures are generally removed between 5 to 7 days postoperatively depending on the strength of the dermal closure and the amount of tension placed on the wound. The type of suture material may also help in determining the timing of suture removal. Nylon and Prolene possess very low antigenicity and can be left in place for 10 to 14 days with minimal tissue reaction. Since silk is braided, absorption of bacteria-containing fluid can occur along the sutures and lead to the development of small microabscesses. For this reason silk needs to be removed in 3 to 7 days.[20]

When repairing a laceration in small children in whom suture removal may be difficult, a fast-absorbing catgut suture (Ethicon) is a reasonable alternative because it will be degraded within 3 to 5 days.[17,21] Mild chromic gut (Davis and Geck) is a comparable alternative. When used in the epidermis, it induces less tissue reaction than when used subcutaneously and it will disappear from the skin surface within 1 week.

Continuous epidermal sutures are usually started at the wound edge farthest away from the surgeon, whereas interrupted sutures are placed by halving the wound and thus avoiding the formation of "dog-ears." The point of the needle is initially placed perpendicular to the skin surface and the suture is introduced into the dermis in a manner so that it lies farthest away from the skin edge at some point below the epidermis (Fig. 1–10). The suture should exit the dermis deeply and enter the dermis of the opposite wound edge at this same depth. Accurate skin edge approximation is aided by taking equal and small bites (about 2 mm) on each side of the wound.[21] A useful rule of thumb is that the depth of the suture placement should roughly approximate the entry and exit points of the suture with respect to the wound edge. If the opposing margins of the wound have uneven thickness before the placement of the skin suture, the discrepancy can be corrected by placing the suture at a deeper level on the side that is lower and at a more superficial level on the side that is higher.[13] Farrior[22] suggests the "spring loop" technique for placement of epidermal interrupted sutures that allow for postoperative swelling to occur without causing strangulation of the wound edges. In the spring loop technique, a double loop knot (surgeon's

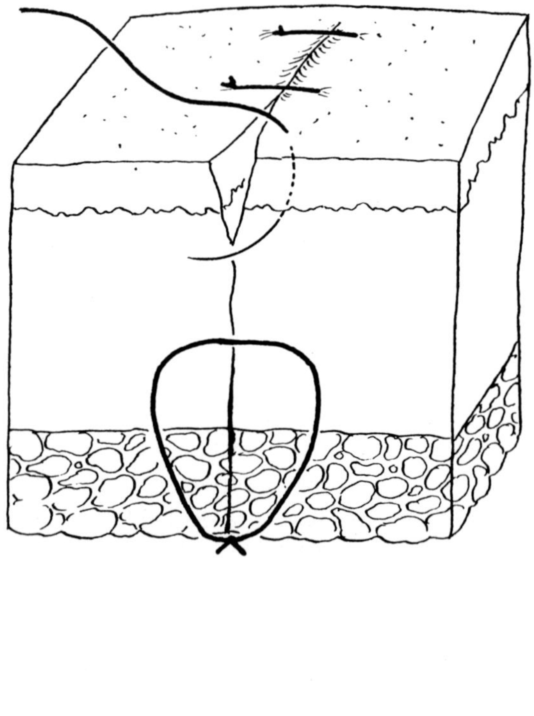

Figure 1–10. Epidermal closure.

knot) is first laid flat, then a small (2 mm) loop is closed with second and third throws placed square to each other (Fig. 1–11.). This loop allows postoperative swelling to open the double loop if necessary, whereas the square knot prevents the stitch from unraveling.

Continuous sutures save time when closing a straight wound and allow a more even distribution of tension along the suture line.[13] However, when approximating irregular edges, or when fluid accumulation is a concern, interrupted sutures are preferred because partial removal may allow for drainage of the wound without disrupting the entire suture line. Also, interrupted sutures tend to allow egress of blood or serum between the sutures whereas the continuous suture tends to be more watertight. In most instances, however, the continuous interlocking or interrupted sutures can be used interchangeably.

The continuous subcuticular suture provides accurate approximation of the skin edges without the threat of stitch marks. A fine three-eighths curved cutting needle with a fine monofilament suture (nylon or Prolene) is generally utilized. The suture is first introduced toward the surgeon, about 1 cm from the end of the incision line, and brought in through the end of the incision. The suture is then passed into the dermis about 1 to 2 mm from the skin surface. After a distance of 3 to 4 mm, the suture is then brought out at the same depth at which it entered the dermis. This is then repeated on the opposite side, at the same depth, and with slight backtracking. Laterally, away from the skin margin, the suture will lie slightly deeper than at the skin margin thereby facilitating wound edge eversion.[22]

When approximating a laceration with a sharp angle, an epidermal suture through the tip of the skin flap may, at least in theory, compromise its blood supply. In this situation, the corner stitch may be used as an alternative. The needle is first passed through the epidermis and out through the dermis in the skin edge opposite the flap. The needle is then passed through the dermis of the flap exiting the opposite dermal edge. The suture is then introduced into the dermis of the contralateral opposing edge, at the same level at which it exited the flap dermis, and brought out through the epidermis. In this manner, the farther into the flap dermis the suture is placed, the more snugly the tip of the flap will fit into the apex of the opposite edge (Fig. 1–12). As an alternative, two simple sutures may be placed

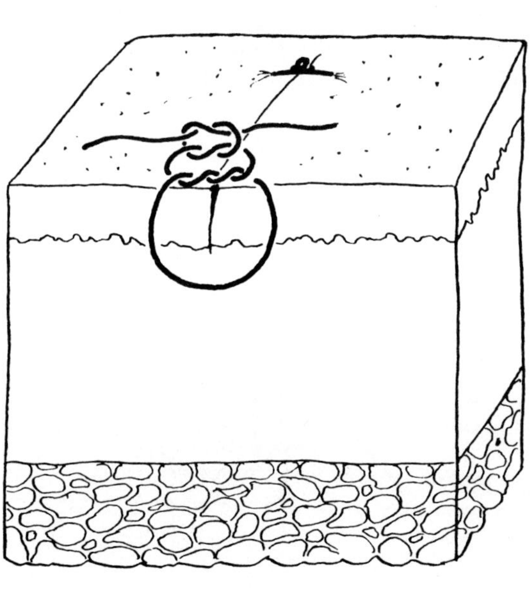

Figure 1–11. Spring loop closure.

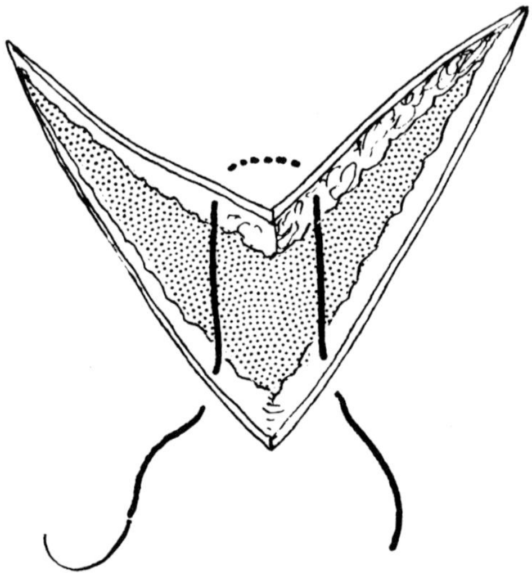

Figure 1–12. Single-stitch corner closure.

on each side of the tip of the flap and also achieve adequate approximation (Fig. 1–13). Additionally, Webster and Smith[23] utilize running interlocking sutures through similar skin flaps when closing geometric broken line scar revisions with reported good results.

Skin staples are fabricated from stainless steel, which is a minimally reactive material that can be left in place for up to 2 weeks. Their use tends to decrease epidermal closure times and is particularly applicable to approximation of neck and hair-bearing wounds. If placed properly, skin staples are capable of producing adequate skin eversion while traumatizing the skin no more than a comparable size suture.[17]

Steri-strips are microporous adhesive tapes used alone or in combination with subcutaneous or skin sutures to increase the strength of the closure by decreasing the tension on the wound edge. The effectiveness of steri-strips depends on a perfectly dry surface along the wound edges to prevent their early detachment. As a result, ideal edge-to-edge approximation is not guaranteed. Steri-strips may be applied in different patterns depending on the anatomic location of the wound and the direction of the wound tension. They are

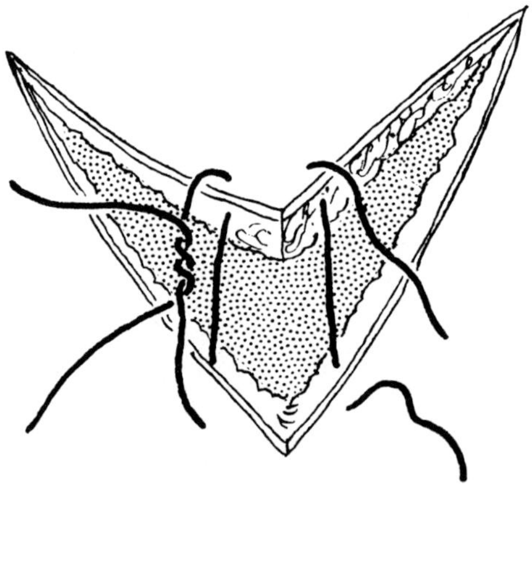

Figure 1–13. Two-stitch corner closure.

most often used after suture removal to provide additional antitension wound support for as long as possible. Other situations in which steri-strips may be useful are in small children where suture removal may be difficult, in tissues in which further suturing may compromise an already marginal blood supply, for epidermal suture reinforcement, and as a wound dressing. Steri- strips are often used after applying mastic (Mastisol) or tinture of benzoin (Tincoben) to improve their adhesive capabilities.[13,17]

CONTUSIONS

A contusion is an injury caused by blunt trauma resulting in a bruise. Oftentimes there may be an underlying hematoma. Contusions usually heal well on their own and hematomas usually spontaneously reabsorb. If a hematoma does not reabsorb and becomes encapsulated, it will need to be drained as soon as possible to avert a potentially permanent subcutaneous deformity.

Removal of hematomas involves either incisional drainage or needle aspiration. The first several days after injury, a hematoma is in the "current jelly" or gelatinous stage of healing and is best treated by incisional drainage. The surgeon should make an incision in the most cosmetically acceptable site, then subcutaneously undermine and drain the hematoma. If the hematoma has liquified it may be drained by needle aspiration. Hematomas undergo liquification between 7 to 10 days after formation. Usually a no. 16 or no. 18 gauge needle is used for aspiration at this stage. The results of untreated hematomas of the nasal septum and ear can result in saddle-nose deformity and cauliflower ear, respectively.

ABRASION

Abrasions are treated by cleaning the wound with a mild nonirritating soap or antiseptic solution. The wound can then be covered with antibiotic ointment and allowed to heal uncovered. When pain is present the wound may be covered with a nonadherent dressing (ie, Opsite, Tegaderm, Telfa, Adaptic), which can usually be removed within a day or two. Healing is usually prompt with minimal scarring, unless the abrasion penetrates the dermal layer or becomes infected.

REFERENCES

1. Schultz RC. Mechanism, characterization and incidence of injury. In: Schultz RC, ed. *Facial Injuries*. 3rd ed. Chicago, Ill: Year Book Medical Publishers. 1988:13–44.
2. Mathog RH, Worman L, Pollak D. Animal Bites to the Head and Neck. In: Sisson GA, Tardy ME, eds. *Proceedings of the Second International Symposium on Plastic and Reconstructive Surgery of the Head and Neck*. Vol II. New York, NY: Grune and Stratton Inc; 1977:105–113.
3. Simpson WR. Physiological principles of therapy in head and neck cutaneous wounds. *Laryngoscope*. 1977; 87:792–816.
4. Fawcett DW. Skin. In: Bloom W, Fawcett. D, eds. *A Textbook of Histology*. 11th ed. Philadelphia, Pa: WB Saunders Co; 1986:543–550.
5. Robson MC. Infected soft tissue wounds. In: Marsh JL, ed. *Current Therapy in Plastic and Reconstructive Surgery*. Vol 1. Toronto: BC Decker Inc; 1989:1–4.
6. Dickinson JT, Jaquis GW, Thompson JN. Soft tissue trauma. *Otolaryngol Clin North Am*. 1976;9:331–360.

7. Robson MC, Heggers JD. Surgical infection II. The beta-hemolytic streptococcus. *J Surg Res*. 1969;9:289–292.
8. Heggers JP, Robson MC, Ristroph JD. A rapid method of performing quantitative wound cultures. *Milit Med*. 1969; 134:666.
9. Robson MC, Duke WF, Krizek TJ. Rapid bacterial screening in the treatment of civilian wounds. *J Surg Res*. 1973; 14:426–430.
10. Krizek TJ, Robson MC, Kho E. Bacterial growth and skin graft survival. *Surg Forum*. 1967; 18:518–519.
11. Holt GR. Treatment of trapdoor scars. In: Thomas JR, Holt GR, eds. *Facial Scars: Incision, Revision, and Camouflage*. St Louis, Mo: CV Mosby; 1989:271–277.
12. Holt GR. Concepts of soft tissue trauma repair. Otolarygol Clin North Am. 1990; 23:1019–1030.
13. Chang WHJ. Wound management. In: Chang WHJ, ed. *Fundamentals of Plastic and Reconstructive Surgery*. Baltimore, Md: Williams & Wilkins; 1980:9–61.
14. Farrior RT. Dermabrasion in facial surgery. *Laryngoscope*. 1985;95:534–545.
15. Bailey BJ, Calhoun KH. Basic principles of plastic surgery in the head and neck. In: Paparella M, Shumrick D, Gluckman J, et al, eds. *Otolaryngology*. 3rd ed. Philadelphia, Pa: WB Saunders Co; 1991:2629–2637.
16. Holt GR, Holt JE. Suture materials and techniques. *Ear Nose Throat J*. 1981; 6:23–30.
17. Thomas JR. Wound closure materials. In: Thomas JR, Holt GR, eds. *Facial Scars: Incision, Revision, and Camouflage*. St Louis, Mo: CV Mosby; 1989:69–74.
18. Donald PJ. The management of soft tissue trauma to the face and neck. In: Paparella M, Shumrick D, Glukman J, et al, eds. *Otolaryngology*. 3rd ed. Philadelphia, Pa: WB Saunders Co; 1991:2883–2896.
19. van Rifssel EJ, Brand R, Amiraal C, et al. Tissue reaction and surgical knots: the effect of suture size, knot configuration, and knot volume. *Obstet Gynecol*. 1989; 74:64–68.
20. Holt GR. Dressings, medications, and post-operative care. In: Thomas JR, Holt GR, eds. *Facial Scars: Incision, Revision, and Camouflage*. St Louis, Mo: CV Mosby; 1989:75–82.
21. Walike JW. Suturing technique in facial soft tissue injuries. *Otolaryngol Clin North Am*. 1979; 12:415–430.
22. Farrior RT. Management of lacerations and scars. *Laryngoscope*. 1977;87:917–933.
23. Webster RC, Smith RC. Scar revision and camouflaging. *Otolaryngol Clin North Am*. 1982; 15:55–68.

2

Diagnosis and Management of Acute Nasal Fracture

DUANE SMITH, M.D.
ROBERT H. MATHOG, M.D.

Injury to the nasal skeleton constitutes the most common facial fracture.[1] Nasal fractures account for up to 50% of total facial fractures[2,3] and are a frequent reason for emergency room visitation. The facial trauma specialist must be astute in the diagnosis and management of acute nasal trauma if this individual is to be responsible for the restoration of premorbid appearance and function.

ANATOMY

The external nasal skeleton or nasal pyramid projects from the midface and supports the investing soft tissues. The nose is commonly divided into an upper bony and lower cartilaginous vault, the latter of which is subdivided further into upper and lower components.[4] The major portion of the bony vault consists of paired rectangularly shaped nasal bones with some contribution from the nasal spine of frontal bone and the frontal processes of the maxilla (Fig. 2–1). The nasal bones articulate with each other in the midline, laterally with the frontal process of the maxilla, and superiorly with the nasal spine. The bony pyramid, although a relatively weak structure, is supported from the nasal spine and somewhat from the underlying midline articulation of the nasal bones with the perpendicular plate of the ethmoid.

The upper cephalic cartilaginous vault consists of two upper lateral cartilages and the quadrilateral cartilage of the septum (Fig. 2–2). All three are enclosed in a common perichondrial sheath.[5] The lateral cephalic borders of the upper lateral cartilages attach to the pyriform aperture by connective tissue. The lower more caudal cartilaginous vault consists of paired lower lateral cartilages, the membranous septum, and columella. This is considered the base of the nose and defines the tip. The lateral crura overlap with the upper lateral cartilages superiorly and are loosely attached to the pyriform aperture laterally. The

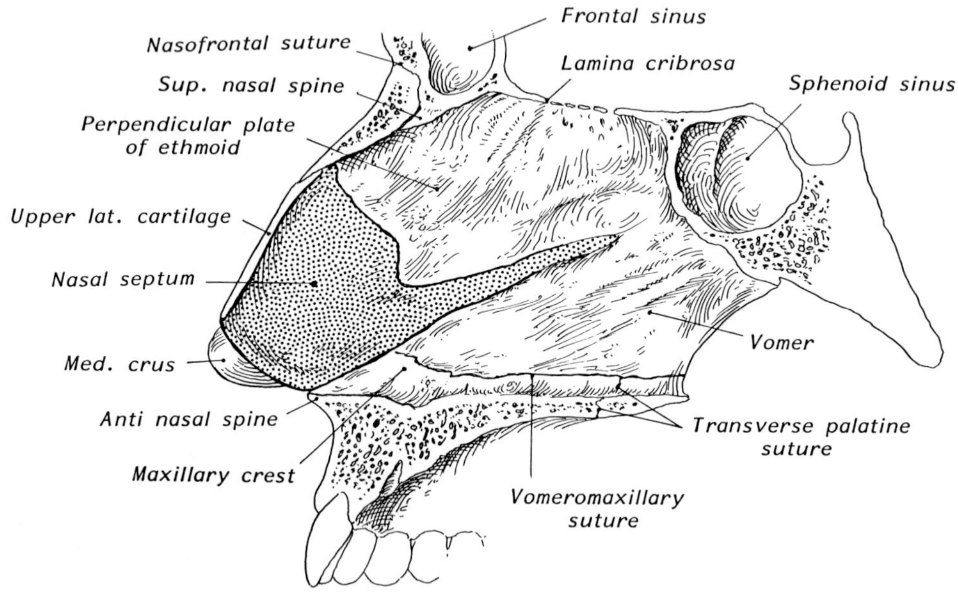

Figure 2–1. External bony nasal skeleton consisting of nasal bones, the nasal spine of the frontal bone, and the frontal processes of the maxilla.

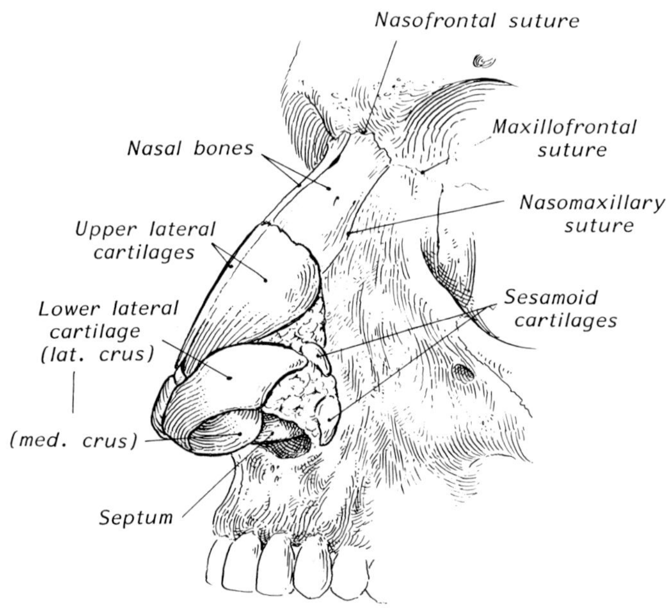

Figure 2–2. Cartilaginous portion of nose consisting of upper lateral cartilages, septum, lower lateral cartilages, and sesamoid cartilages.

paired medial crura are invested by the columellar soft tissue anteriorly and flare posteriorly to articulate with the caudal septum.

The septal framework consists of bony contributions from the perpendicular plate of the ethmoid, which articulates with the vertical crest of the nasal bones anteriorly and the sphenoid crest and vomer posteriorly. The vomer in turn articulates inferiorly with the maxillary crest ending posteriorly with the choana. The quadrilateral septal cartilage has a fibrous attachment to the maxillary crest and anterior nasal spine. It begins posterior to the medial crura and then extends superiorly and posteriorly to articulate with the nasal bones, ethmoid, and vomer. There exists a strong osteochondral junction where a sleeve of the quadrilateral cartilage is interposed between the perpendicular plate of the ethmoid and the vomer. The anatomic interplay between the nasal skeleton and the septum is of utmost importance and it should be considered together when attempting to diagnose and manage nasal fractures.

There are significant anatomic differences between pediatric and adult age groups.[6,7] The nasal bones are relatively shorter in children and there is a greater proportion of soft pliable cartilage. The nasal structure projects less than in the adult nose making it less susceptible to injury. The nasal bones also have more protection from bulkier soft tissue and a prominent midfacial skeleton. This helps protect the nasal structures by absorbing and dispersing the force of the trauma over a greater area. On the other hand, several anatomic growth centers in the pediatric nasal skeleton may be adversely affected. These differences have importance in terms of the nature of the injury and long-term sequela.

EPIDEMIOLOGY

The nose, being a prominent facial feature, is a frequent recipient of trauma, incidentally and intentionally. There are numerous reports of a high incidence of nasal fractures in both the pediatric and adult population.[8–11] A prospective study by Lundin et al[3] reported that nasal fractures constituted 39% of maxillofacial fractures. This percentage is notably higher in other studies[1] such as that in Denmark, which reported the incidence of nasal fractures to be 53 per 100,000.[12]

There is a clear sexual predilection for males greater than females at a ratio of 2:1 with a significant incidence in the 15 to 25-year-old male population.[2,13] The highest incidence in females is in women in the over 60 category and usually this is a result of personal injury, most commonly falls.[13] Most adult nasal fractures are the result of interpersonal altercations and sporting injuries with a smaller number resulting from motor vehicle accidents and falls.

The incidence of facial trauma in children is lower than in adults.[14] Although there are anatomic differences between the child and adult, the injury in the child is often overlooked or underestimated by the examining physician.[7] Sexual predilection is less clear-cut in the pediatric population.[15] The most common causative factors are falls and contact sports.[7] The examining physician should be cognizant that 30 to 50% of all child abuse victims present with facial trauma.[16]

PATHOPHYSIOLOGY

The nose, being prominent and centrally located on the face, can serve as an energy absorber, thus acting as a protective buffer of the cranial vault. The cartilaginous components have springlike flexibility and can be subjected to small amounts of trauma without significant injury. In general, the greater the force, the more severe the injury to the nasoseptal and possibly the surrounding structures. The amount of force required to fracture the nasal pyramid is believed to be small (25 to 75 lb) as compared with the surrounding midfacial structures.[17,18] The thicker portions of the nasal bones superiorly with support from the nasal spine of the frontal bone are resistant to injury whereas the thinner parts distally tend to fracture. The groove for the anterior ethmoidal arteries is also a potential area of weakness.[19] The osseous density of the nasal bones will impact on the type of fracture as the elderly patient with osteoporotic bones often has comminuted fractures. Because the nasal skeleton of the child is much more flexible, injury to the cartilaginous structures is more common and these cartilages usually spring back to a normal location after trauma or suffer a greenstick-type fracture.[20] With pediatric trauma there are potential derangements in growth and development of the nasoseptal and midfacial tissues.

CLASSIFICATION

The nature and extent of the injury to the nose will depend on the direction, degree, and concentration of the force. Most classification schemes take these issues into consideration. In a series of loading experiments on human skulls, Clark and Wallace[19] noted that nasal bones are more likely to break with lateral than frontal impact blows. Likewise less force is necessary to cause significant injury from a lateral blow than a frontal impact because there is less skeletal support to help absorb the trauma.

Lateral injuries are the more common pattern. Illum et al.,[12] in a study of 173 consecutive nasal fractures, reported that 66% of nasal fractures were of a lateral type as compared with 13% of frontal type. Stranc and Robertson[21] divided lateral oblique injuries into three planes based on the force of impact. Plane 1 injuries involve just the ipsilateral nasal bone characterized by a depression of the bone usually at the junction of its upper two thirds and lower one third (Fig. 2–3). This was noted to be the likely fracture site 80% of the time based on a study by Kazanjian and Converse in 1959.[22] Greater force will lead to a Plane 2 type injury, which in addition to the ipsilateral depression, the contralateral nasal bone is outfractured and/or impacted into the frontal process of the maxilla. In Plane 3 injuries, forces are great enough to fracture the frontal process of the maxilla and the lacrimal bone with possible injury to the lacrimal collecting system. There may be multiple fragments involved in this type of injury or alternatively, the entire nasal pyramid may be fracture dislocated to the side opposite the injury force. The septum may or may not be injured with mild impact forces but is usually dislocated, fractured, or fracture dislocated with greater degrees of injury.[10] A variable amount of injury can occur to the lateral cartilages including dislocation and avulsion from their loose connective tissue attachments to bone.[23]

The less commonly occurring frontal type injury may require more impact force but can also be more severe in nature.[24] Stranc and Robertson[21] again divided this type of injury into planes based on the depth of injury in the coronal plane. Plane 1 injuries do not extend beyond a line joining the lower end of the nasal bone to the anterior nasal spine. The majority of the force is transmitted to the cartilaginous vault with fractures of the bony nasal tip and separation or avulsion of the lateral cartilages from their attachments.

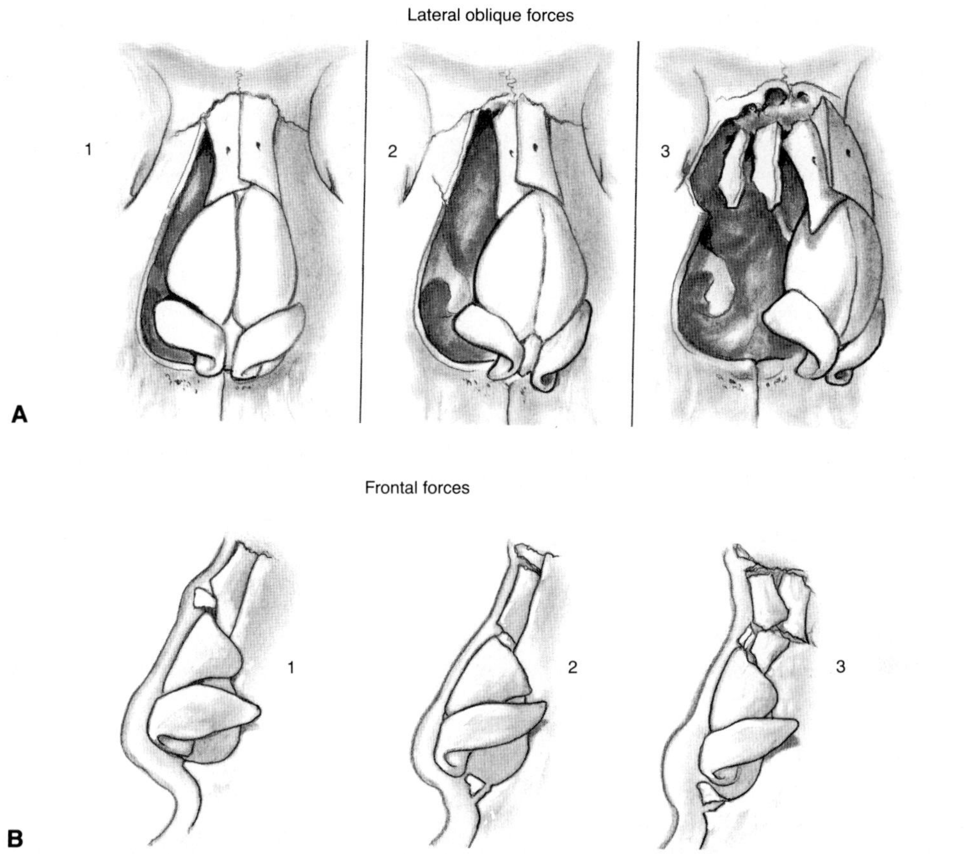

Figure 2–3. (A). Nasal fractures demonstrating planes of injury as a result of lateral oblique forces. (B). Nasal fractures demonstrating planes of injury as a result of frontal forces. (Reprinted with permission from Mathog.[62(p227)])

Posterior dislocations of the septal and alar cartilages are also seen infrequently. Plane 2 injuries are still limited to the external nose but are more extensive with flattening and splaying of the nasal bones, segmental overriding of septal cartilage with mucosal tears, and fractures of the anterior nasal spine. The injuries do not transgress the orbital rims. Plane 3 nasal injuries are extensive and involve orbital and possibly intracranial structures. Comminution of the nasal bones (ie, the open book fracture) with fracture of the frontal processes of the maxilla, ethmoid labyrinths, and lacrimal bones can occur. The cribriform plate and the orbital plate of the frontal bone may be fractured. The septum is severely injured resulting in dorsal collapse and anteroposterior telescoping of the septal fragments.

According to Holt[10] significant septal injury occurs in approximately 20% of nasal fractures. Numerous investigators have attempted to classify septal injuries to guide treatment regiments. It has been shown that inadequate septal management can lead to a delayed nasal pyramid deviation and thus a poor result. Cadaveric studies by Murray et al[24,25] demonstrated that laterally directed forces will produce a cartilaginous septal fracture below the nasal bones extending posteriorly into the perpendicular plate of the ethmoid toward but not involving the cribriform plate. Greater impact forces regardless of the direction will create a more or less constant C- shaped fracture.[23] This type of fracture begins just posterior to the anterior nasal spine, extends running 2 to 3 mm above the cartilaginous interface with the vomer and passes backward and upward into the perpendicular plate from turning forward below the cribriform plate just behind the upper aspect of the nasal bones (Fig. 2–4). Characteristically intranasal examination will reveal a buckling of the posterior septum into the airway on one side with a displacement of the caudal septum to the opposite side.

DIAGNOSIS

Determining the etiologic agent of the nasal injury is important for estimation of the extent of the injury. The direction and amount of force will relate to the injury type. For example, a person suffering nasal trauma as a result of a motor vehicle accident will potentially have a greater injury than that sustained from a simple fall. Information regarding the premorbid appearance and nasal fraction should be ascertained as studies have demonstrated a significant percentage of preexisting nasal deformity.[26] A history of epistaxis indicates the presence of mucosal tears usually occurring on the septum. If there is a history of new onset nasal obstruction this may imply edematous mucosa, obstructing bloody debris, a new onset anatomic deformity, or possibly septal hematoma. Although anosmia may be secondary to edema, bloody debris, or internal derangements, injury to the cribriform plate should be considered.

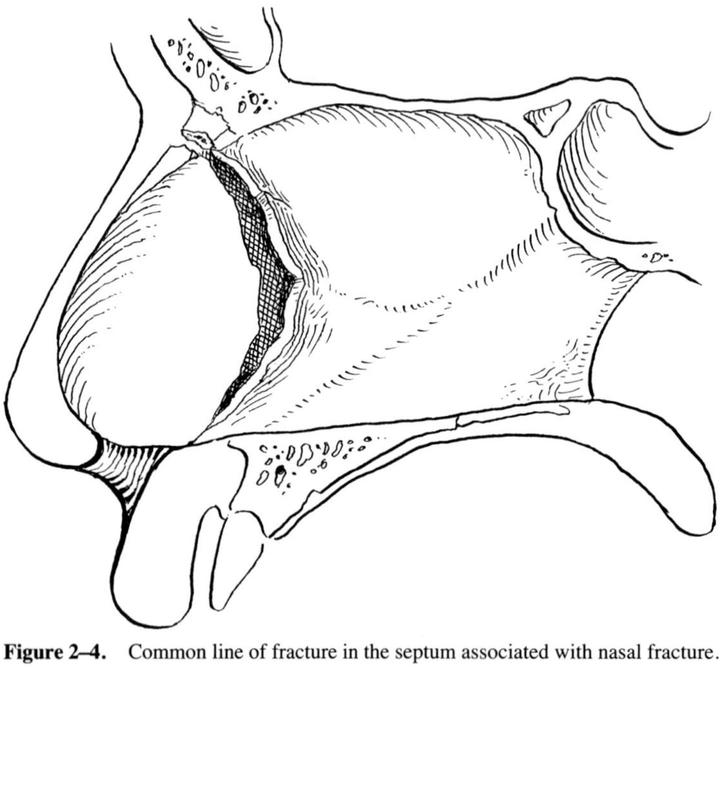

Figure 2–4. Common line of fracture in the septum associated with nasal fracture.

Nasal trauma may on occasion be associated with other craniofacial and systemic injury. Questioning should include a review of systems with special reference to brain, eyes, and cranial nerves. Preexisting sinus and allergic history should be ascertained.

PHYSICAL EXAM

A complete physical examination of the external nasal pyramid, the internal nose, and associated craniofacial structures is essential. The external nasal pyramid should be assessed for obvious deformity such as an S or C-shaped deformity. Crepitence is often considered to be a sine quanon of nasal fracture.[27] Tenderness, mobility, or step-offs are also indicators of injury. Flattening of the bony pyramid with widening of the nasal base indicates a severe impact with probable septal involvement. The profile view may show collapse of the nasal dorsum with tip elevation and retracted columella, all signs of telescoping septal injury and loss of dorsal support.

The skin should be assessed for lacerations and hematomas. Naso-orbital injuries and possible nasal lacrimal injuries should be ruled out. Loss of the glabellar angle and the presence of telecanthus usually indicate a naso-orbital injury. Paskert and Manson[28] described a method of bimanual examination utilizing a Kelly clamp to assess the stability of the naso-orbital ethmoid complex. A cerebrospinal fluid (CSF) leak may be present if cribriform or frontal sinus fracture is present. Medial maxillary fractures should be differentiated as they can also present with a C-shaped nasal deformity, but additionally there is an associated depression of the medial maxillary wall and occasionally a depression of the frontal process of the maxilla and inferior orbit. The physical exam should elicit whether or not there are more extensive midfacial fractures or whether mandible fractures are present.

Careful examination of the internal nose requires patient cooperation, adequate lighting, and mucosal decongestion. All clots should be removed and epistaxis controlled with vasoconstrictors such as phenylephrine hydrochloride (Neo-Synephrine). Cocaine 4% or tetracaine (Pontocaine) 0.5% soaked cotton pledgets can be placed intranasally to provide topical anesthesia and vasoconstriction. The nasal speculum should be used to inspect each nasal cavity. The addition of endoscopic instrumentation may be beneficial. The cartilages should be examined for position, stability, and for hematoma. The septal exam should note dislocation, abnormal mucosal swelling, mucosal tears, or exposed structural components. Because 40% of adults have a septal deflection as a result of prior trauma, tenderness and motion on bimanual palpation are good indicators of acute injury. A tender or dislocated anterior nasal spine (by sublabial palpation) also implies septal trauma.[29]

Septal hematoma may be present unilaterally or bilaterally usually only involving the cartilaginous septum.[10] It is manifested by septal widening with bluish discoloration that persists after mucosal decongestion. Bogginess of the septal mucosa from edema may be difficult to distinguish from hematoma, but the latter can be ruled out with an aspiration or incision of the septal mucosa.

RADIOGRAPHIC EVALUATION

The use of radiography in evaluating nasal fractures is controversial and most practitioners will treat according to the severity of the cosmetic and functional impairment. Still, x-rays may be useful and may demonstrate fractures unsuspected from clinical evaluation. Standard x-rays include the lateral and Waters view. The lateral view is specific for evaluating nasal trauma whereas the Waters view has potential value for evaluating other maxillofacial injuries.

One criticism is the high incidence of both false-positive and false-negative interpretations of plain films. A recent retrospective review noted a disagreement of approximately 25% of cases between x-ray findings and clinical exam.[30] Another investigation demonstrated that the Waters view was of no diagnostic value in terms of nasal fractures because of misinterpretation of the normal midline and nasal maxillary sutures as fractures. The lateral view films were more accurate in their assessment but offered no information with respect to the lateral displacement of the nasal bones.[31]

Another point of contention is the lack of predictive value in terms of clinical management. In a recent prospective study of 54 patients it was shown that radiographs of the nasal bones had no influence on the treatment that patients received.[30]

In children standard films may be even of less value. The bones are smaller and fractures are of a greenstick variety, and the common cartilaginous injuries are not apparent on plain films. In both adults and children, tomograms and computed tomographic scans play a significant role when more extensive craniofacial trauma is suspected.

MANAGEMENT

Epistaxis

Epistaxis is commonly associated with nasal trauma and may be brisk requiring immediate attention. Adequate lighting, suction equipment, and patient cooperation are essential for effective management. A topical vasoconstrictor such as phenylephrine soaked on cotton pledgets and placed intranasally will usually slow or stop hemorrhage and facilitate visualization. Cocaine or tetracaine applied to the mucus membranes will provide topical analgesia and allow instrumentation, cauterization, and/or packing.

If bleeding persists despite these measures then ligation of the ethmoidal vessels or the internal maxillary artery should be considered. If nasal packing is successful it can be left in place for a period of 2 to 5 days and removed when fracture reduction is carried out. Antibiotics with adequate antistaphylococcal coverage should be instituted to lessen the possibility of paranasal sinus infection, otitis media, or toxic shock syndrome with nasal packing.

Lacerations

Lacerations involving the skin and soft tissue of the nasal dorsum should be cleansed, minimally debrided, and repaired with a nonabsorbable fine suture. Alternatively, laceration repair may be delayed if immediate open reduction of fractured nasal segments is anticipated.

Hematoma/Abscess

Septal hematoma develops as a result of submucoperichondrial bleeding and accumulation of blood, often associated with trauma to the intervening cartilage. A septal hematoma usually occurs unilaterally but it can be bilateral if a cartilaginous fracture allows for the passage of blood to the contralateral side. In children in whom the cartilage is more pliable and likely to buckle, separation of the perichondrium from the underlying cartilage leads to hematoma formation.[20] Because the blood supply for the cartilage arises from the perichondrium, an intervening hematoma interrupts the blood supply to the cartilage and may lead to avascular necrosis. This may occur as early as 3 to 4 days after the development of a hematoma.[32] Untreated, a hematoma may develop sequelae of a septal abscess, dense and/or fibrous scarring, and thickening of the septum. Cartilage can be destroyed resulting in loss of nasal dorsal support.

Immediate intervention of septal hematoma is desirable and includes making mucosal incisions low on the septum to facilitate drainage or removal of hematoma by aspiration (Fig. 2–5). Drains are sometimes placed and packing is useful to prevent reaccumulation postoperatively. Transseptal mattress sutures to hold the mucoperichondrial flaps in place or intranasal or extranasal septal splints can also be applied. If a septal abscess is present on evacuation then aggressive antibiotic therapy is instituted.

Dorsal hematomas can also develop as a result of a direct blow and tearing of the upper lateral cartilages from the nasal bones.[9] Pressure necrosis of the cartilaginous structures may occur so immediate intranasal drainage should be accomplished.

Timing of the Fracture Repair

In certain limited situations the reduction of the nasal fracture may be performed in the emergency room using local anesthesia. In this case swelling should be minimal (usually in

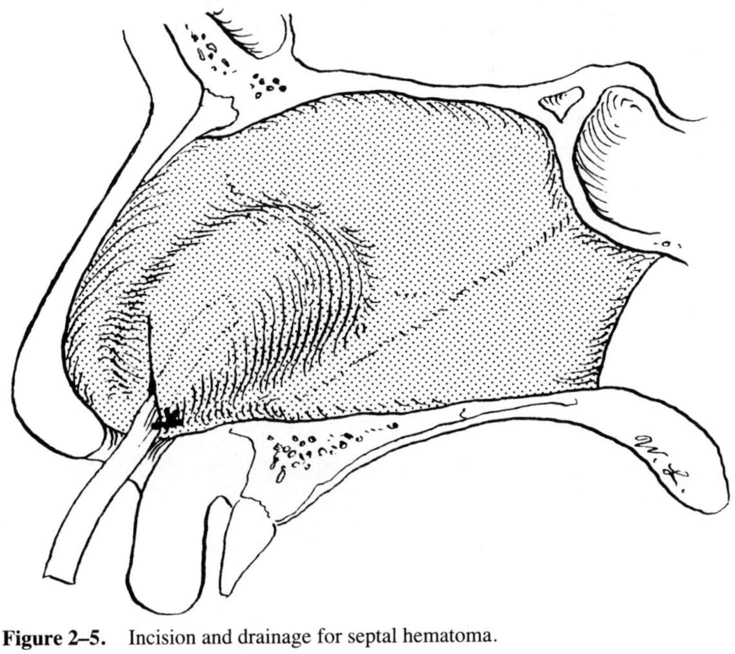

Figure 2–5. Incision and drainage for septal hematoma.

the first 2 to 3 hours of injury), fractures should be simple, and patient cooperation is required. Invariably this ideal situation does not often exist and extensive swelling or more life- threatening injury precludes early definitive management of the fracture. Usually edema will resolve within 3 to 5 days. The utilization of ice and head of bed elevation will facilitate the resolution of nasal swelling. The obvious risk of fracture reduction that is delayed is a malunion as bony fixation can occur as early as 2 to 3 weeks especially in young healthy patients. Ideally fracture reduction should proceed within 5 to 7 days for children and within 7 to 10 days for adults.

ANESTHESIA

Local and general anesthesia have both been used to treat nasal fractures. In the majority of situations local anesthesia with sedation can be used in adults whereas general anesthesia appears to work better with the younger patients. The choice of anesthesia is also dependent on the severity of the nasal injury and on the degree of patient apprehension and pain tolerance. Local anesthesia with or without sedation is considered the safest approach but if this modality precludes an adequate reduction of the nasal fracture then general anesthesia should be considered. There have been criticism that local anesthesia and patient intolerance may prevent the clinician from utilizing the necessary force required for reduction and that final outcome may be suboptimal for that patient. Recent literature however in comparing manipulation of the fractured nose under local and general anesthesia found no obvious advantage in clinical outcome.[33,34]

Regardless of the anesthetic choice the nose is usually prepared topically and locally. The vibrissae should be trimmed and a topical anesthetic agent such as cocaine 4% on cotton pledgets is placed in strategic locations intranasally (Fig. 2–6). Adding five drops of 1000 epinephrine to 8 mL of 4% cocaine will increase the vasoconstrictive effects. The pledgets are usually placed beneath the nasal dorsum, at the posterior edge of the middle turbinate, on the septum and on the floor of the nose, and left in place for a period of 10 minutes. If cocaine is not desirable, phenylephrine hydrochloride or oxymetazoline hydrochloride or (Afrin®) nasal spray can be used as the vasoconstricting agent.

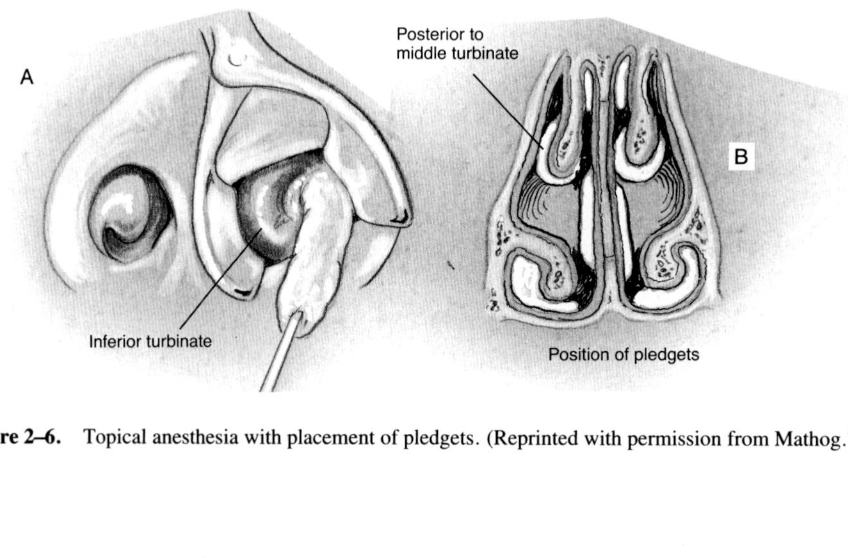

Figure 2–6. Topical anesthesia with placement of pledgets. (Reprinted with permission from Mathog.[62(p231)])

After applying the topical anesthesia the nose should be blocked with a local anesthetic agent such as xylocaine 1 to 2% with 1/100,000 adrenaline (Fig. 2–7). The injections should be intranasally placed on the dorsum to block the infratrochlear and anterior ethmoidal nerves, along the superior maxilla to block the infraorbital nerve, and at the base of the caudal septum to block the nasopalatine nerve, superior alveolar nerve, and branches of other nerves to the midface.

CLOSED VERSUS OPEN REDUCTION

The repair of acute nasal fractures can be managed by closed or open techniques. The choice of which technique should be used primarily has been the subject of controversy in the literature.

Closed nasal reduction is generally safe and easy to perform with a low morbidity and if a trial of manipulation is unsuccessful open reduction or delayed reconstructive techniques can be used. Kurihara and Kim[35] reported that 82% of nasal fracture patients were managed successfully with manipulation of the nasal segments alone. Illum[36] reported that 90% of patients treated with closed nasal reduction were fully satisfied with the results and that 82% of these patients had no cosmetic complaints. This study as well as others did not support the concept that a large number of nasal fractures should be treated with open reduction.[35] Alternatively, Harrison[23] demonstrated in a retrospective study of 40 patients that only 13 had perfect results following manipulation. Evaluating their own success rate, Murray and Maran[13] noted a 30 to 42% failure rate of closed nasal reduction.

The significant failure rate is a major criticism of closed nasal reduction techniques and advocates of open methods believe that a better result can be obtained primarily with

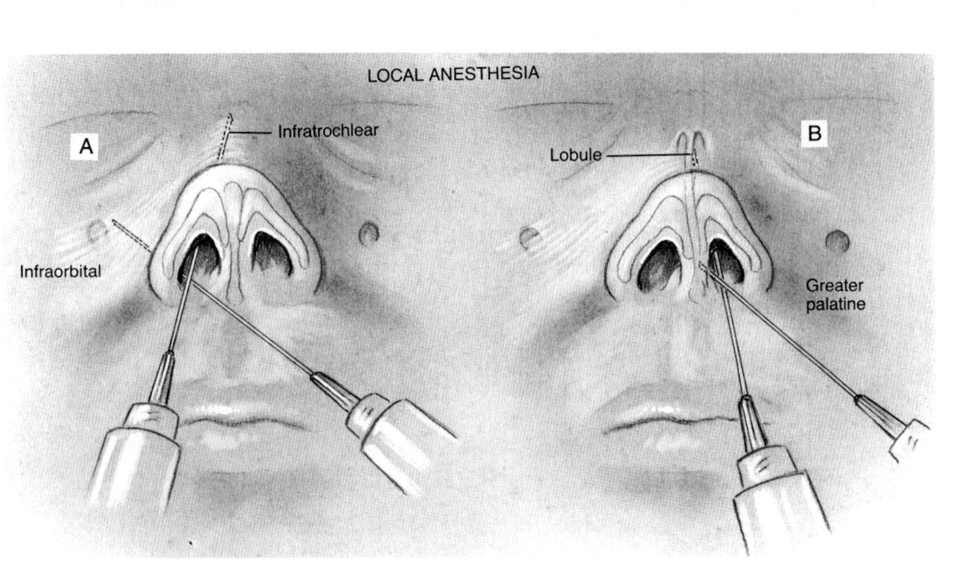

Figure 2–7. (A). Local anesthesia applied to infratrochlear and infraorbital nerves. (B). Local anesthesia applied to lobule and greater palatine nerve. (Reprinted with permission from Mathog.[62(p231)])

open reduction thus obviating later reconstructive techniques. The proposed advantage is better visualization of the fractured segments allowing a more accurate repositioning and fixation.[23,37,38] Hematomas can be directly addressed through open techniques as well.

Ideally the least invasive technique that provides the best long-term results should be used. A trial of closed nasoseptal manipulation appears reasonable for most acute fractures. If reduction is inadequate or if there is significant instability of the reduced nasoseptal segments then it is logical to proceed to open reduction techniques.

Septal Considerations

The literature has shown that despite successful management of the nasal pyramid an inadequately managed acute septal dislocation can produce a late external nasal deformity. The adage of "as goes the septum goes the nose" is a valid one in that late distortion of the nasal pyramid is secondary to progressive deviation of the septum.

Fry[39] believes that this progressive deformity is the result of a release of interlocked stresses on the septal cartilage when an incomplete fracture occurs in this cartilage. This situation creates an imbalance in cartilaginous stresses and thus a progressive deviation occurs away from the fractured side.

Harrison[23] in cadaveric work refuted Fry's concept of delayed septal distortion due to release of internal stresses. He theorized that recurring deformity arises from failure to centralize the displaced septal fracture. The anterior cartilaginous segment can be replaced in the midline position but the unrepaired displaced rigid bony posterior portion of the C-shaped fracture will ultimately redisplace this anterior cartilaginous segment. The concept of progressive anterior septal deformity as a result of an unrepaired posterior bony fragment was reinforced by Murray et al.[24]

Guidelines for acute septal management regarding technique considerations are also unclear. Murray et al[24] in an attempt to alleviate this controversy did a cadaveric study on nasal fractures. They noted that after trauma, if the nasal bones were deviated greater than one half the bridge width then a concomitant C-shaped fracture of the bony cartilaginous septum was likely present. They concluded that open management of the septum (a limited resection of the cartilaginous bony deformity at their interface) at the time of nasal pyramid reduction provides significantly superior results over manipulation alone. If the fracture displacement is less than one half the bridge width without obvious septal fracture, then traditional realignment with manipulation provides acceptable repositioning.

Nevertheless the general rule is conservatism. Open reduction of the septum either with septoplasty or submucous resection techniques can be associated with complications such as perforation of already traumatized mucosa. Determining the adequacy of cartilaginous nasal support may be difficult and overzealous resection of septal skeleton can lead to saddling and/or columella retraction.

Closed Technique

Manual reduction is the method of choice for most presentations. The ideal patient is one with a normal preoperative appearance that presents with a tip fracture or an ipsilateral depressed nasal bone fracture (the Stranc and Robertson Plane 1 injuries). In the closed technique, typically the fractured external pyramid is first reduced followed by the septum. The reduction of septal fractures is sometimes accomplished as a result of a nasal pyramid reduction alone.[35]

After adequate vasoconstriction and anesthesia, a smooth straight elevator (eg, a Boies) is inserted into the nose under the depressed fragments (Fig. 2–8). The depth of insertion is controlled by measuring the distance from the point just inferior to the glabellar angle to the tip of the nose and then applying the elevator just short of that depth. After insertion and using slowly increasing outward and anterior pressure, the depressed fractures are reduced. The opposite hand, with external pressure on the nasal dorsum, controls the degree of elevation; it also helps to mold the fragments into the appropriate position. If there is a contralateral outwardly displaced nasal bone, the depressed side is elevated first followed by digital pressure on the lateralized segment for its reduction. Occasionally, the edges of the fractured bones may override, become impacted, and produce a "locked" effect compromising the closed nasal reduction.[40] A Walsham forceps can be used to grasp and directly manipulate the nasal bones, disimpacting and facilitating their reduction. If the nasal tip is fractured, direct elevation with the Boies elevator at the front part of the septum just under the dorsum of the nose should be performed. Bilateral elevation is required for comminuted fractures. If inspection of the septum reveals inadequate reduction, one can simultaneously elevate the dorsum and place the septum back in its normal anatomic position with an Asch forceps.

Once reduction is deemed satisfactory, it may be necessary to maintain correction with internal and/or external splinting techniques until healing begins. An internal packing of ribbon gauze impregnated with antibiotic ointment with or without incorporating polyethylene septal splints can be used. Certain authors believe that internal packing should be reserved for unstable reductions as nasal packing is uncomfortable, it macerates mucosa, and if inappropriately placed may actually displace the reduced segments.[2,41] If applied bilaterally and symmetrically internal nasal packing or alternatively nasal tampons may be used for nasoseptal support and hemostasis. Polyethylene splints should be instituted for

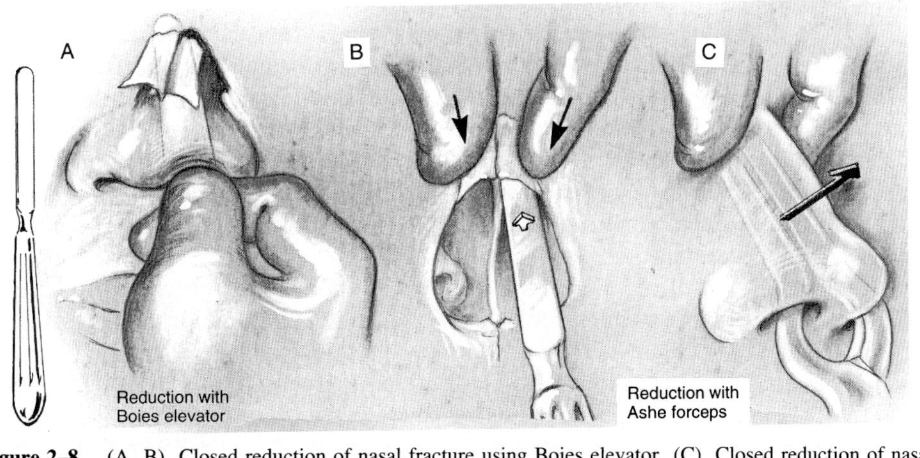

Figure 2–8. (A, B). Closed reduction of nasal fracture using Boies elevator. (C). Closed reduction of nasal fracture using Asch forceps. (Reprinted with permission from Mathog.[62(p232)])

open and/or unstable septal reductions. The packing is usually maintained for a period of 3 to 5 days with appropriate antibiotic coverage. Subsequent crusting should be removed and prophylactically treated with ointment and nasal saline douches.

The external nose should be protected by first applying steri-strips or cloth tape to the external skin. Pressure from the tape will inhibit hematoma formation and allow for symmetrical swelling to occur. An external splint made from pliable metal, plaster, or thermoplastic material may then be applied and molded to properly fit the nasal bones. It is removed 7 to 14 days after nasoseptal reduction.

In the event of suspected CSF rhinorrhea nasal packing is contraindicated. Septal splints in combination with external splinting may be sufficient. Alternative techniques utilizing external lead retention plates,[42] external halo fixation devices,[43] or orthodontic appliances[44] may be used. The "semiclosed" techniques require a closed nasal reduction and additionally, perforation of the nasal bones with pins or wires with attachment of external fixation or traction appliances. Other than CSF leakage, indications for these techniques include situations where the nasal dorsum is unstable and cannot be maintained with traditional splinting and packing techniques.

Open Reduction Techniques

Open techniques are indicated for nasal fractures that have failed closed nasal reduction either because severe comminution precludes adequate reduction and stabilization or early malunion has occurred.[38] Fractures that involve associated soft tissue and bony structures of the Stranc and Robertson Plane 3 fractures, naso-orbital fractures, medial maxillary, or Le Fort fractures are usually treated with open techniques.

Several approaches for open reduction are available. Standard endonasal rhinoplasty techniques can be of cosmetic benefit and allow direct fragment manipulation and reduction. Exposure is limited and may be inadequate if fixation is required[40] or if primary bone grafting is being considered. Intra or intercartilaginous incisions with conversion to transfixion incisions are used in conjunction with elevation of soft tissues of the nasal dorsum. Judicious undermining of soft tissue lateral to the fractures will help provide a degree of external stabilization afforded by soft tissue periosteal attachments.[45] Fragments can then be gently mobilized and reduced under direct vision. External approaches, although requiring skin incisions, provide exposure for fixation of fracture segments and repair of associated injuries as well. If already present, a laceration of the nasal dorsum may be used or extended for exposure. Alternatively a transverse glabellar incision may be placed with addition of Lynch incisions as needed for lateral exposure. This "open sky" approach is applicable for exploring naso-orbital or associated frontal sinus injuries.[46] Coronal, lateral rhinotomy, and degloving approaches are also available in certain circumstances. With exposure, the mucosal periosteum or perichondrium should be preserved and left attached to the bony segments. Unstable fragments can be secured with internal wire fixation techniques. Small caliber stainless steel wire is passed through l-mm drill holes and then secured in a figure of 8 configuration. To avoid wires being palpable or visible under thin nasal skin Renner[40] utilizes a slowly absorbing suture in a figure eight pattern. Reconstructive plates have been used in selected cases but have greater cosmetic limitations than wire. Although good results can be obtained with open techniques, late reconstructive efforts may be more difficult in the face of a placed wire or plate.

SEPTUM

Septal injuries can be managed via open methods with submucous resection or septoplasty techniques through Killian or intramembranous incisions. Mucosal flaps are elevated carefully to avoid mucosal tears that could lead to septal perforation. Hematomas are removed and if present, the bony cartilaginous skeletal framework can be examined. Conservative resection of a damaged skeletal septal framework is performed as overzealous removal of cartilage can cause saddle deformity secondary to the loss of dorsal support. Submucous resection involves the excision of buckled or telescoped portions of the nasoseptum and then returns the remainder to the midline. If a C-shaped deformity is present Harrison[23] recommends a low horizontal resection at the quadrilateral-vomerine groove interface, as well as removal of the fractured vertical component of the septum. Septoplasty techniques, on the other hand, involve minimal resection and replacement of displaced components. Scoring of the cartilage, figure eight suturing, and wiring techniques are utilized to facilitate reduction. Polyethylene splints should be applied during the healing period.

Pediatric Considerations

Injuries to the pediatric nasoseptal skeleton raise controversial management issues because of the impact on nasal and midfacial growth and development. Significant delayed aesthetic and functional abnormalities may develop. Significant delayed aesthetic and functional abnormalities may result as a consequence of disruption to the growth centers within the developing nasoseptal skeleton.[47] Growth center disruption occurs as a result of inciting trauma and may also be secondary to aggressive reparative efforts.[48,49] Therefore, careful considerations regarding the severity of injury and the treatment advocated must be weighed against the effects on nasal development.

Septal integrity, especially that of the quadrilateral cartilage, appears to be vital for proper nasal and anterior maxillary growth.[40,50] The loss of septal skeletal integrity leads to progressive bowing and septal spur formation as unequal forces act during growth. The sequelae of nasal obstruction, external deformity with loss of dorsal nasal support (secondary to abnormal septal development), and retarded midfacial development may occur. The importance of the nasoseptum for growth and development has been demonstrated in animal models but researchers cannot agree on the precise location of growth centers in humans.[51–53]

A conservative approach is advocated in pediatric nasal trauma. The nasoseptal skeleton of the child being proportionately cartilaginous tends to buckle and twist rather than fracture with injury.[7,54] Minimal impact may result in a returning to the normal anatomic position of the nasal skeleton or result in a greenstick-type injury with minimal or no obvious deformity. In this situation, the external nose should be protected with a splint during the healing process. If displacement is noted on examination, then reduction should be performed. During birth, trauma to the neonatal nasal skeleton can result in nasal obstruction, which can be life-threatening as newborns are obligate nasal breathers. Reduction with improvement of nasal airflow can usually be accomplished by external digital pressure alone without the need for anesthesia.[54]

Older children will require general anesthesia and closed nasal techniques for displaced nasal fractures. Stucker et al[54] advocate a trial of external digital compression for 15 minutes to realign the dislocated segments. If this will not suffice standard intranasal reduction instrumentation should be implemented and external splints and/or intranasal packing placed once reduction is deemed adequate.

Those fracture dislocations not responding to closed nasal reduction may require open techniques utilizing the utmost conservatism-preserving and reestablishing the integrity of the nasoseptal skeleton and protecting the investing soft tissues. Aggressive septoplasty or submucous resection techniques are contraindicated as well as the correction of congenital abnormalities in this setting. The goal is to correct the deformity and to recreate a functional airway as can be accomplished without harming growth and development. The resilience of cartilage to reduction and the unpredictability of long-term results can make this difficult. Chimielik et al[55] in evaluating treatment efficacy noted that 71% of children treated with closed nasal reduction techniques had adequate outcome with respect to aesthetics and function. It is generally agreed that any secondary reconstructive septorhinoplasty procedure should be postponed until at least the midteen years in most instances.[56]

COMPLICATIONS

Late septonasal deformities with or without associated obstruction as a result of suboptimal reduction or secondary to lack of intervention can be managed by a reconstructive septorhinoplasty techniques. Any reconstructive measures beyond the acute phase should be delayed for at least 6 months from the time of the initial injury. S-shaped, C-shaped, and twisted nasal deformities can result from malunion. The saddle-nose deformity characterized by a loss of dorsal nasal support is the result of a loss of septal skeletal framework either by resorption or telescoping injury. This produces a shortened flat nose with depressed nasal tip, retracted columella, and constricted soft tissue envelope.[57] Open or closed septorhinoplasty techniques with the incorporation of bone or cartilage grafting are employed for reconstructive efforts.[58, 61]

REFERENCES

1. Facer GW. A blow to the nose. *Postgrad Med.* 1981;70:83–93.
2. Schultz RC,DeVillers YT. Nasal fractures. *J Trauma.* 1975;15:319–327.
3. Lundin K. Ridell A, Sandberg N, Ohman A. One thousand maxillofacial and related fractures at the ENT clinic in Gothenberg. A two year prospective study. *Acta Otolaryngol.* 1972;75:359–361.
4. Hinderer KH. *Fundamentals of Anatomy and Surgery of the Nose.* Birmingham, Ala: Aecsculapius Publishing Co., 1971.
5. Bernstein L. Surgical anatomy in rhinoplasty. *Otolaryngol Clin North Am.* 1975;8:549–558.
6. Martinez SA. Nasal fractures. What to do for a successful outcome. *Postgrad Med.* 1987;82:71–77.
7. East CA, O'Donaghue G. Acute nasal trauma in children. *J Pediatr Surg.* 1987;22:308–310.
8. Courtiss EH. Septorhinoplasty of the traumatically deformed nose. *Ann Plast Surg.* 1978;5:443–449.
9. Hinderer KH. Nasal problems in children. *Pediatr Ann.* 1976;5:499–509.
10. Holt GR. Immediate open reduction of nasal septal injuries. *Ear Nose Throat J.* 1978;57:345–354.
11. Schultz RC. The management of common facial fractures. *Surg Clin North Am.* 1973;53:3–32.
12. Illum P, Kristensen KS, Jorgensen R, Pedersen CB. Role of fixation in the treatment of nasal fractures. *Clin Otolaryngol.* 1983;8:191–195.
13. Murray JAM, Maran AGD. The treatment of nasal injuries by manipulation. *J Laryngol Oto.* 1980;94:1405–1410.

14. James D. Maxillofacial injuries in children. In: Rowe NL, Williams JL, eds. *Maxillofacial Injuries*. New York, NY: Longman (Churchill Livingstone); 1985:538.
15. Dommerby H, Tos M. Nasal fractures in children long term results. *ORL J Otorhinolaryngol Relat Spec*. 1985;47:272–277.
16. Becker DB, Needleman H, Kotelchuck M. Child abuse orofacial trauma and its recognition by dentists. *J Am Dent Assoc*. 1978;97:24–28.
17. Nahum AM. The biomechanics of maxillofacial trauma. *Clin Plast Surg*. 1975;2:59–64.
18. Swearinger JJ. *Tolerance of the Human Face to Crash Impact*. Oklahoma City, Okla: Office of Aviation Medicine, Federal Aviation Administration, Civil Aeromedic Research Institute; July 1965.
19. Clark GM, Wallace CS. Analysis of nasal support. *Arch Otolaryngol*. 1970;92:118–123.
20. Moran WB. Nasal trauma in children. *Otolaryngol Clin North Am*. 1977;10:95–101.
21. Stranc MI, Robertson GA. A classification of injuries of the nasal skeleton. *Ann Plast Surg*. 1979;2:468–474.
22. Kazanjian VH, Converse JM. *The Surgical Treatment of Facial Injuries*. Baltimore, Md: Williams & Wilkins; 1959.
23. Harrison DH. Nasal injuries: their pathogenesis and treatment. *Br J Plast Surg*. 1979;32:57–64.
24. Murray JAM, Maran AGD, Mackenzie IJ, Raab G. Open vs closed reduction of the fractured nose. *Arch Otolaryngol*. 1984;110:797–802.
25. Murray JAM, Maran AGD. A pathologic classification of nasal fractures. *Injury*. 1986;17:338–344.
26. Mayell MF. Nasal fractures: their occurrence, management and some late results, *J R Coll Surg Edinb*. 1973;18:31–36.
27. Goode RL, Spooner TR. Management of nasal fractures in children. A review of current practices. *Clin Pediatr*. 1972;11:526–529.
28. Paskert JP, Manson PN. The bimanual examination for assessing instability in naso-orbito-ethmoida injuries. *Plas Reconstr Surg*. 1989;83:165–167.
29. Clark WD. Nasal and nasal septal fractures. *Ear Nose Throat J*. 1983;62:352–356.
30. Clayton MI, Lesse THJ. The role of radiography in the management of nose fractures. *J Laryngol Otolaryngol*. 1986;100:797–801.
31. deLacey GJ, Wignall BR, Hussain S, Reidy JR. The radiology of nasal injuries: problems of interpretation and clinical relevance. *Br J Radiol*. 1977;50:412–414.
32. Fry H. The pathology and treatment of hematoma of the nasal septum. *Br J Plast Surg*. 1969;22:331–335.
33. Cook JA, McRae RDR, Irving RM, Dowie LN. A randomized comparison of manipulation of the fractured nose under local and general anesthesia, *Clin Otolaryngol*. 1990;15:343–346.
34. Waldron J, Mitchell DB, Ford G. Reduction of fractured nasal bones; local vs general anesthesia. *Clin Otolaryngol*. 1989;14:357–359.
35. Kurihara K, Kim K. Open reduction and interfragment wire fixation of comminuted nasal fractures. *Ann Plast Surg*. 1990;24:179–185.
36. Illum P. Long term results after treatment of nasal fractures. *J Laryngol Otol*. 1986;100:273–277.
37. Kane NP, Kane LA. Open reduction of nasal fractures. *J Otolaryngol*. 1978;7:183–186.
38. Peerless SA. Nasal and septal reconstruction in acute nasal trauma. Presented to the middle section meeting, American Academy of Facial Plastic and Reconstructive Surgery; January 20, 1984; Madison, Wis.
39. Fry HJH. Nasal skeleton trauma and the interlocked stresses on the nasal septal cartilage. *Br J Plast Surg*. 1967;20:146–158.
40. Renner GJ. Management of nasal fractures. *Otolaryngol Clin North Am*. 1991;24:195–213.
41. Dingman RO, Natvig P. *Surgery of Facial Fractures*. Philadelphia, Pa: WB Saunders Co; 1964:267–294.
42. Mathog RH. *Atlas of Maxillofacial Trauma*. Philadelphia, Pa: WB Saunders Co; 1992:234–237.
43. Wurman LH, Sack GJ, Flannery JV. Halo external fixation of nasal fractures. *Laryngoscope*. 1983;93:1212–1216.
44. Lai S. Suspension and traction appliance for nasal, zygomaticomaxillary complex and zygomatic arch fractures. *J Oral Maxillofac Surg*. 1983;41:133–134.
45. Arden RL, Mathog RH. Nasal fractures. In: Cummings CW, Fredrickson JM, Harker LE, Crause JK, Shuller DE, eds. *Otolaryngology—Head and Neck Surgery*. St. Louis, Mo: Mosby-Year Book Inc; 1993:737–753.
46. Converse JM, Hogan VM. Open Sky approach for reduction of naso-orbital fractures. *Plast Reconstr Surg*. 1970;46:396.
47. Grymer LF, Gutierrez C, Stoksted P. Nasal fractures in children: influence on the development of the nose. *J Laryngol Otol*. 1985;99:735–739.
48. Pirsig W, Lehman I. The influence of trauma on the growing septal cartilage. *Rhinology* 1975;13:39–46.
49. Pirsig W. Septoplasty in children: influence on nasal growth. *Rhinology*. 1977;15:193–204.
50. Kemble JVH. The importance of the nasal septum in facial development. *J Laryngol Otol*. 1973;87:379–386.
51. Sarnat BG, Wexler MR. Growth of the face and jaws after resection of the septal cartilage in the rabbit. *Am J Anat*. 1966;118:755–768.

52. Wexler MR, Sarnat BG. Rabbit snout growth after dislocation of nasal septum. *Arch Otolaryngol*. 1965;81: 68–71.
53. Wexler MR, Sarnat BG. Rabbit snout growth: effect of injury to septonasal region. *Arch Otolaryngol*. 1961;74:305–313.
54. Stucker FJ, Bryarly RC, Shockley WW. Management of nasal trauma in children. *Arch Otolaryngol*. 1984;110:190–192.
55. Chmielik M, Gutkowska J, Kossowska E, Praglowska B. Reduction of nasal fractures in children. *Int J Pediatr Otorhinolaryngol*. 1986;11:1–4.
56. Farrior R. Management of late sequelae of nasal fractures. In: Mathog RH, ed. *Maxillofacial Trauma*. Baltimore, Md: Williams & Wilkins; 1984:266–279.
57. Stuzin JM, Kawamoto HK. Saddle nose deformity. *Clin Plast Surg*. 1988;15:83–93.
58. Olsen KD, Carpenter RJ, Kern E. Nasal septal injury in children. *Arch Otolaryngol*. 1980;106:317–320.
59. Wexler MR. Reconstructive surgery of the injuried nose. *Otolaryngol Clin North Am*. 1975;8:663–677.
60. Mathog RH. *Atlas of Craniofacial Surgery*. Philadelphia, Pa: WB Saunders Co; 1992:245–254.
61. David DJ, Moore MH. Cantilever nasal bone grafting with miniscrew fixation. *Plast Reconstr Surg*. 1987;83:728–732.
62. Mathog RH. *Atlas of Craniofacial Trauma*. Philadelphia, Pa: WB Saunders Co; 1992.

3

Management of Frontal Sinus Fractures

JAMES K. DZIADZIOLA, JR., M.D.
STEVEN C. MARKS, M.D.

Frontal sinus fractures are challenging and frequently complex injuries. Management may need to include soft tissue, bone, and dural repair and must take into consideration frontal sinus drainage and the possibility of long-term complications. Frontal sinus fractures are relatively uncommon accounting for 5 to 12% of maxillofacial injuries.[1] However, when including injury to the frontal drainage this rate rises to nearly 30% of patients treated for facial fractures.[2] Injury to the frontal sinus most often occurs from high-velocity impacts secondary to motor vehicle accidents with a high incidence of associated trauma.[3] Considering the amount of energy required to fracture the frontal bone it is not surprising that there is a significant amount of associated maxillofacial trauma as well as a high incidence of intracranial injury.[2,4]

Appropriate management of frontal sinus fractures is based on application of specific techniques according to the type of injury. Many factors are important in that decision-making process including soft tissue trauma, location of the fracture, degree of displacement of fractured segments, the presence of a cerebrospinal fluid (CSF) leak, and status of the nasofrontal drainage. Combined team approaches utilizing a maxillofacial surgeon and a neurosurgeon are often required for the creation of a safe sinus with low likelihood for long-term complications.

ANATOMY/EMBRYOLOGY

The frontal sinuses do not begin to develop until 2 years of age.[5] They are derived from the frontal recess as an invagination of the middle meatus. Alternately, they may arise from the ethmoid air cells. Aeration develops slowly during childhood. They do not assume their adult form until the teenage years with full development by the end of the second decade.[6] Unilateral frontal sinus development is seen in approximately 10% of people and bilateral agenesis is seen in 4 to 5%.[7]

The frontal sinus is situated between the anterior and posterior lamellae of the frontal bone. The anterior boundary of the sinus is the strong anterior wall. It is arched and much thicker than the posterior wall and is capable of withstanding between 800 and 2200 lb of pressure before fracturing.[8] The posterior wall is thin and delicate and intimately related to the underlying dura and cribriform plate. The inferior border is the roof of the orbit and the frontal sinus ostium. The ostium lies at the posteromedial aspect of the sinus floor. In most sinuses a true nasofrontal duct is not present, rather the frontal sinus opens by an ostium into the frontal recess of the ethmoid sinus or occasionally the ethmoidal infundibulum. The frontal sinuses are divided by a midline bony septum. It is not uncommon to find additional incomplete septa within each sinus.

Histologically, the sinus is lined by a pseudostratified ciliated columnar epithelium. Drainage of the sinus is facilitated by the unidirectional sweeping motion of the ciliated epithelium. The mucosa extends into the foramina of Breschet, which are the points of penetration for the diploic veins.[9] These veins connect the mucosal capillaries to the marrow cavity of the frontal bone. They also drain into the dural veins and are the mode for bacterial access from the sinus to the meninges.

DIAGNOSIS

Physical Exam

A high degree of suspicion for frontal sinus fracture is maintained when high-energy blunt trauma occurs to the face or when a local penetrating injury is seen. Typical signs indicating a frontal sinus fracture are anesthesia over the distribution of the supraorbital nerve, laceration over the lower forehead, supraorbital ridge or glabella, or a palpable depression over the frontal sinus.[10] The presence of a CSF leak may indicate a posterior table fracture, and the exact location of the leak must be sought out if it persists. Other less specific signs of fracture may include subconjunctival hemorrhage and periorbital emphysema. A late sign for a missed fracture may be the early development of frontal sinusitis following trauma.

A frontal sinus fracture is frequently accompanied by other multisystem trauma. Management of the airway and other potentially life-threatening conditions takes first priority. Owing to proximity of systems and the tremendous energy required to damage the anterior frontal sinus wall there is also frequently associated midfacial and orbital injuries. The full extent of neurotrauma must be quickly determined and the cervical spine must be cleared of injury. Full ophthalmologic examination is essential. Other associated facial injuries must be investigated.

Radiological Exam

Plain radiographs still play a screening role in the diagnosis of frontal sinus fractures. Caldwell and lateral views are generally the most useful.[11] Fracture lines are usually detected on the anterior wall especially if displaced. Pneumocephalus is indicative of posterior table involvement.[10,12] Any sign of sinus involvement should prompt further radiographic evaluation by computed tomography (CT). Both axial and coronal sections are preferred; however, a severely injured patient may not be able to tolerate positioning for coronal sections. The majority of these patients will require CT evaluation for intracranial pathology; concomitant evaluation of the frontal sinus can usually be performed.

CLASSIFICATION

Frontal sinus fractures can be classified according to location of injury. Incidence of fractures involving the anterior table alone range between 18 to 67% depending on the author.[4,13] The remaining injuries involve the posterior table or the frontal sinus floor with or without involvement of the anterior table. The posterior table is rarely involved without a concurrent fracture of the anterior table. Treatment strategies are based on three categories of involvement: (1) anterior table injury only; (2) posterior table injury with or without anterior table involvement; and (3) nasofrontal drainage compromise with or without either anterior or posterior table involvement.

MANAGEMENT

Acute management of frontal sinus injury is postponed until other life-threatening injuries are addressed. However, once a patient is stabilized complete evaluation of the sinus must proceed in a stepwise and expedient fashion to avoid complications of delayed treatment. Surgical management when indicated should proceed as soon as the patient is neurologically and medically stable.

In the remainder of this chapter, a systematic approach to the management of frontal sinus fractures based on the nature of the injury will be presented. The discussion begins with surgical approaches to the frontal sinus followed by anterior wall fractures, nasofrontal drainage, and finally posterior wall fractures.

Approaches

The bicoronal approach is preferred for greatest exposure and can be used for other midfacial trauma or as an extension of a neurosurgical approach.[10,12] It is indicated for nearly all frontal sinus surgery except in patients with preexisting lacerations in the forehead and male patients with frontal baldness. The bicoronal incision is placed 2 to 3 cm behind the hairline, extending from the preauricular crease on one side across the vertex to the preauricular crease on the opposite side (Fig. 3–1). The flap is elevated in the subgaleal plane on the surface of the pericranium and temporalis fascia. It is usually reflected inferiorly to the level of the orbital rims without difficulty. If greater exposure is needed inferiorly, the dissection must course below the temporalis fascia starting 1.5 to 2 cm above the zygomatic arch to avoid damaging the frontal branch of the facial nerve. The periosteum of the zygomatic arch can then be incised and elevation continued inferiorly to completely expose the zygomatic arch and lateral orbital rim.

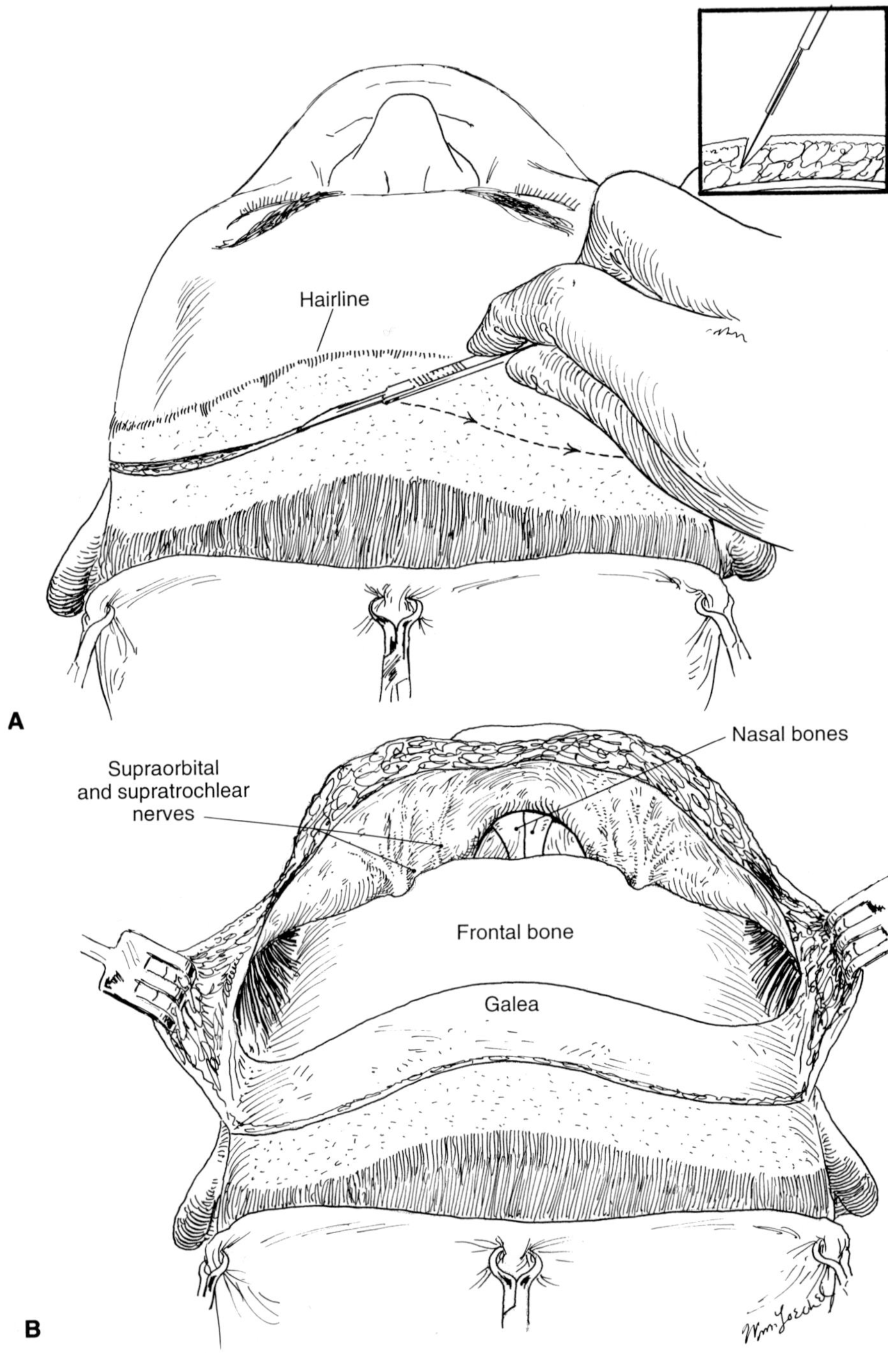

Figure 3–1. Bicoronal incision. (A). Incision is placed 1 to 2 cm behind hairline and beveled to avoid cutting across hair follicles. (B). Inferior exposure to the nasal dorsum achieved by elevating the supraorbital nerves from the bony canals.

Medially, the exposure is limited by the supraorbital nerves. By releasing the supraorbital nerves from their bony canals inferior exposure can be extended to the nasal dorsum.

Alternatively, the frontal sinus can be exposed through a unilateral or bilateral subbrow incision or a butterfly incision connecting bilateral subbrow incisions through a glabellar crease (Fig. 3–2). A third approach using a midforehead incision through an existing furrow is also possible. The brow incision should be considered in patients with frontal baldness but requires sacrifice of the supraorbital nerves and therefore is not routinely used. The midforehead approach is usually reserved for patients with lacerations or baldness with deep forehead creases as it is cosmetically inferior.

Anterior Wall Fractures

Nondisplaced anterior wall fractures do not require surgical management as the likelihood of obstruction to sinus drainage is low without sinus floor involvement.[6,14] Observation includes interval plain radiographs to demonstrate reaeration of an opacified sinus and to rule out mucocele.

Simple depressed fractures can be treated by elevation of the fragment alone. The fragments will usually remain in reduction owing to a lack of muscular pull. These can be temporarily supported by placing a Gelfoam sponge in the sinus. However, internal fixation with interfragment wires or microfixation plates adds a degree of stability and can be placed with little or no additional morbidity.

Comminuted depressed fractures are treated with interfragment wiring or microplating because periosteal closure over bony fragments without fixation can lead to loss of reduction and resultant deformity.[15] The sinus is inspected for damaged mucosa, with careful removal of loose fragments. The sinus is then copiously irrigated to remove residual debris. This is necessary to prevent mucosa from becoming trapped in the fracture repair leading to late mucocele formation.

The decision to use wires or plates is made on the basis of the degree of comminution. The microplates are easily applied and add stability. However, in cases with extensive comminution, the fragments may be too small and numerous to utilize plating. In these cases interfragment wiring or a combination of wires and plates is used to piece the anterior wall together.

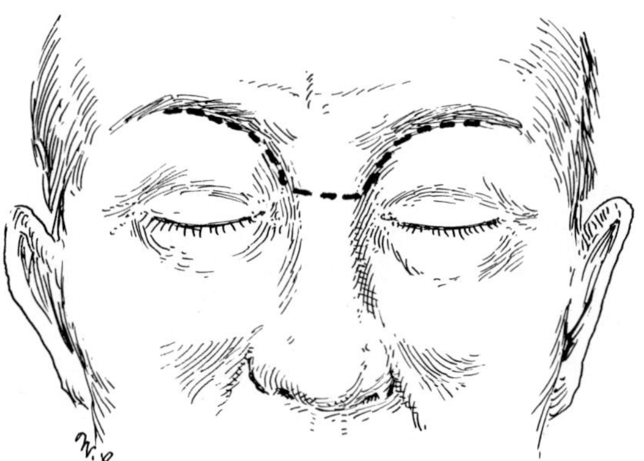

Figure 3–2. Bilateral subbrow incision connected through a glabellar crease.

There are various approaches to the problem of missing segments of bone. Defects smaller than 1.5 cm in diameter can be tolerated as residual deformity is minimal.[6] Split calvarial grafts, rib grafts, and methyl methacrylate can be used for reconstruction of larger defects.[6,10] Split calvarial grafts are preferred because they can be harvested locally with minimal donor site morbidity and have been associated with less late resorption.[16] Grafts are trimmed to span the defect and then secured with microfixation plates or wires (Fig. 3–3).

If the anterior wall cannot be adequately reconstructed, the frontal sinus can be ablated. The sinus mucosa is denuded and the inner cortex is burred down to extirpate the mucosa in the foramina of Breschet. The nasofrontal drainage is closed by invaginating the mucosa into the frontal recess. Care must be taken to remove as much of the mucosa from the drainage area as possible to decrease the likelihood of ingrowth of mucosa into the sinus. The sinus is then permanently blocked with a temporalis muscle and fascia graft. The cosmetic defect is then addressed with either bone grafts or methyl methacrylate implants.

Nasofrontal Recess Involvement

Nasofrontal drainage is exposed to injury whenever there is an anterior frontal wall fracture. The additional presence of a supraorbital fracture, a nasoethmoid fracture, or a

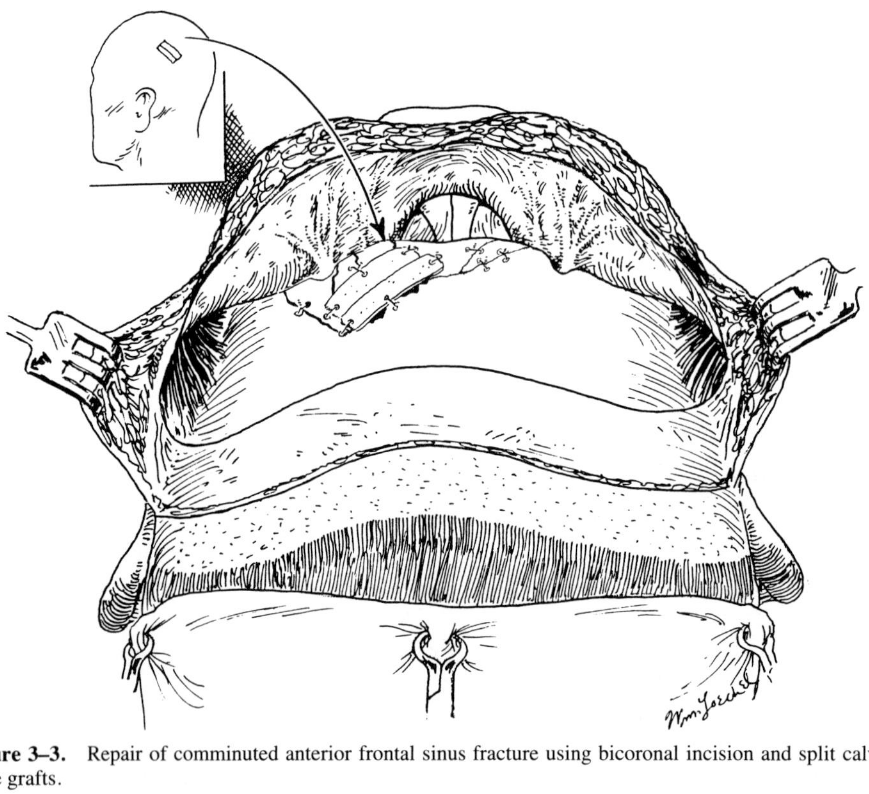

Figure 3–3. Repair of comminuted anterior frontal sinus fracture using bicoronal incision and split calvarial bone grafts.

fracture of the sinus floor increases the likelihood of drainage involvement.[17] Combined posterior and anterior wall fractures almost uniformly involve the sinus floor causing drainage injury.[17]

Preoperatively, plain radiographic findings of a persistent sinus opacification or air-fluid level suggest obstruction.[18] Computed tomographic findings of anterior ethmoid involvement and fracture of the frontal sinus floor are strongly suspicious of nasofrontal drainage compromise.[19] Failure to diagnose an obstruction may lead to formation of a mucocele or a mucopyocele.[10] All patients suspected of having a nasofrontal obstruction should undergo evaluation. Fractures through the duct require operative intervention. In cases that are suspicious for injury the nasofrontal drainage system can be evaluated for patency by injecting either methylene blue or fluorescein into the sinus and observing the nasal cavity for presence of these solutions.[6,10] Failure of these substances to enter the nasal cavity indicates an obstruction. The goal of treatment of an obstruction is to restore patency of the duct or to remove the sinus as a functional unit.

Removal of the intersinus septum in the presence of a unilateral nasofrontal drainage injury theoretically may allow drainage from the injured sinus to the contralateral uninjured side. However, this has been found to be inadequate.[6,14]

Reconstruction of the duct can be attempted. This may require mucosal flaps and long-term stenting, and is associated with a high rate of eventual stricture.[18] Close long-term follow-up is required to evaluate for late obstruction.

Obliteration of the sinus is a safer procedure for this injury and has been our practice. There are three basic principles for safe obliteration of the frontal sinus. The entire sinus mucosa must first be removed, the nasofrontal drainage must be occluded, and the sinus must be packed.

Exposure of the sinus after initial incision and flap elevation is either through existing anterior wall fractures or by creating a template from a preoperative Caldwell view radiograph taken with a coin taped to the forehead. The coin is utilized to assure accurate one-to-one reproduction. The outline of the frontal sinus is then cut out and traced onto the patient's frontal bone. An oscillating sagittal saw is used at shallow angles to outline the bony flap. Slight back cuts are formed at the supraorbital rims to allow clean flap elevation. Osteotomes are used to divide the intersinus septum and elevate the flap. (Fig. 3–4).

Once the sinus cavity is exposed, great care is taken to completely remove all mucosa. Initial dissection with an elevator is followed by drilling down the entire interior surface of the sinus to remove any microinvaginations into the foramina of Breschet.

The mucosa of the frontal recess is then invaginated onto the ethmoid and the recess obstructed with temporalis muscle or bone. A useful technique that has been successful in our hands is to occlude the recess with muscle and then overly this with a temporalis fascia graft (Fig. 3–5). This has the theoretical advantage of adding multiple layers as well as providing a platform for the obliteration.

The sinus itself can be obliterated with muscle, pericranium, autogenous bone, or fat.[6,14] Fat is usually utilized because it can be harvested with minimal donor site morbidity and resists reabsorption.[20] Another advantage of using fat is that is creates a distinctive signal on a magnetic resonance image scan, which facilitates postoperative follow-up.[21]

Immediate complications associated with obliteration are infection, dural lacerations, forehead dysesthesia, and imperfect forehead contour. Late complications include frontal bossing.[22] As reported by Hardy and Montgomery[23] the long-term success rate of frontal sinus obliteration is about 95% with very few complications when performed carefully.

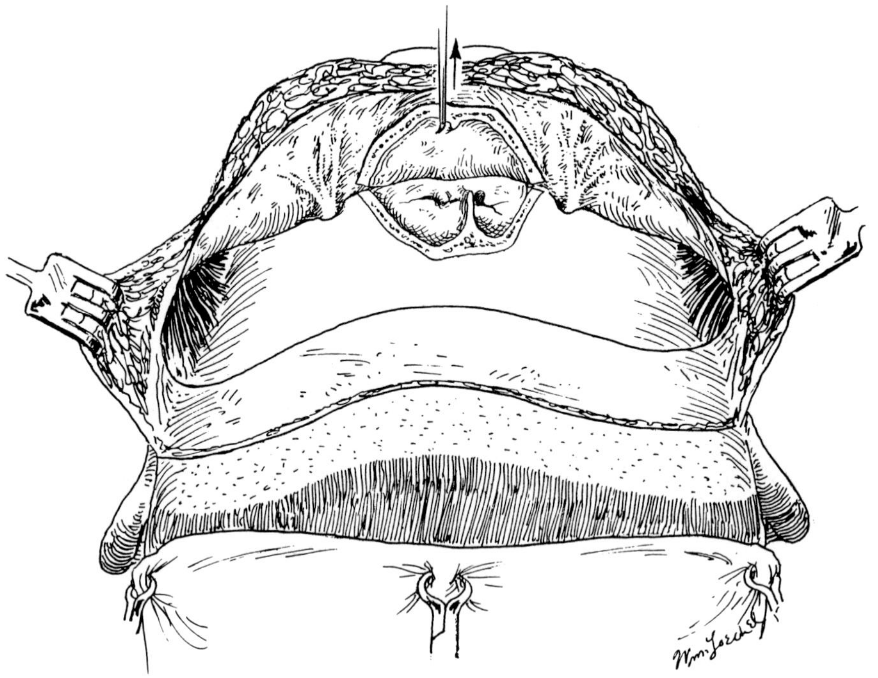

Figure 3–4. Exposure of fracture through the floor of the frontal sinus by bicoronal incision and osteoplastic flap.

Posterior Table Involvement

Management of posterior table fractures remains controversial. Some authors would advise observation of patients with minimal (less than one table width) or no displacement.[10,18] However, the risk of long-term complications in these injuries is high and continued observation for up to 10 to 20 years may be necessary.[24] Furthermore, plain radiographs and even CT scans are frequently unable to completely and accurately assess the degree of posterior table involvement. It has, therefore, been the practice of these authors to explore all cases of frontal sinus fractures in which there is either a combined anterior and posterior table fracture or a potentially unreliable patient with an isolated posterior table fracture.

Exploration is usually performed through a bicoronal flap and osteoplastic frontal sinusotomy. If there is no displacement and no CSF leak, the sinus is irrigated and closed. If there is displacement or leak, the posterior table fragments are carefully elevated and reduced. If impacted, the surrounding bone may need to be burred down to allow disimpaction without dural laceration. As previously described mucosa within the sinus is completely removed and all bony surfaces are polished down to allow obliteration to be performed.

When dural laceration is discovered direct suturing is preferred. However, if not possible, repair with fascia lata, temporalis fascia, or lyophilized dura is required. The use of fibrin glue if available can facilitate this closure.

In cases with severe comminution and bone loss, cranialization is required. The sinus is prepared as for obliteration and the posterior wall is removed. Then the sinus floor is

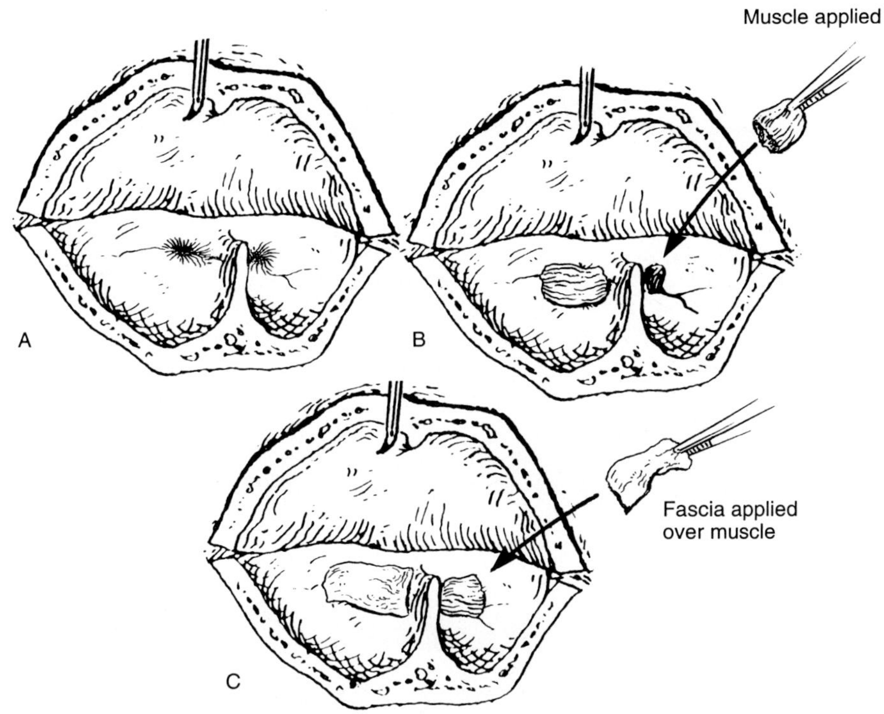

Figure 3–5. Blockage of nasal frontal drainage. (A). Mucosal flaps are turned in toward the nose. (B). A muscle plug obliterates the opening. (C). A temporalis fascia graft is laid over the muscle plugs.

supported by a pericranial flap, fat graft or a fascial patch, and the frontal lobe allowed to advance to fill the sinus cavity (Fig. 3–6).

COMPLICATIONS

The mechanism of action for most major complications stems from infectious causes related to nasofrontal drainage obstruction and communication to the intracranial contents. Meningitis has been found to be as high as 6% in some series following treatment for frontal sinus fracture.[2,4] Immediate exploration with repair of dural tears and obliteration or cranialization of the sinus are recommended in these cases.

Sinus obstruction has been shown to cause development of pyocele or mucopyocele.[25] After obliteration, residual mucosa from within the foramina of Breschet or from the nasofrontal recess can reepithelialize the frontal sinus to cause mucocele formation. Partial loss of the bony sinus walls appears to increase the likelihood of mucocele formation.[26] Mucoceles can develop within 6 months of initial exploration or can manifest as late as 40 years after injury.[27] Unchecked these can lead to meningitis or brain abscess by bacterial migration via the diploic veins as well as lead to pressure osteonecrosis.[9,24]

Frontal sinusitis following conservative sinus surgery is common and can initially be treated medically with antibiotics and decongestants. Failure to respond to therapy or

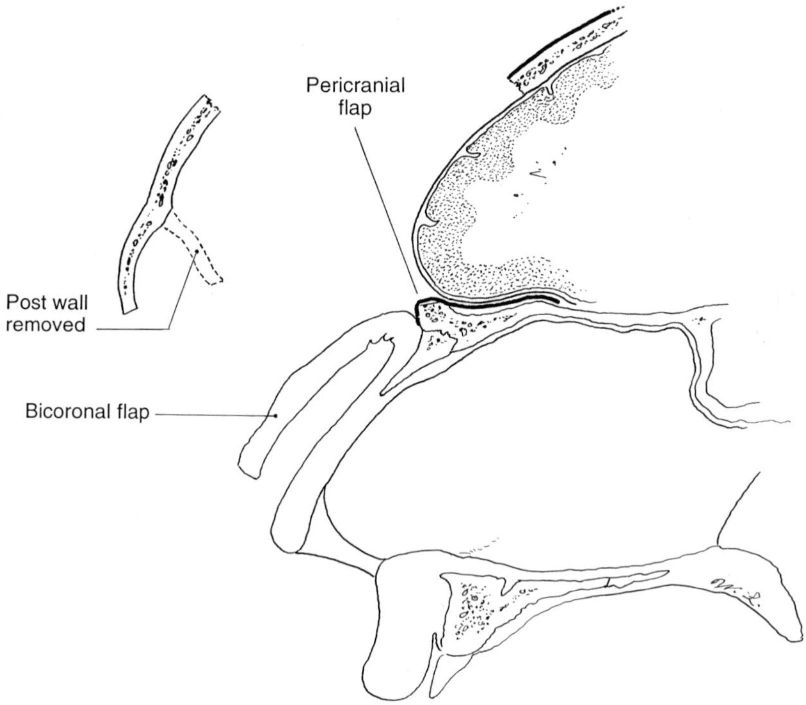

Figure 3–6. Cranialization of the frontal sinus. The posterior wall of the sinus is removed and the floor and drainage pathway covered by a pericranial flap from the frontal bone.

evidence of continued sinus opacification should prompt early reexploration with obliteration of the sinus.

Minor complications are often related to local infection, which is reported to be up to 10% when the frontal sinus is injured.[2,4,28] The majority of patients respond adequately to local care and antibiotics. Infrequently, fat grafts have been reported as a source of infection requiring reexploration and debridement.[29]

Persistent frontal headache and pain postoperatively have been reported when infections causes were absent in up to 5% of patients.[2] Etiology is not known. Dysesthesias of the supraorbital nerve are frequent with lacerations over the glabellar region and when the butterfly incision is used for approach to the sinus. The supraorbital nerve is generally preserved when the bicoronal approach is used however.[10]

Major bony deformities were frequent late complications after frontal sinus fracture.[10,18] Reabsorption of frontal bone due to loss of reduction was predominantly the cause. Since the advent of rigid fixators and the use of interfragment wiring, massive loss of bone is infrequently seen. Presently contour defects can be corrected at the time of repair with bone grafting or with methyl methacrylate in clean cases.[6,10]

SUMMARY

A systematic approach to frontal sinus fractures including thorough physical examination and CT imaging will minimize complications and lead to the reconstruction of a safe sinus.

Decision points in treatment hinge on the degree of bony displacement, the presence of CSF leak, and the likelihood of nasofrontal obstruction. Severe displacement requires reduction. Nasofrontal obstruction requires obliteration of the sinus. Persistant CSF leak requires dural repair. Complications are often manifested late and prompt recognition through long-term follow-up is mandatory.

REFERENCES

1. May M. Nasofrontal duct in frontal sinus fractures. *Arch Otolaryngol*. 1970;92:534–538.
2. Wilson BC, Davidson B. Comparison of complications following frontal sinus fractures managed with exploration with or without obliteration over 10 years. *Laryngoscope*. 1988;98:516–520.
3. Schultz RC. Frontal sinus and supraorbital fractures from vehicle accidents. *Clin Plast Surg*. 1975;2:93–106.
4. Wallis A, Donald PJ. Frontal sinus fractures: a review of 72 cases. *Laryngoscope*. 1988;98:593–598.
5. Ritter F. *The Paranasal Sinuses: Anatomy and Surgical Technique*. 2nd-ed. St Louis, Mo: CV Mosby Co; 1978:34.
6. Donald PJ. Frontal Sinus Fractures. In: Cummings CW, Fredrickson JM, Harker LA, eds. *Otolaryngology, Head and Neck Surgery*. St Louis, Mo: CV Mosby Co; 1986:901–21.
7. Harris L, Marano GD, McCorkle D. Nasofrontal dust: CT in frontal sinus trauma. *Radiology*. 1987;165: 195–198.
8. Nahum AM. The biomechanics of maxillofacial trauma. *Clin Plast Surg*. 1975;2:59–64.
9. Donald PJ. The tenacity of the frontal sinus mucosa. *Otolaryngol Head Neck Surg*. 1979;87:557–566.
10. Luce EA. Frontal sinus fractures: guidelines to management. *Plast Reconstr Surg*. 1987;80:500–508.
11. Vasconez HC, Luce EH. Frontoethmoidal fractures. In: Habal MB, Ariyan S, eds. *Facial Fractures*. Philadelphia, Pa: BC Dreher; 1989:568.
12. Pollack K, Payne EE. Fractures of the frontal sinus. *Otolaryngol Clin North Am*. 1976;9:517–522.
13. Shockley WW, Stucker FJ, Gage-White L, Antony SO. Frontal sinus fractures: some problems and some solutions. *Laryngoscope*. 1988;98:18–22.
14. Owens OT, Mathog RH. Frontal sinus fractures. In: Foster CA, Sherman JE, eds. *Surgery of Facial Bone Fractures*. New York, NY: Churchill Livingstone; 1987:13.
15. Gruss JS. Fronto-naso-orbital trauma. *Clin Plast Surg*. 1982;9:577–589.
16. Maves DM, Matt BH. Calvarial bone grafting of facial defects. *Otolaryngol Head Neck Surg*. 1986;95:464–474.
17. Stanley RB, Becker TS. Injuries of the nasofrontal orifaces in frontal sinus fractures. *Laryngoscope*. 1987;97:728–731.
18. Rohrich RJ, Hollier LH. Management of frontal sinus fractures. *Adv Craniomaxillofac Fracture Mgmt*. 1992;19:219–232.
19. Harris L, Marano GD, McCorkle D. Nasofrontal duct: CT in frontal sinus trauma. *Radiology*. 1987;165: 195–198.
20. Montgomery WW. The fate of adipose implants in a bony cavity. *Laryngoscope*. 1964;74:816–827.
21. Catalano PJ, Lawson W, Som P, Biller HF. Radiographic evaluation and diagnosis of the failed frontal osteoplastic flap with fat obliteration. *Otolaryngol Head Neck Surg*. 1991;104:225–234.
22. Nichols RD. Treatment of frontal sinus fractures. In: Mathog RH, ed. *Maxillofacial Trauma*. Baltimore, Md: Williams & Wilkins; 1984:288.
23. Hardy JM, Montgomery WW. Osteoplastic frontal sinusotomy: an analysis of 250 operations. *Ann Otol Rhinol Laryngol*. 1976;84:523–532.
24. Denneny JC, Davidson WD. Combined otolaryngological and neurosurgical approach in treating sinus fractures. *Laryngoscope* 1987;97:633–637.
25. Schenck NL, Rauchbach E, Ogura JH. Frontal sinus disease II, development of the frontal sinus model: occlusion of the nasofrontal duct. *Laryngoscope*. 1974;84:728–731.
26. Hybels RL, Newman MH. Posterior table fractures of the frontal sinus: an experimental study. *Laryngoscope*. 1977;87:171–179.
27. Bordley JE, Bosley WR. Mucoceles of the frontal sinus: causes and treatment. *Ann Otol Rhinol Laryngol*. 1973;82:696–702.
28. Nadell J, Kline D. Primary reconstruction of depressed frontal skull fractures including those involving the sinus, orbit and cribiform plate. *J Neurosurg*. 1974;41:200–207.
29. Larrabee WF, Travis LW. Frontal sinus fractures their supparative complications and surgical management. *Laryngoscope*. 1980;90:1810–1813.

4

Maxillary Trauma

KEVIN L. ROBINSON, M.D.
STEVEN C. MARKS, M.D.

The maxilla is frequently involved in traumatic injuries. It is the focal point of the bony architecture of the face and links the frontoethmoid and cranial base superiorly to the occlusal plane inferiorly. Moreover, it has important relationships to the orbit and nasal and oral cavities. Trauma to the maxilla may therefore have serious functional consequences including disorders of lacrimation and smell, loss of nasal airway, malocclusion, as well as cosmetic deformities. The modern understanding of maxillary trauma begins with an understanding of the premorbid anatomy and mechanisms that lead to maxillary fractures. Le Fort[1] applied low-velocity impact forces to the skull to describe the great lines of weakness in the face and classified the fractures based on the most superior level fracture line. He recognized that the primary fracture sites could occur in combination or in association with any number of different lesser fracture lines. His work, in addition to characterizing fracture patterns, brought clinical attention to these injuries. Today many maxillary fractures are the sequelae of high-energy impact forces resulting from motor vehicle accidents and violent assaults.[2] Most occur in combination with fractures extending into the nasoethmoid and orbital regions.

INCIDENCE

Maxillary fractures are less common than mandibular, malar, or nasal fractures, and only comprise 10 to 20% of all facial fractures.[3–7] Males outnumber females by a ratio of 5:1. This is thought to occur secondary to a greater number of males involved in at-risk behaviors. Seventy-five percent of victims are between the ages of 10 and 40 years. Assaults and motor vehicle accidents are the most common causes. Other causes include industrial accidents, falls, and sports-related injuries. The most frequently encountered concomitant injuries are lacerations and abrasions (75) followed by concurrent facial bone injuries and neurological injuries.[3–7] In most series Le Fort II fractures were the most common occurring in 38 to 50% of individuals whereas Le Fort III fractures were the least common occurring in 9 to 12%.[3–7]

In a series of experiments by Nahum[8] force tolerance ranges were determined for facial bones. Relatively low forces were found to disrupt the maxilla (150 to 300 lb) in comparison with the frontal bone (800 to 1600 lb) and mandible (550 to 900 lb). Tolerance values were found to be slightly lower in the female skeleton. Motor vehicle accidents continue to account for the greatest number of Le Fort fractures despite the instituting of mandatory seat belt laws in many states. Forward collisions account for approximately one half of all motorist injuries. It is readily appreciated that a soft yielding surface absorbs and dissipates forces on impact (ie, a padded dashboard) much more effectively than a solid rigid structure (ie, steering wheel or windshield). Obviously, the unrestrained driver and passenger place themselves at a greater risk for severe head, chest, neck, and abdominal injuries. Side collisions, unlike frontal restrained motor vehicle accidents, can cause the head to strike any object in the compartment of the vehicle. Depending on the angle and direction of impact, the head may strike the oncoming vehicle, window, or other nearby occupants. These types of injuries are more likely to involve the temporo-parietal skull, zygoma, and possibly mandible. The use of lap belts combined with shoulder restraints should lower the incidence of midfacial fractures. As driver and passenger airbags become standard in motor vehicles, it should help to drastically reduce the number and severity of facial fractures secondary to motor vehicle accidents.

ANATOMY

The maxillary bones are paired structures that contribute much to the vertical facial skeleton. The maxilla consists of a body and four processes, the alveolar, frontal, palatine, and zygomatic (Fig. 4–1). The maxillary sinus is contained in the body and is thought to protect the craniofacial structures and absorb the forces of mastication. The alveolar process of the maxilla is dependent on the dentition for strength and support. When teeth are present, the alveolar process is strong and provides adequate support for the upper component of the maxilla. Alveolar atrophy and bony recession are common in edentulous patients, which predispose them to Le Fort I fractures.

The maxilla attaches to the cranial base via a series of pillars or buttresses. The buttresses maintain the relative position of the maxilla to the mandible and skull base in addition to dissipating the forces of mastication. There are four vertical buttresses as described by Manson et al,[9] three of which are paired: the nasomaxillary (anterior), the zygomaticomaxillary (lateral), and the pterygomaxillary (posterior) buttress. The fronto-ethmoidal-vomerine pillar is the unpaired median buttress. The nasomaxillary buttress extends from the anterior part of the alveolus along the piriform aperture, to attach to the frontal base at the superior orbital rim. The lateral buttress extends from the lateral alveolus above the anterior molars to the zygomatic process of the frontal bone superiorly and the zygomatic arch laterally. The posterior buttress extends from the maxillary tuberosity to the cranial base via the pyramidal process of the palatine bone and medial pterygoid plate. The frontoethmoidal-vomerine pillar is composed of the median process of the frontal bone, the crista galli, the lamina perpendicularis of the ethmoid, and the nasoseptum.

There is little protection from horizontal forces as demonstrated in a study by Stanley and Nowak[10] in 1985, which showed forces directly perpendicular to the axis of the vertical pillars caused midfacial sheer in a posteroinferior direction along the sloping incline of the basisphenoid. Muscular forces are relatively insignificant in determining the maxillofacial complex displacement.

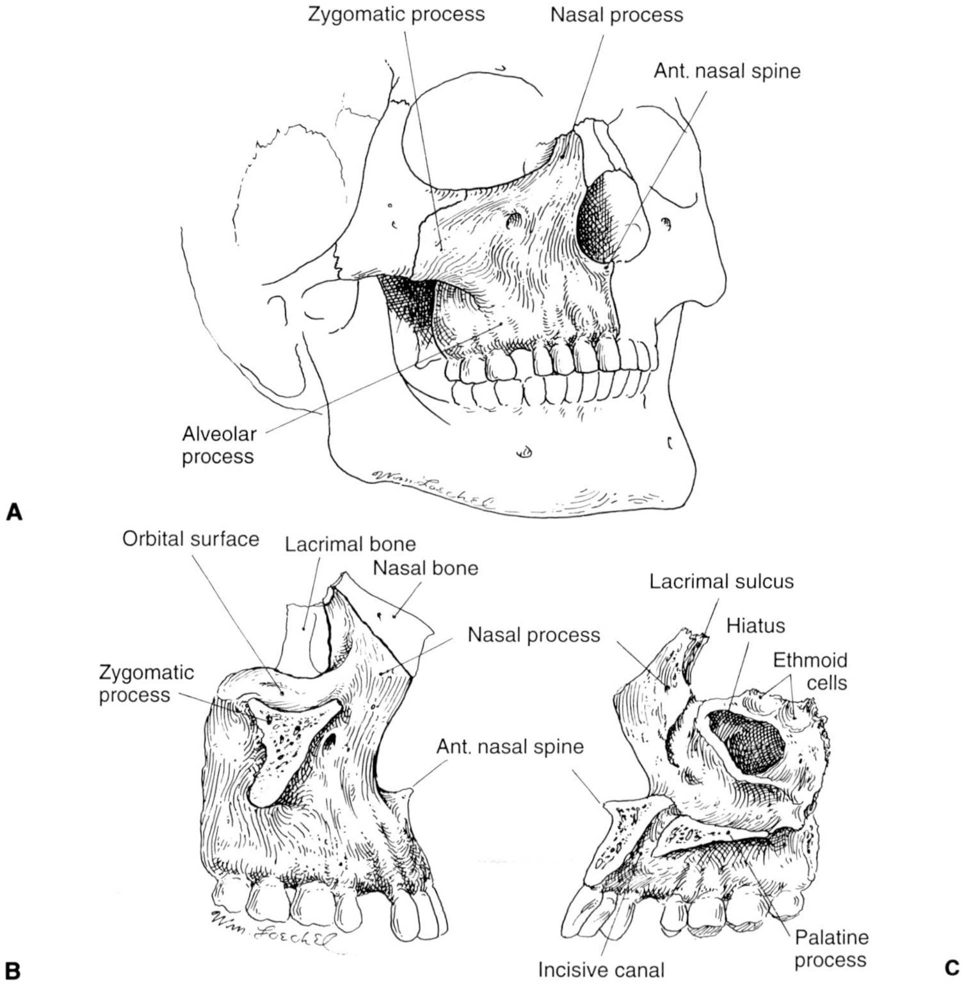

Figure 4–1. Anatomy of the maxilla. (A). Anterior view showing the nasal, zygomatic and alveolar processes, the anterior nasal spine, and the infraorbital foramen. (B). Lateral view. Note the relationship between the nasal process and the lacrimal and nasal bones. (C). Medial view showing the palatine process and the incisive canal. Note with the soft tissues removed the medial wall of the maxillary sinus forms a large opening—the maxillary meatus.

EVALUATION

General Considerations

Maxillary fractures should be considered after any severe blow to the midface. Initial presentation will vary with the nature of the injury and the degree of associated trauma. Evaluation of maxillary and facial trauma should proceed after the patient has been fully evaluated and stabilized from life-threatening injuries.

The evaluation of the facial skeleton should proceed in an orderly fashion. Initial inspection is performed followed by a detailed examination. The initial screen usually reveals extensive facial edema, ecchymosis, and possibly lacerations. The patient may have an obvious skeletal deformity, epistaxis, or malocclusion. On more detailed assessment the frontal and periorbital areas are palpated and examined for fractures, depressions, and asymmetry. Telecanthus when present is not always readily appreciated secondary to acute edema, but should be assessed. The eyelids may be severely edematous, limiting a thorough ophthalmologic examination, however, a careful examination must be performed to rule out concurrent eye injuries. Usually an ophthalmologic consultation is required but visual acuity and extraocular mobility should be immediately assessed. Epiphora is noted when present and may be secondary to posttraumatic tissue edema or an injury to the lacrimal apparatus. Intraoral examination may reveal blood clots, broken teeth, or mucosal lacerations.

After the physical examination is complete, a standard facial radiographic series is usually obtained. These radiographs were once the mainstay of preoperative evaluation and still have much to offer in terms of preliminary diagnosis. However, the current standard of care utilizes high resolution computed tomography (CT). This is usually performed with both soft tissue and bone windows in both the axial and coronal planes. Sufficiently thin cuts (2 mm) to delineate the anatomy are required. In some centers three- dimensional rendering of these scans is now available. This technique may be useful in developing a three-dimensional appreciation of the fracture pattern, especially in the more comminuted cases.

The CT scan should be closely evaluated for the fracture pattern, degree of displacement, and comminution. In addition, soft tissue relationships and orbital injury can be assessed on the same scan. Following careful review of the CT, it is almost always possible to classify the injury into one of several recurring patterns.

Le Fort I

Fractures of the maxilla can be classified conveniently into Le Fort and non-Le Fort fractures. Although the Le Fort fractures are usually described in their pure form, in clinical practice they are often mixed or comminuted. The Le Fort I or Guerin fracture is a low-transverse fracture that describes the separation of the palate from the body of the maxilla. The fracture line traverses the inferior nasoseptum along the floor of the nose and passes through the lateral piriform aperture, canine fossa, and the lateral wall of the maxilla (Fig. 4–2A). The fracture may also involve the inferior portion of the pterygoid plates. The resulting traumatic separation is also described as a "floating palate."

Clinically this can be diagnosed by grasping the most anterior stable maxillary teeth between the thumb and forefinger and rocking the maxilla. Motion of the anterior nasal spine and palate without motion of the nasal bones or maxilla is characteristic for this fracture. In contrast to the findings in the Le Fort II and III fractures, midface elongation and edema are not common. In addition, there is no circumorbital or subconjunctival hemorrhage.

Le Fort II

The Le Fort II or pyramidal fracture is the most common, and is frequently seen in association with the Le Fort I fracture. The fracture line passes through the nasal bones and descends a short way down the frontal process of the maxilla and lacrimal bones. It then courses through the orbital rim (the only Le Fort fracture to do so) close to the zygomaticomaxillary suture line. Finally, it traverses the lateral wall of the maxillary sinus and pterygoid plates via the pterygomaxillary fossa (Fig. 4–2B). This injury results in a "floating maxilla."

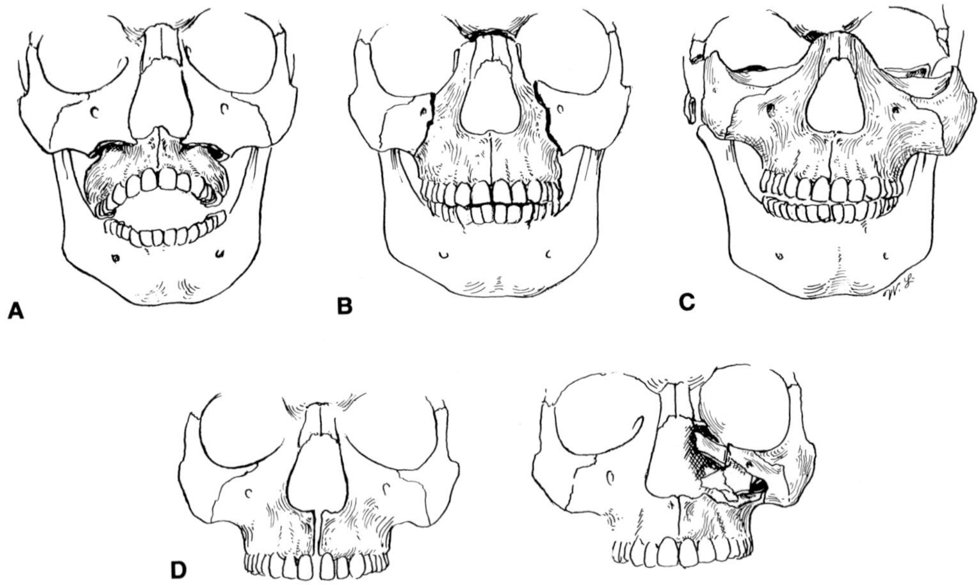

Figure 4–2. Maxillary fracture patterns. (A). Le Fort I. (B). Le Fort II. (C). Le Fort III. (D). Paramedian sagittal. (E). Medial maxillary.

Clinically this can be diagnosed by grasping the most anterior stable maxillary teeth between the thumb and forefinger and rocking the maxilla. This will elicit motion of the nasal pyramid but the zygoma and zygomaticofrontal region will remain fixed. Associated step deformities of the inferior orbital rims, circumorbital ecchymosis, and infraorbital nerve anesthesia are common features. Anosmia, which is common to Le Fort II and III fractures, may be secondary to tissue edema and hemorrhage, however it may persist if damage to the cribriform plate has occurred.

Examination of the face may reveal several appearances in the Le Fort II and III fractures. A "balloon" face is described when the normal facial contour is hidden secondary to severe edema and subcutaneous emphysema. This is contrasted with the "flat" or "pan" face, which is secondary to retrodisplacement of the maxilla, and should be viewed looking from above downward.

Le Fort III

The Le Fort III fracture, also referred to as craniofacial disjunction, is the most severe form of the traumatic maxillary fractures. In contrast to the Le Fort I and II fractures, these fractures result from impact forces angled obliquely to the horizontal buttresses. The fracture line originates just on the nasal side of the frontonasal suture line. It fractures the nasal bones and crosses the upper portion of the frontal process of the maxilla and lacrimal bone just before passing through the lamina papyracea and ethmoid sinuses. The fracture line extends laterally across the orbital floor, posterior to the inferior orbital fissure and divides in two directions. One extends across the lateral orbital wall near the sphenozygomatic junction whereas the other descends across the posterior maxilla passing through the upper aspect of the pterygoid plate near the basisphenoid (Fig. 4–2C).

The triad of raccoon facies (circumorbital ecchymosis), severe midfacial edema, and marked lengthening of the face is typical for the Le Fort III fracture. In craniofacial disjunction the entire midface will move and is appreciated with palpation of the zygomaticofrontal, zygomaticotemporal, and nasofrontal sutures. A thorough complete physical examination of patients with Le Fort III fractures must be carried out. Multiple organ system involvement is not uncommon in patients with Le Fort III fractures. In a series by Spector et al,[11] 4 of 26 patients expired before care could be provided.

Non-Le Fort Fractures

Sagittal Maxillary Fractures. Sagittal fractures of the palate are not common in facial trauma. It can occur with a palatoalveolar fracture or with a comminuted Le Fort fracture. Almost all midfacial fractures with sagittal splitting of the palate are comminuted. More than three fourths of these patients present with other concurrent facial fractures. These are most commonly the result of motor vehicle accidents and falls from excessive heights. Clinically, a step deformity with or without palatal mucosal laceration is seen. The fracture is usually off the midline because the vomer reinforces the palate in the midline (Fig. 4–2D). In cases where the mucosa is intact it is critical that the palate be palpated to avoid missing this diagnosis. Late posttraumatic sequelae include oronasal fistula and malocclusion.

Medial Maxillary Fractures. Medial maxillary fractures mimic nasal fractures, but they involve the maxilla and orbital rim (Fig. 4–2E). Patients often sustain this injury secondary to an object striking the side of the nose and medial maxillary wall. Presenting symptoms usually include epistaxis, nasal obstruction, and on occasion epiphora. In most patients there is a characteristic C- shaped deviation of the dorsum of the nose. Failure to recognize this injury can result in facial deformity and functional problems of the nasal cavity and eyelids. Medial maxillary fractures usually involve the medial buttress, anteromedial and superior aspects of the body, the frontal, and occasionally the palatine processes. The anteromedial wall of the maxilla provides a major support and, if affected, can cause an alteration in the vertical and projected dimensions of the face. Injury to the infraorbital nerve is common and results in paresthesia or hypesthesia of the cheek and upper dentition. Extensive fractures can result in damage to the lacrimal apparatus.

Anterior Maxillary Sinus Fractures. In addition to the involvement of the maxilla in complex Le Fort fractures, the maxillary sinus may have an isolated anterior wall injury. The mechanisms of injury may occur secondary to blunt, penetrating, or iatrogenic trauma. It is interesting to note that the sinus most commonly involved in penetrating injuries is the maxillary antrum. Complications from anterior maxillary sinus fractures include permanent infraorbital nerve hypoesthesia, loose teeth, and mucopyoceles.

TREATMENT

General Considerations

The greatest threat to the patient with serious maxillofacial trauma is airway obstruction. Causes leading to airway obstruction include intraoral bleeding, edema, hematoma formation, posterior displacement of the maxilla, or dislodged teeth or dentures. Although some patients require intubation or tracheostomy (less than 1%),[12] the airway can usually be managed by clearance of loose debris, suctioning, and placement of the patient in an upright forward position. If severe intranasal bleeding can usually be controlled with anterior or posterior nasal packing techniques.

Facial fractures are also commonly associated with cerebral injury. Approximately 52% of patients with facial fractures have an associated closed head injury.[3,5] Great emphasis has been placed on the immediate correction of facial fractures, secondary to the aesthetic and functional results when compared with a delayed surgical approach.[9,13] However, many individuals are at an increased risk for further cerebral injury when proceeding with an early surgical intervention. Dilating anesthetics, intraoperative fluid shifts, and supine positioning may exacerbate cerebral edema and negatively affect outcome. This risk was clarified by Derdyn et al[14] by correlating the Glasgow coma scale (GCS) to outcome. They demonstrated that (1) those patients with scores of less than 5 uniformly did poorly, either expiring or having severe disability; (2) 61% of patients with GCS scores of 6 to 8 recovered with minimal disability; and (3) 86% of patients with scores of 9 to 14 at initial presentation did well achieving good recovery. Low GCS scores and CT evidence of intracranial hemorrhage, with shift of midline structures, are associated with a poor prognosis. In these patients definitive repair should be delayed until the patient is medically stable. However, in patients with favorable GCS scores, repair can usually be done in the acute stage.

The goals of the definitive repair should include correction of midfacial height and projection with restoration of normal occlusion. After restoring the pretraumatic dental occlusive relationships, usually the repair is accomplished from a cranial to caudal direction. The general rule is to reconstruct from stable to unstable.

Common to all Le Fort fracture repairs is the initial placement of intermaxillary fixation (IMF). This is necessary to assure that the patient's natural occlusion is restored and maintained during fracture repair. The preferred method is by placement of Erich arch bars. However, in patients with inadequate dentition, Ivy loops or occlusal splints may be required.

Erich arch bars are applied with the hooks directed toward the gingiva on each dental arch (Fig. 4–3A). The first bar can be placed on the upper or lower dental arch. The bar is initially secured onto the first premolar tooth. Six-inch 25- or 26-gauge stainless steel wire is passed above the bar and between the teeth onto the lingual surface (Fig. 4–3B). The wire is then fed back between the adjacent interdental space below the bar so that both free ends of the wire are on the buccal surface (Fig. 4–3C). The wire is secured on the crown as high as possible by maintaining placement with a Freer elevator and twisting in a clockwise direction (Fig. 4–3C). After the bar has been secured on the first premolars, the remainder of the bar can be affixed to the remaining teeth. The arch bar should be secured to a minimum of four teeth on each side of each dental arch (Fig. 4–3D). Because the canine is cone shaped, a Dingman loop must be applied to secure the bar on this tooth to avoid slippage. The wire is passed around the canine as previously described; however one free end is looped around the arch bar before it is secured by twisting (Fig. 4–4). This technique can also be used on an isolated molar that sits adjacent to an edentulous area. The arch bars can be secured to each other by stainless steel wire or elastic bands (thin cut no. 14 elastic catheter). As the wires or elastics are placed, occlusion must be restored and maintained in its normal alignment.

The Ivy loop provides an alternative method to the Erich arch bar and is indicated in

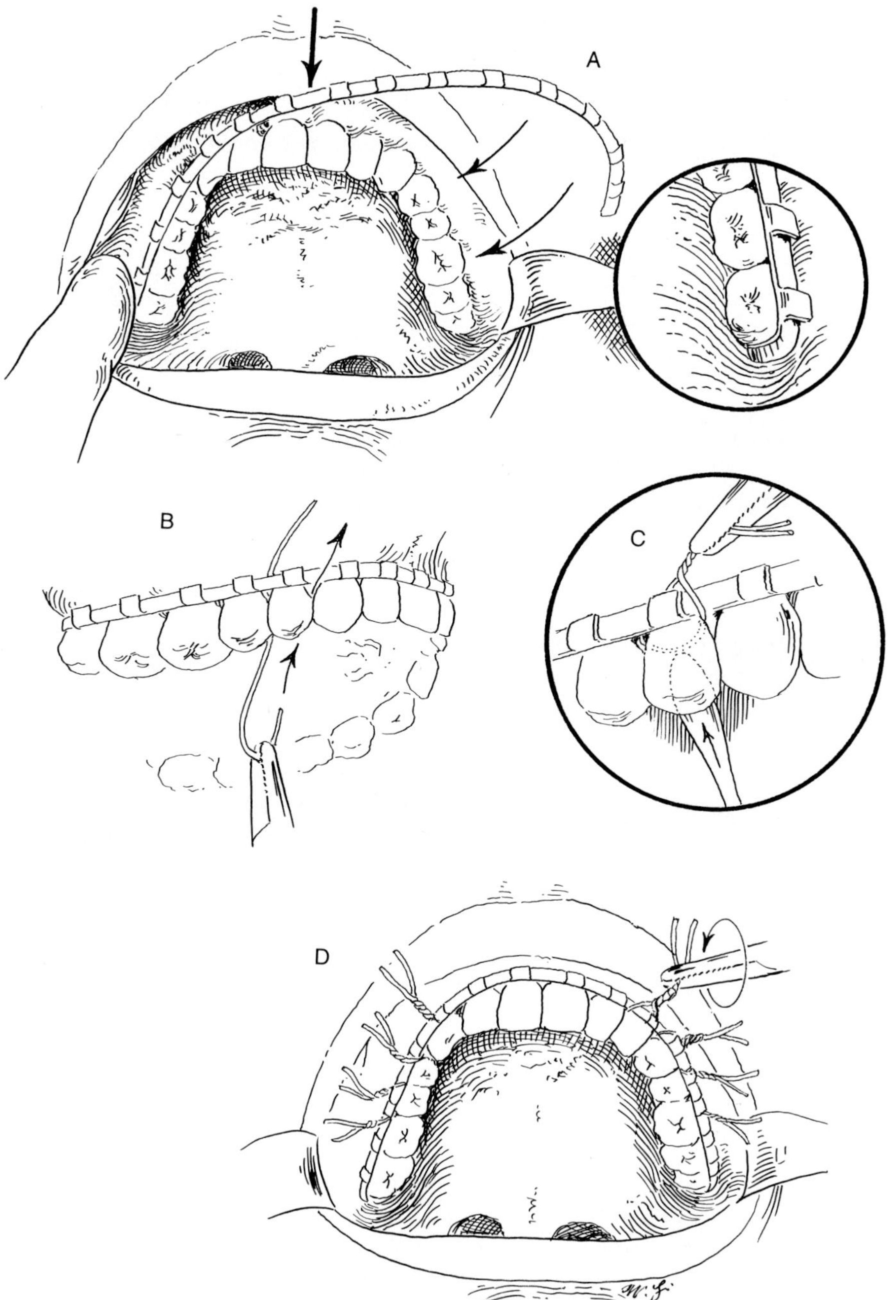

Figure 4–3. Application of Erich arch bars. (A). Sizing the arch bar. (B). Placing the wire. (C). Securing the wire. (D). Completing the application.

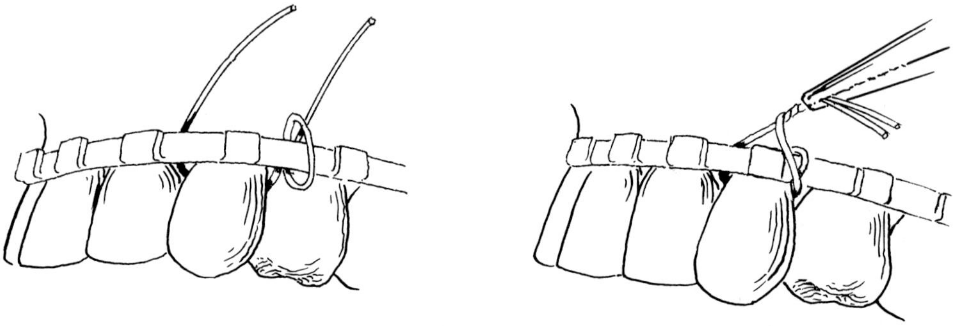

Figure 4–4. Dingman loop. Placed around the canine teeth. The wire loops around the bar before being secured around the tooth.

pediatric patients with mixed dentition, partially edentulous patients who will have additional forms of fixation, and in individuals requiring temporary occlusion while other methods are being applied (ie, biphase and plates). The Ivy loop is assembled by utilizing 25- or 26-gauge stainless steel wire. A small loop is created by folding the wire (12 to 16-cm length) in half and performing two to three twists (Fig. 4–5A). The two free ends

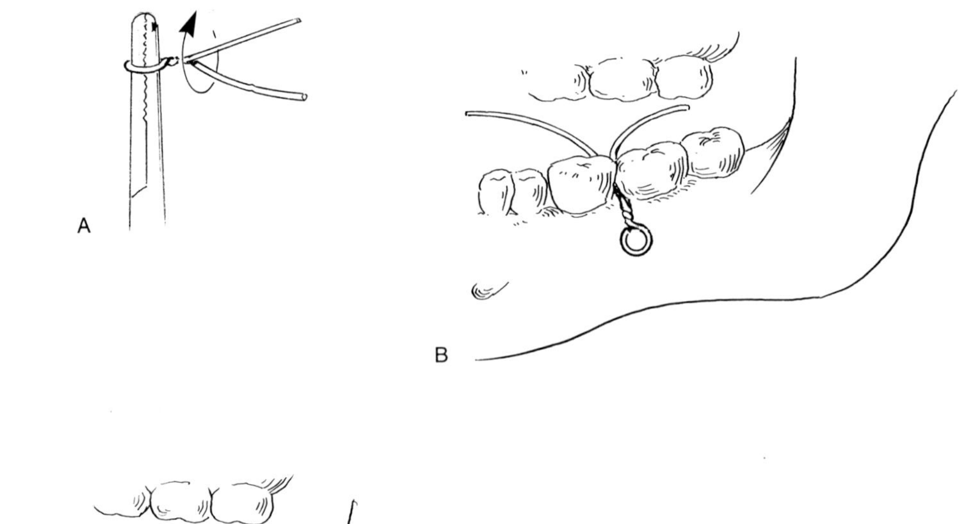

Figure 4–5. Ivy loop. (A). A loop is created by twisting around a clamp. (B). Both free ends are passed through the same interdental space. (C). The free ends are passed back around adjacent teeth. (D). The wire is secured through the loop.

are then placed from a buccal to lingual direction between two suitable teeth (Fig. 4–5B). The wire is then wrapped around the neck of each tooth and brought out to the buccal/labial surface (Fig. 4–5C). The wire is secured high on the crown by using a Freer elevator. The mesial wire is then inserted through the loop and both free ends are twisted around the more distal tooth (Fig. 4–5D).

In edentulous patients or patients with inadequate dentition for arch bars or Ivy loops, maxillary-mandibular relationships can be reestablished using occlusal splints or dentures. If dentures are available and intact, they can be affixed with circummandibular and circumzygomatic wires or alternatively by direct fixation to underlying bone by screws. Once secured to the patient, the splints or dentures are placed in occlusion and wired together by preplaced arch bars or specially added studs.

Le Fort I

The goals in the treatment of Le Fort I fractures is to restore normal occlusion, reduce and stabilize the palatal segment, and repair septal dislocations. If the fracture is impacted, reduction may be achieved with digital manipulation or Rowe disimpaction forceps. Intermaxillary fixation is accomplished as described above. Traditionally, Le Fort I fractures are managed with IMF with or without suspension wires. Stable fractures after reductions may only require IMF. In contrast, unstable fractures require internal suspension. This is usually accomplished via wiring from the zygomatic arch (Fig. 4–6). The

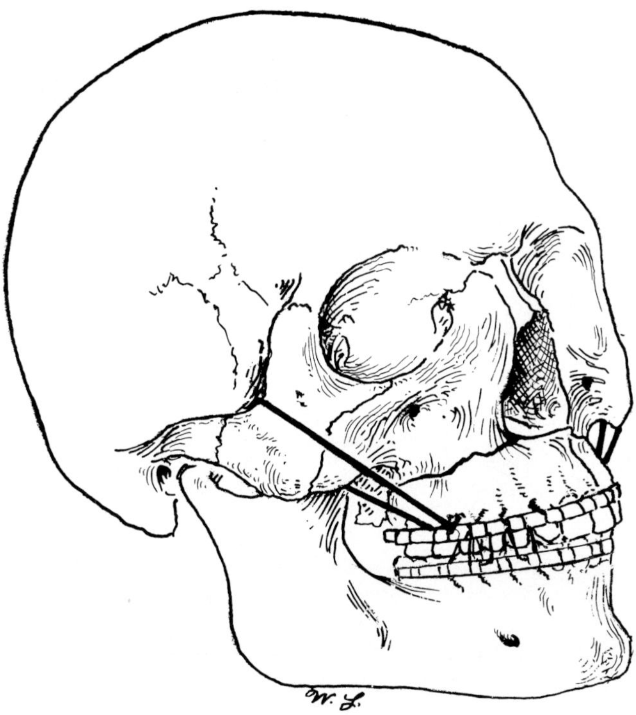

Figure 4–6. Repair of Le Fort I fracture by IMF and circumzygomatic wires.

nasoseptum is reduced after treatment of the palate, and if it is unstable may be splinted with Silastic splints. Patients are maintained on a liquid diet until the suspension wires and IMF are released at 4 to 6 weeks.

Currently, interosseous fixation using direct wiring or plating of the fracture is favored owing to early release of IMF and return to masticatory function. This has advantages of minimizing the effects of prolonged IMF on dentition and temporomandibular joint function. Direct repair is achieved after IMF through sublabial incisions and facial degloving. The incision is made through the mucosa 0.5 to 1 cm to the labial side of the gingival-labial sulcus. This is carried down to the alveolus and the periosteum incised. The fractures are exposed by elevating the facial soft tissues in the subperiosteal plane. Interosseous fixation can then be achieved by wiring across the fracture lines or applying fixation plates (Fig. 4–7). Mini or microfixation plates are preferred for their low contour and rigid fixation. With this technique IMF can usually be removed immediately or by 2 weeks after surgery. Soft diet is maintained for 6 weeks with full mastication allowed in 6 to 8 weeks.

Le Fort II

Disimpaction, IMF, and fracture exposure are carried out as described above. Exposure of these fractures requires a longer incision and more extensive degloving laterally to adequately visualize the fracture lines. Repair of Le Fort II fractures requires fixation of the

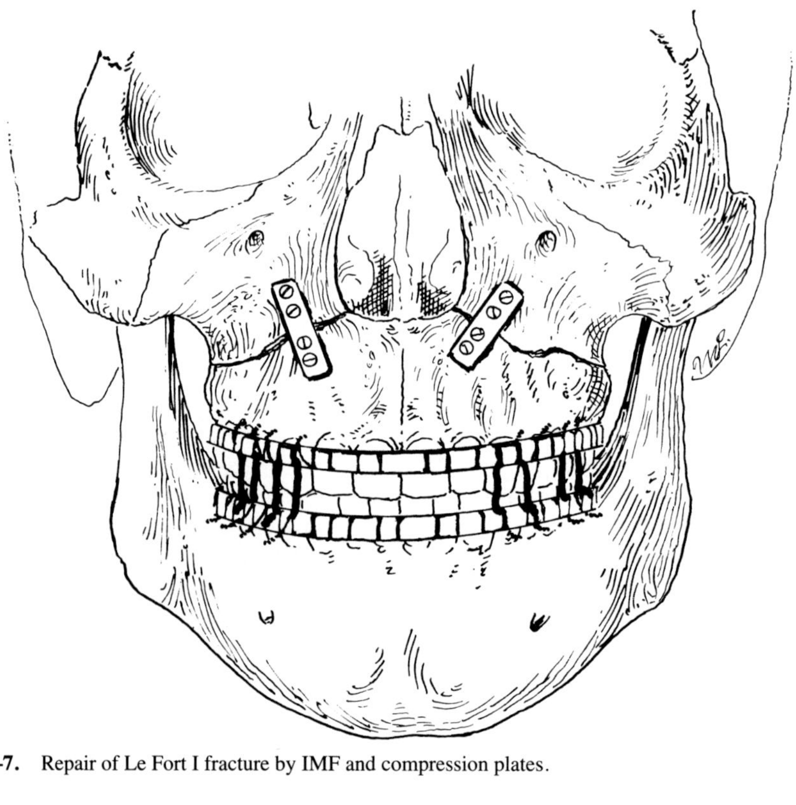

Figure 4–7. Repair of Le Fort I fracture by IMF and compression plates.

alveolar ridge to the malar eminence laterally (Fig. 4–8). When fixation plates are used this usually requires extensive manipulation of the plate to match the bony contour in this area. Typically, exploration of the orbital floor and rim is necessary and can be accomplished through either a transconjunctival or subciliary incision. The subciliary incision generally provides superior medial exposure and is favored for Le Fort II repairs. The fracture of the orbital rim can be repaired with wires or plates depending on the severity of comminution but the mini or microplates are favored. Concurrent nasoethmoid fractures need to be addressed but will be covered in another chapter.

In cases with severe comminution or bone loss, repair with lay bone grafts is advocated. Split calvarial grafts are usually employed, but rib grafts may be substituted if extensive grafting is required and insufficient calvarial bone is harvested. The grafts are laid across the defects to recreate the lateral and anterior buttresses and then secured with fixation plates (Fig. 4–9). As with Le Fort I fractures, when adequate stabilization by rigid fixation is accomplished, IMF may be removed after 2 weeks with regular diet resumed 6 weeks after repair.

Le Fort III

The basic principle in repairing Le Fort III fractures is to stabilize from cranial to caudal. To begin, the maxilla is disimpacted and IMF placed. In most cases both the frontonasal

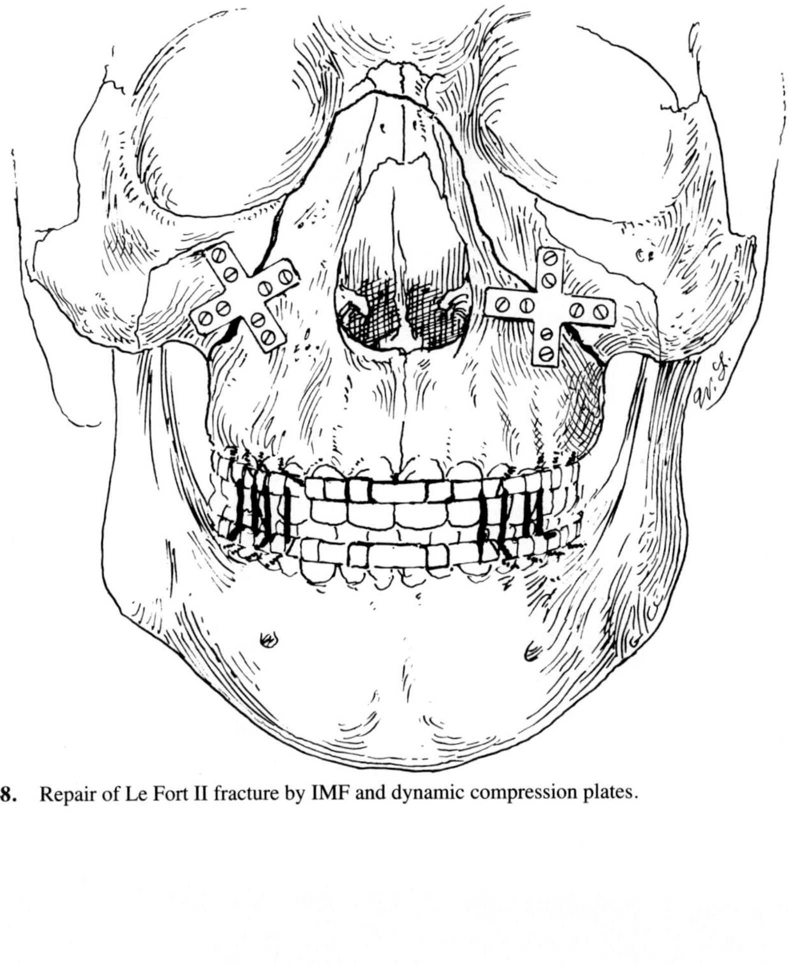

Figure 4–8. Repair of Le Fort II fracture by IMF and dynamic compression plates.

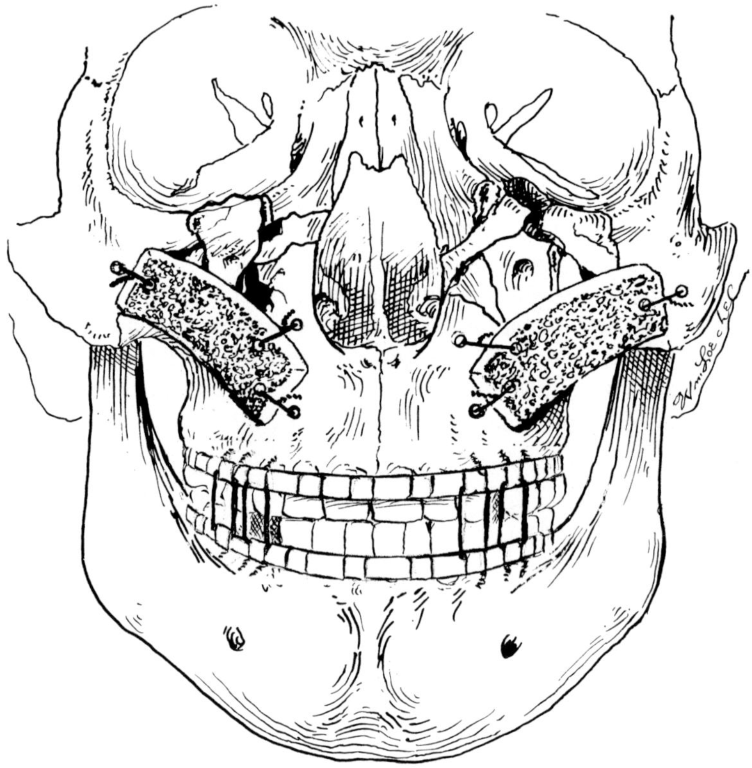

Figure 4–9. Repair of Le Fort II fracture by free cortical bone grafts.

and frontozygomatic buttress will need to be reestablished first. This may be accomplished through lateral brow incisions with a combined incision in a glabellar fold or may be approached through a bicoronal flap. If the bicoronal flap is selected, special attention is given to the pathway of the frontal branch of the facial nerve. To avoid injury of the nerve during elevation of this flap, the temporalis fascia is incised 1.5 to 2 cm above the zygomatic arch with continued elevation on the subfascial plane down to the arch. The fascia is then reincised on the medial surface of the arch to expose the bone allowing subperiosteal elevation from the arch itself. The frontozygomatic, frontonasal, and zygomatic arch fractures can then be secured with mini or microfixation plates (Fig. 4–10).

If necessary reconstruction of the orbital rims should then be performed as previously described. The face is then exposed through the sublabial approach with repair of any fractures in the Le Fort I or II distribution with bone grafts used as necessary. Intermaxillary fixation and diet are managed as described for the Le Fort I and II patients.

Other Maxillary Fractures

In the repair of medial maxillary fractures, fixation with 28-gauge wire is preferred because plates are often palpable beneath the skin in this area. Open reduction with fixation is recommended as opposed to a closed technique because there is a higher

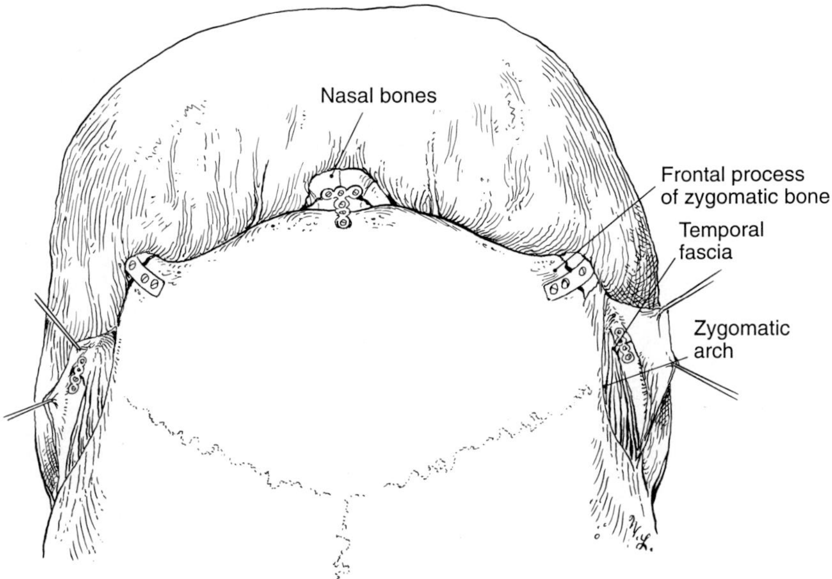

Figure 4–10. Repair of Le Fort III fracture through bicoronal approach. Microfixation plates are applied across the nasofrontal fracture and the zygomatic arch fractures. Minicompression plates are placed across the fractured zygomaticofrontal suture line.

incidence of nasolacrimal obstruction. Most fractures can be managed with facial degloving approaches in combination with periorbital incisions.[15] Delayed or late treatment requires osteotomies with or without bone grafting techniques. Paramedian or sagittal fractures of the maxilla are repaired with IMF and miniplates or cranial suspension wires. Palatal splints are recommended in severely comminuted cases.[16,17]

Pediatric Considerations

Maxillofacial trauma in pediatric patients is an infrequent occurrence with estimates in the range of 5% of all fractures and less than 1% in those younger than 6 years of age.[18–21] This low incidence is thought to occur secondary to the large craniofacial ratio in children as compared with adults. The infant's face is small in proportion to the overall head size, with a small, flat midface and prominent frontal cranium. Thus, the facial skeleton is protected from injury by the cranium and forehead in infants and young children. In addition, the osseous suture lines are flexible, and there is a relative increase in the soft tissue covering the facial skeleton. With the maturation process, the paranasal sinuses grow and pneumatize, making the midface more susceptible to fractures. In a large series by McGraw[18] it was found that Le Fort and unclassified maxillary sinus fractures occurred in less than 10% of the total pediatric cases. Le Fort fractures more commonly occurred in older children as pneumatization of the paranasal sinuses increased. The cause of injury was most commonly secondary to motor vehicle (42%) and auto–pedestrian accidents (25%).[18]

Radiographic diagnosis is more difficult in this age group secondary to underdeveloped and poorly pneumatized sinuses offering less contrast. In addition the presence of teeth and tooth buds can hide fracture lines. Moreover greenstick fractures occur commonly with minimal or no displacement. Because union of a displaced fracture occurs earlier in pediatric patients, reduction and immobilization must be performed early, with 7 days postinjury. A conservative attitude and conscience toward interruption of dental and facial growth centers should always be maintained. Young children with nondisplaced low maxillary fractures can be immobilized with a Barton bandage for 2 to 3 weeks. In contrast, displaced low maxillary fractures may be treated by maxillary arch bars with suspension. Treatment of high maxillary fractures is the same as for adults.

REFERENCES

1. Le Fort R. Experimental study of fractures to the upper jaw. *Rev Chir*. 1908;23:208–227, 360–379.
2. Council Report: Automobile-related injuries: components, trends, prevention. *JAMA*. 1983;249:3216–3222.
3. Haug RH, Savage JD, Likavec MJ, Conforti PJ. A review of 100 closed head injuries associated with facial fractures. *J Oral Maxillofac Surg*. 1992;50:218–222.
4. Adekeye EO. The pattern of fractures of facial skeleton in Kaduna, Nigeria. *Oral Surg Oral Med Oral Pathol*. 1980;49:491–495.
5. Haug R. An epidemiologic survey of facial fractures and concomitant injuries. *Oral Maxillofac Surg*. 1990;48:926–932.
6. Kelley DE, Harrigan WF. A survey of facial fractures: Bellevue Hospital 1948–1974. *J Oral Surg*. 1975;33:146.
7. Morgan BD, Madan DK, Bergerot JP. Fractures of the middle third of the face: a review of 300 cases. *Br J Plast Surg*. 1972;25:147–151.
8. Nahum AM. The biomechanics of maxillofacial trauma. *Clin Plast Surg*. 1975;2:59–64.
9. Manson PN, Crawley WA, Yaremchuk MJ, et al. Midfacial fractures: advantages of immediate extended open reduction and bone grafting. *Plast Reconstr Surg*. 1980;66:54–61.
10. Stanley RB, Nowak GM. Midfacial fractures: importance of angle of impact to horizontal craniofacial buttresses. *Otolaryngol Head Neck Surg*. 1985;93:186–192.
11. Spector GL, Alonso WA, Berkowitz WP. Craniofacial dysjunction: otolaryngological point of view. *Laryngoscope*. 1974;84:1297–1309.
12. Duckert LG. Management of middle third facial fractures. *Otolaryngol Clin North Am*. 1991;24:103–118.
13. Gruss JS, Mackinnon SE. Complex maxillary fractures: role of buttress reconstruction and immediate bone grafts. *Plast Reconstr Surg*. 1986;78:9–23.
14. Derdyn C, Persing JA, Broaddus WC. Craniofacial trauma: an assessment of risk related to timing of surgery. *Plast Reconstr Surg*. 1990;86:238–247.
15. Hillstrom R. Medial maxillary fractures. *Otolaryngol Head Neck Surg*. 1991;104:270–275.
16. Manson PN, Glassman D, Vanderkolk C, Petty P, Crawley WA. Rigid stabilization of sagittal fractures of the maxilla and palate. *Plast Reconstr Surg*. 1990;85:711–717.
17. Werther JR. Fixation of sagittal fractures of the maxilla. *Plast Reconstr Surg*. 1991;87:198–199.
18. McGraw B. Pediatric maxillofacial trauma age-related variations in injury. *Arch Otolaryngol Head Neck Surg*. 1990;116:41–45.
19. Converse JM, Dingman RO. Facial injuries in children. *Reconstr Plast Surg*. 1977;2:794–821.
20. Maniglia A, Kline S. Maxillofacial trauma in the pediatric age group. *Otolaryngol Clin North Am*. 1983;16:717–730.
21. Stylogianni L, Arsenopoulos A, Patrikiou A. Fractures of the facial skeleton in children. *Br J Oral Maxillofac Surg*. 1991;29:9–11.

5

Diagnosis and Treatment of Naso-Orbital Fractures

ROBERT J. MELECA, M.D.
ROBERT H. MATHOG, M.D.

Fractures of the naso-orbital complex resulting from trauma to the anteromedial wall of the orbit pose considerable diagnostic and treatment challenges. Because the naso-orbital complex occupies a central location on the facial skeleton, injury to this area may cause significant cosmetic and functional abnormalities. Early diagnosis and successful treatment of this type of injury depends on the physicians' thorough knowledge of the normal bony and soft tissue anatomy and function, as well as an understanding of the pathophysiology associated with trauma to this vital region.

ANATOMY

The naso-orbital complex occupies a position in the upper central portion of the facial skeleton and is often referred to as the interorbital space or compartment (Fig. 5–1).[1–19] This compartment contains the two ethmoid air cell systems and represents a meeting point of the anterior cranial fossa, frontal bones, orbits, maxillae, and nasal bones.

The facial skeleton is supported by a framework of horizontal and vertical buttresses, of which the naso-orbital complex represents an important central component (Fig. 5–2).[4,5] The horizontal buttresses project the complex and are represented superiorly and inferiorly by the superior and inferior orbital rims, respectively. The principal vertical buttress consists of the frontal process of the maxilla, together with the thickened, proximal portion of the nasal bones, as well as that area of the frontal bone that articulates with these structures. This buttress provides a central skeletal framework to which more delicate facial bones are joined.

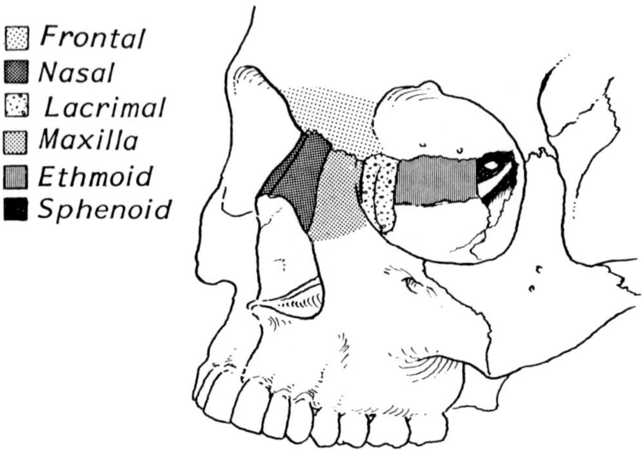

Figure 5–1. Bony contributions to the interorbital compartment.

The medial orbital wall represents the lateral extent of the interorbital compartment and lies immediately posterior to the vertical buttress (Fig. 5–3). It is a delicate wall composed of the lacrimal bone, housing the lacrimal sac, located just behind the frontal process of the maxilla. Posterior to the lacrimal bone is the papery-thin orbital plate (lamina papyracea) of the ethmoid bone. The anterior and posterior ethmoid foramina are found along the upper border of the ethmoid bone, within the frontoethmoid suture. This suture marks the level of the cribriform plate. The anterior ethmoidal foramen transmits the nasociliary nerve of V_1 and the anterior ethmoidal artery whereas the posterior ethmoidal nerve and vessels pass through the posterior foramen. The junction of the maxilla, lacri-

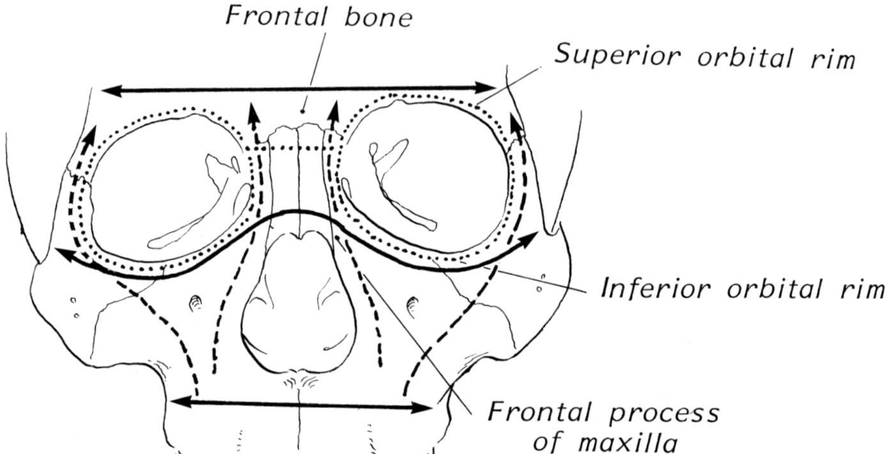

Figure 5–2. The naso-orbital complex provides a framework of horizontal and vertical buttresses to which more delicate facial bones are attached.

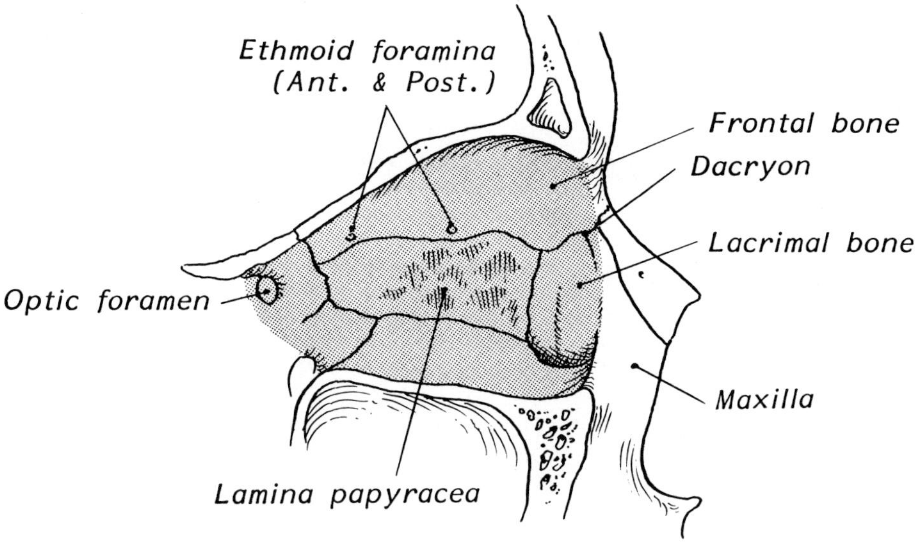

Figure 5–3. Bony anatomy of the medial wall of the orbit.

mal, and frontal bones is known as the dacryon. The most posterior portion of the medial orbital wall is formed by the lesser wing of the sphenoid through which the optic nerve exits. The medial boundary of the interorbital compartment, dividing the ethmoid sinus into equal halves, is the perpendicular plate of the ethmoid (Fig. 5–4). It has an intracranial extension, the crista galli, and it articulates inferiorly and anteriorly with the vomer and cartilaginous nasoseptum, respectively. The superior limit of the interorbital compartment is defined medially by the cribriform plate and laterally by the roof of the ethmoid sinuses. The ethmoid air cells occupy the upper lateral wall of the nose, project about 2 mm above the level of the cribriform laterally, and drain into the middle meatus of the nose. The inferior border of the ethmoid air cells outlines the inferior extent of the interorbital compartment. The anterior limits of the compartment include the frontal and nasal bones, and more laterally, the frontal processes of the maxillae. The sphenoid bone and its sinus occupy the posterior extent of the interorbital compartment.

Because of its close anatomic relationship to the naso-orbital complex, the lacrimal collecting system is often involved with injury to this region. The collecting portion of the lacrimal system includes the upper and lower eyelid puncta, the upper and lower canaliculi, the common canaliculus, the lacrimal sac, and the nasolacrimal duct (Fig. 5–5).[20–24] Each punctum is located along the medial free border of each eyelid, with the lower punctum located slightly lateral to the upper punctum. Each punctum opens into a canaliculus that has an approximate 2-mm vertical limb and an 8-mm horizontal limb. The canaliculi join to form a common canaliculus, which in turn enters the upper one third of the lacrimal sac between the fundus and body. The lacrimal fossa is a bony depression that houses the lacrimal sac. Anteriorly, the frontal process of the maxilla contributes to the anterior lacrimal crest whereas the posterior lacrimal crest is formed by the lacrimal bone. The lacrimal sac measures approximately 15 mm in vertical dimension and lies posterior to the medial canthal tendon. The inferior aspect of the lacrimal sac tapers where it joins with

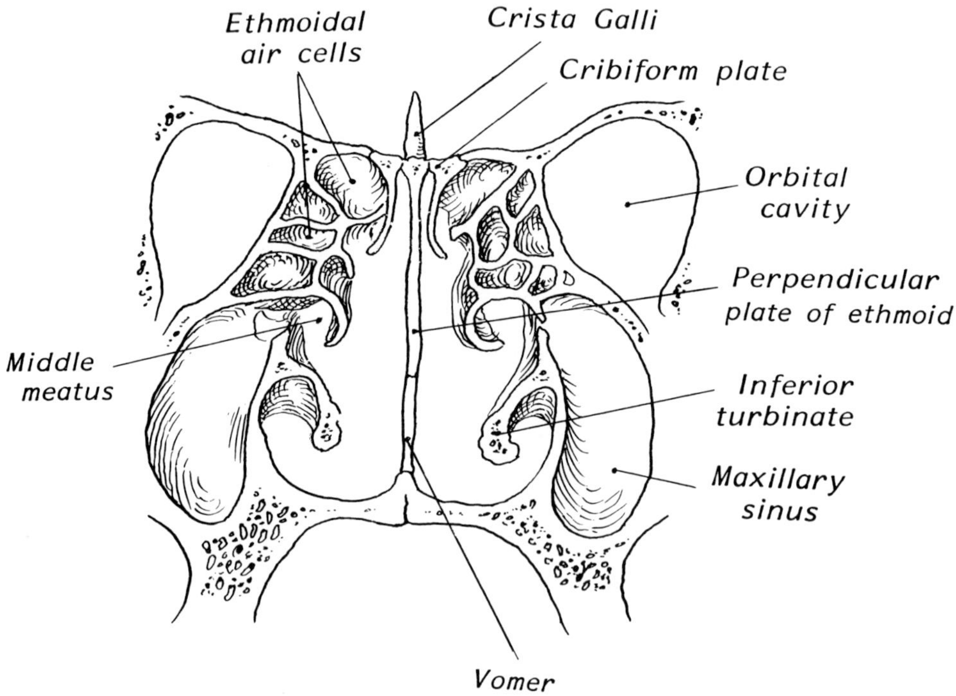

Figure 5–4. Coronal section through the orbit demonstrating the superior and inferior extent of the interorbital compartment.

the nasolacrimal duct. The duct descends through a bony canal in the frontal process of the maxilla and opens beneath the inferior turbinate in the anterior one third of the inferior meatus.

The medial canthal tendon defines the palpebral opening and provides crucial medial globe support as part of an ill-defined suspensory system called Lockwood's ligament (Fig. 5–6). This ligament acts as a hammock to give inferior support to the globe as it lies in continuity between extensions from the medial and lateral canthal tendons. Contributing to the structural anatomy of the ligament are extensions from the sheaths of the inferior oblique, inferior, medial, and lateral rectus muscles, and the inferior tarsal plate. The medial canthal tendon has an anterior and posterior limb that insert along the anterior and posterior crests of the lacrimal bone, respectively. With its attachment to the upper and lower tarsal plates, the medial canthal tendon is instrumental in keeping the eyelids tangent to the globe. The lateral canthal tendon attaches to Whitnall's tubercle, located on the lateral orbital wall.

TEAR FUNCTION

The lacrimal collecting system, medial canthal tendon, and orbicularis oculi muscle are intimately associated structures. Through their coordinated interaction tears are collected and transported from the eye to the nose by a well-described process called the Jones

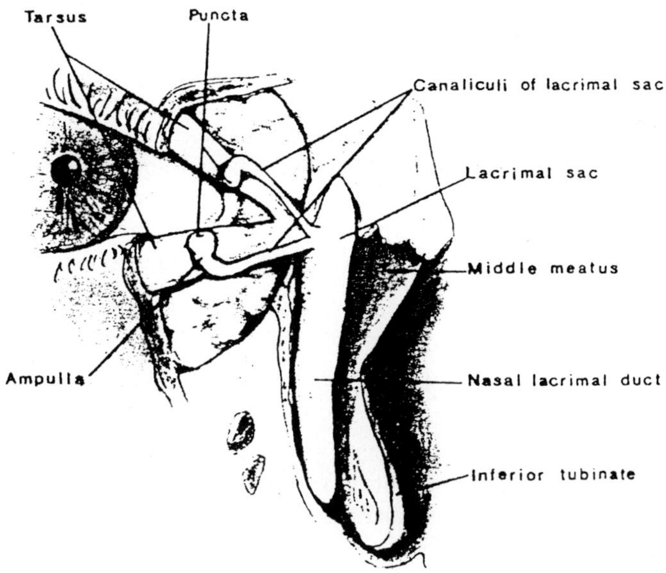

Figure 5–5. The lacrimal collecting system anatomy. Damage to any portion of this collecting system may result in pump failure and epiphora. (Reprinted with permission from Della Rocca et al.[23])

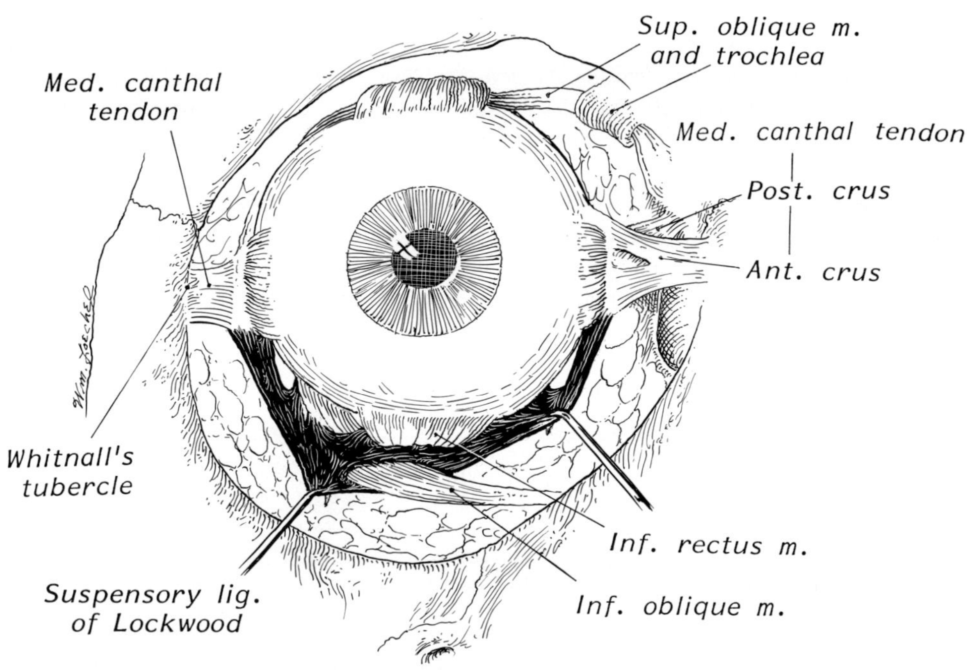

Figure 5–6. Anatomy of the medial canthal tendon demonstrating its anterior and posterior limbs. Lockwood's suspensory ligament provides crucial inferior globe support.

pump.[25] Tears normally enter the puncta at the medial free edge of the upper and lower eyelids and are transported through upper and lower canaliculi to a common canaliculus, and in turn enter the lacrimal sac at the junction of the fundus and body. Tears exit through the nasolacrimal duct. The collection of tears is facilitated by a posterior extension of the orbicularis oculi muscle called Horner's muscle (or pars lacrimalis), which attaches to the posterior crest and pulls the puncta against the globe. The opening and closing action of the eyelids causes the orbicularis oculi muscle to squeeze the tissues surrounding the lacrimal system, therefore producing alternating positive and negative pressures that help collect and transport the tears (Jones pump). Damage to any portion of this collecting system may result in pump failure and epiphora.[20–24]

PATHOPHYSIOLOGY OF INJURY

Naso-orbital complex fractures result from a posteriorly directed force over the upper portion of the nasal bridge (Fig. 5–7). This type of injury usually occurs when the face is projected against the automobile dashboard, steering column, or windshield in a crash stop, or when the face suffers blunt trauma in an altercation. A crushing injury is produced often resulting in comminuted fractures. Soft tissue lacerations may occur due to the severity of the impact and may transform the closed fracture into a compound fracture.[1–19,24]

The most anteriorly projecting and weakest bones of the facial skeleton are the nasal bones. Forces directed posteriorly drive the nasal bones through their underlying buttresses. Once these strong abutments are disrupted, little further resistance is offered by the papery-thin structures of the ethmoid air cell system. As the nasal bones are pushed posteriorly the septal cartilage and perpendicular plate of the ethmoid telescope backwards with subsequent dislodgment of the septum from the maxillary crest. A patient suffering this type injury often presents with a characteristic "pig-snout" deformity.

Naso-orbital trauma affecting the medial wall and floor of the orbit may cause a blow-out fracture with symptoms such as enophthalmos, entrapment with diplopia, decreased visual acuity, and infraorbital nerve anesthesia. Because of its anatomic relationship to the optic nerve, medial orbital wall injuries may cause blindness. In addition, the medial canthal tendon may be disrupted causing telecanthus[26] with resultant epiphora, a narrowed palpebral fissure, a blunted angle, or laxity of the eyelids (Fig. 5–8). This constellation of symptoms is known as posttraumatic telecanthus and is more specifically

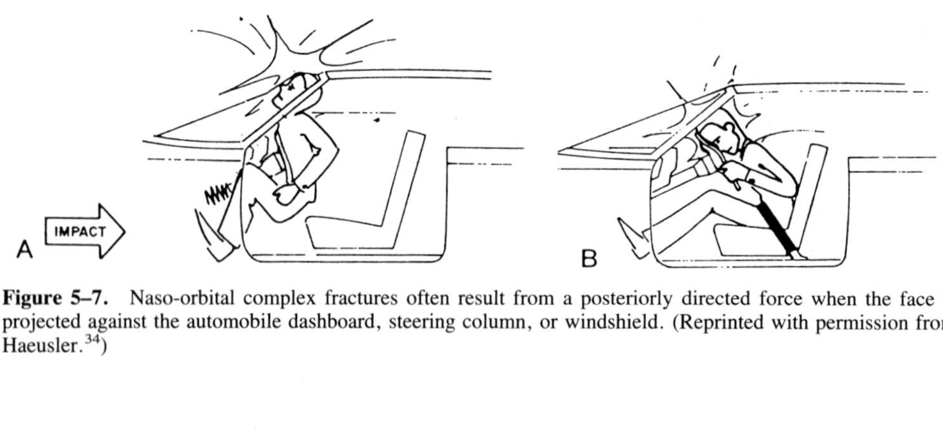

Figure 5–7. Naso-orbital complex fractures often result from a posteriorly directed force when the face is projected against the automobile dashboard, steering column, or windshield. (Reprinted with permission from Haeusler.[34])

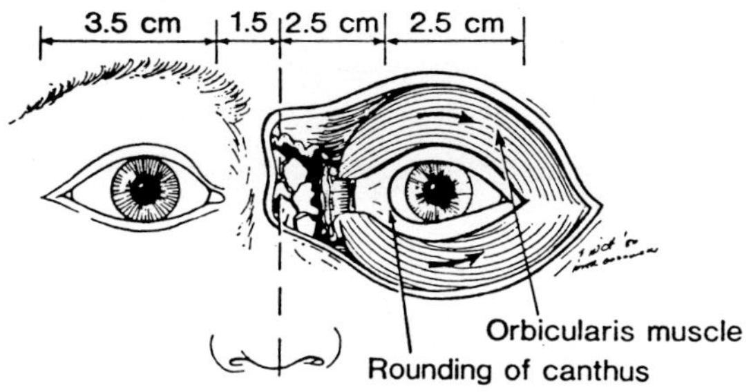

Figure 5–8. Telecanthus results in narrowing of the palpebral fissure, blunting (rounding) of the medial canthal angle, and laxity of the eyelids. (Reprinted with permission from Duval et al.[14])

defined as an increase in the intercanthal distance without an accompanying increase in interpupillary distance because of lateral displacement of the medial canthal tendon (Fig. 5–9B).

Because of its location just beneath the medial canthal tendon the lacrimal collecting system may be lacerated or crushed. Disruption of any portion of the lacrimal collecting system, or improper puncta-canalicular position resulting from eyelid laxity, will cause epiphora.

Any fracture involving the cribriform plate and anterior cranial fossa may cause cerebrospinal fluid (CSF) leaks, pneumocephalus, and/or brain damage. Other commonly associated injuries include fractures to the frontal bone, maxilla, or mandible.

CLASSIFICATION OF NASO-ORBITAL FRACTURES

The naso-orbital fracture pattern typically seen results from fractures that occur along weaker bones, and therefore areas of least resistance. These predictable patterns have been generally categorized as unilateral, bilateral, simple, or comminuted. A number of classification systems have been described[7–9,27] and we choose to use a simple system where three types of injury tend to occur along a continuum related to progressive severity of trauma (Fig. 5–9). A number of surgical techniques have been described for treatment of these specific injury types.[1–24]

Type I injuries (Fig. 5–9C) are unilateral and are of two types: those where the medial canthal tendon is displaced together with a piece of attached lacrimal bone and those where the medial canthal tendon is completely avulsed from its attachment to the medial orbital wall. These injuries result in telecanthus, epiphora, blunting of the inner angle, narrowing of the palpebral fissure, and laxity of the eyelids. Blunt trauma to the naso-orbital region rarely results in avulsion of the medial canthal tendon from its bony insertion. Rather, the medial canthal tendon and its bony attachment are often displaced as a unit. Proper positioning of this "central" unit or fragment is of utmost importance for securing good aesthetic results.[8,10]

Type II injuries (Fig. 5–9D) usually result from more severe trauma and may involve the nasomaxillary buttress and maxilla. The injury is unilateral with comminution and displacement of the medial orbital wall. Depending on the extent of injury the superior and inferior orbital walls may be involved. Fractures of this type often present with signs similar to type I injuries, as well as symptoms associated with orbital blow-out fractures, CSF leaks, and/or damage to the optic nerve.

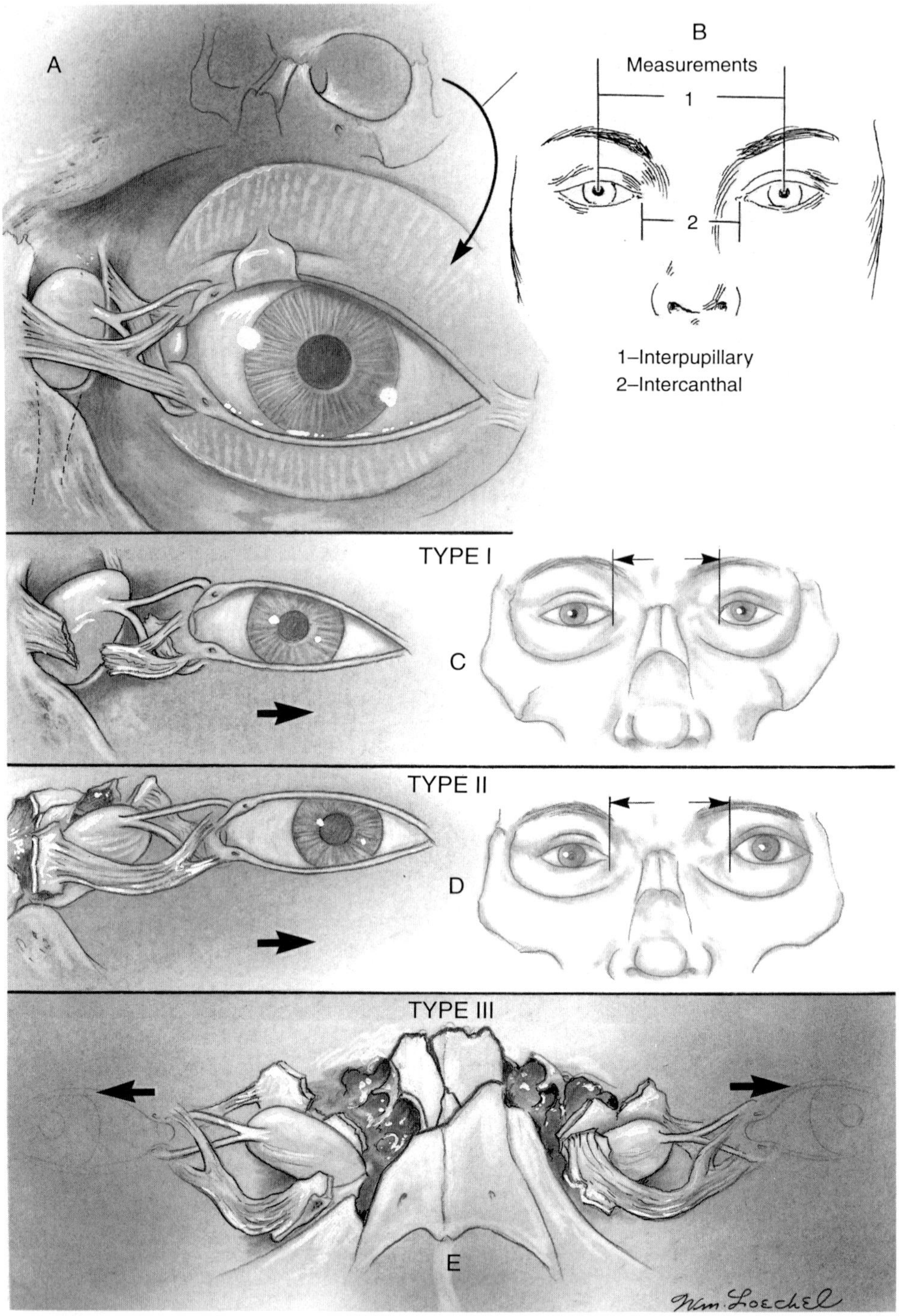

Figure 5–9. Posttraumatic telecanthus is defined as an increase in the intercanthal distance without an accompanying increase in interpupillary distance. Naso-orbital fractures may be classified as type I, II, or III according to the severity of the injury. (Reprinted with permission from Mathog.[24])

Type III injuries (Fig. 5–9E) are bilateral, comminuted, and displaced medial orbital wall fractures. The injury involves the nasoethmoid complex, including the nasal bones, septum, and frontal sinus. Because of the large forces generated to cause such an injury, a number of associated deformities may be seen, including those symptoms desired for the class I or II injuries, as well as flattening and widening of the nasal dorsum, nasal obstruction with epistaxis, depression of the maxilla, orbital and ocular dystopia, and cerebral damage.

PHYSICAL EXAM/DIAGNOSIS

Any patient sustaining blunt midfacial trauma should be suspected of having a naso-orbital complex injury. Of all facial skeletal injuries, naso-orbital fractures may be the most difficult to properly diagnose and treat. Diffuse edema and ecchymosis, often combined with patient noncompliance, make the physical exam extremely difficult. Also, intracranial injury may preclude early otolaryngological consultation, as neurosurgical intervention is of primary importance acutely. Despite these problems the history and physical exam remain the most important first steps in evaluating those patients suspected of having sustained naso-orbital fractures.

The diagnosis of a naso-orbital complex fracture is suggested by any of the signs and symptoms described earlier. Edema, ecchymosis, and pain with palpation are signs of acute injury. Palpation of the medial orbital rim may reveal crepitus or movement suggesting instability of the region. The eyelid traction test described by Furnas and Bircoll in 1973[28] describes lack of a bowstring sign with palpation over the medial canthal tendon when stretching the eyelids laterally, and therefore suggests medial canthal tendon displacement (Fig. 5–10). Paskert et al[8] claim this maneuver is inaccurate and will miss all but the most comminuted injuries (Fig. 5–11). Paskert and Manson[29] described a bimanual examination for detecting those naso-orbital complex injuries not found with external palpation alone. The

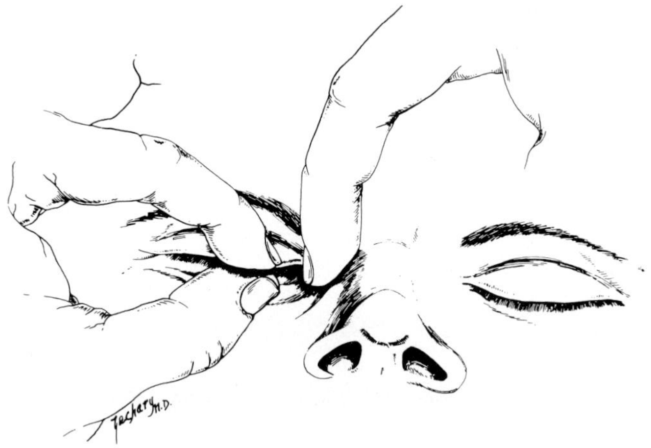

Figure 5–10. The eyelid traction test for detection of medial canthal tendon displacement was originally described by Furnas and Bircoll[28] in 1973. (Reprinted with permission from Mathog and Rosenberg.[35])

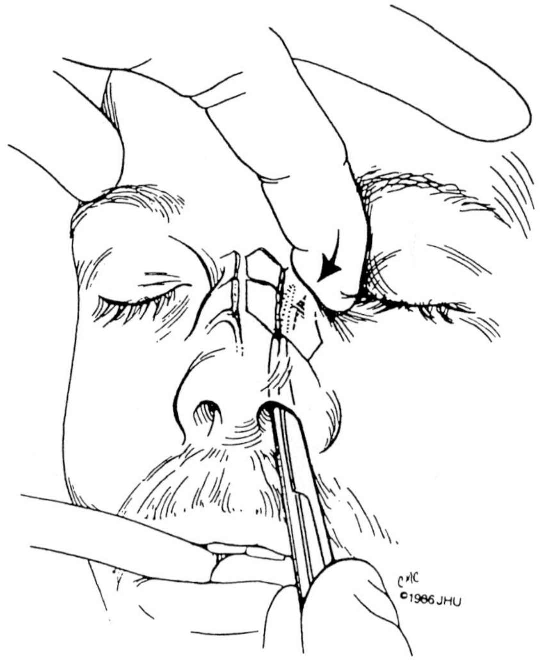

Figure 5–11. Paskert and Manson[29] describe a bimanual exam for detecting medial canthal tendon displacement (Reprinted with permission from Paskert and Manson.[29])

maneuver includes placing a Kelly clamp into the nose and under the frontal process of the maxilla, and then externally palpating the medial central tendon with the opposite index finger in an attempt to move the canthal insertion between the clamp and index finger.

Although plain film examination serves as the initial emergency room radiological assessment for blunt facial trauma, computed tomography (CT) has essentially replaced the once conventional tomograms in the evaluation of naso-orbital complex injury. Plain films may show clouding of the sinuses and more isolated facial bone fractures but are not sensitive enough to detect the extent of naso-orbital complex injury. Combining axial and coronal CT scans has greatly enhanced our ability to accurately diagnose such fractures, as well as other associated facial bone injuries. The CT scan, however, remains less sensitive for questionable, nondisplaced fractures of this region and therefore a careful physical exam remains an intricate component of any diagnostic workup.[30–33]

The integrity of the lacrimal collection system is easily evaluated using saline irrigation and asking patients whether they detect fluid entering the nose. The Jones dye test can be used to localize the type and site of injury and to differentiate an obstructive from a functional abnormality (see "Repair of the Lacrimal Collecting System," later in this chapter). The excretory lacrimal system can be visualized radiographically using a dacryocystogram in conjunction with serial radiographs.[20–22]

OPEN REPAIR OF TYPE I NASO-ORBITAL INJURY

Patients with type I naso-orbital injury, either caused by a sharp, penetrating blow to the medial canthus region with avulsion of the medial canthal tendon or blunt trauma with displacement of the medial canthal tendon and its bony insertion, may present with telecanthus, blunting of the medial canthal angle, a decreased palpebral fissure, upper and lower eyelid laxity, and epiphora. Clinically, the symptoms vary depending on the severity of the injury. Early diagnosis and treatment of these injuries are important for good results because those undergoing delayed treatment face increased risk of surgical and postoperative morbidity as a result of increased scarring and retraction of soft tissues. Once the diagnosis has been made utilizing a thorough history, physical exam, and appropriate radiological studies an open surgical procedure can be performed to correct the deformities associated with this injury (Fig. 5–12).

Under general anesthesia the patient's face is prepared and draped in a sterile fashion. Before making any incisions, an estimate of the correction needed is taken by comparing measurements of the palpebral fissure opening and nasocanthal distance from both the injured and normal sides. Medial canthal and lateral brow incisions are utilized and are outlined with a sterile marking pen at the onset of the procedure (Fig. 5–12A). Both incision sites are then infiltrated with 1% lidocaine containing 1:100,000 epinephrine to help provide hemostasis. After waiting an appropriate time for the epinephrine to effect vasoconstriction an incision is made over the medial canthal region, halfway between the nasal dorsum and caruncle (Fig. 5–12B,C). The angular vessels coursing in the subcutaneous tissue are ligated or cauterized. The dissection is carried down to the periosteum overlying the frontal process of the maxilla. The periosteum is incised and a Joseph elevator is used to bluntly elevate the tissue to the medial orbital rim. The trochlea and its muscle attachment are identified, detached, and retracted laterally. The tissues along the medial orbital wall are elevated exposing the medial canthal tendon, lacrimal fossa, both crests, and lacrimal collecting system. As the dissection is carried posteriorly along the medial orbital wall, additional exposure can be obtained by ligating the anterior ethmoid vessels and then retracting the periorbital tissues laterally using malleable retractors. The medial canthal tendon should be carefully isolated from the lacrimal sac and associated structures. Care must be taken not to strip the medial canthal tendon from its insertion site, as the gradual transition from periosteum to tendon is often difficult to visualize. A thorough evaluation for any lacrimal collecting system injury should be conducted with particular attention to the lacrimal sac.

Before repairing the medial canthal tendon, relaxation of the lateral canthal tendon is performed ipsilaterally using an approach through a lateral brow incision (Fig. 5–12D). This procedure will release tension on the medial canthal tendon repair and allow for overcorrection of the medial canthal tendon insertion site. Release of the lateral canthal tendon has shown no adverse effects with respect to eyelid position and lacrimal collecting system function postoperatively.[24] As the dissection is carried through the lateral eyebrow incision, the orbicularis oculi muscle is visualized and its fibers are separated. The periosteum overlying the frontal process of the zygoma is incised and elevated along the lateral wall and rim of the orbit using a Freer elevator, thereby releasing the lateral canthal tendon insertion. A standard layered closure is performed using 4-0 chromic suture for the subcuticular layer and 5-0 nylon suture for the skin closure. An antibiotic ointment is applied to the wound.

The medial canthal tendon repair technique employed depends on the particular injury pattern. If a piece of lacrimal bone is displaced along with the attached tendon the fragment can be wired into its natural position using 28-gauge stainless steel wires. If the frontal process of the maxilla is involved, small miniplates should be considered. If the tendon is

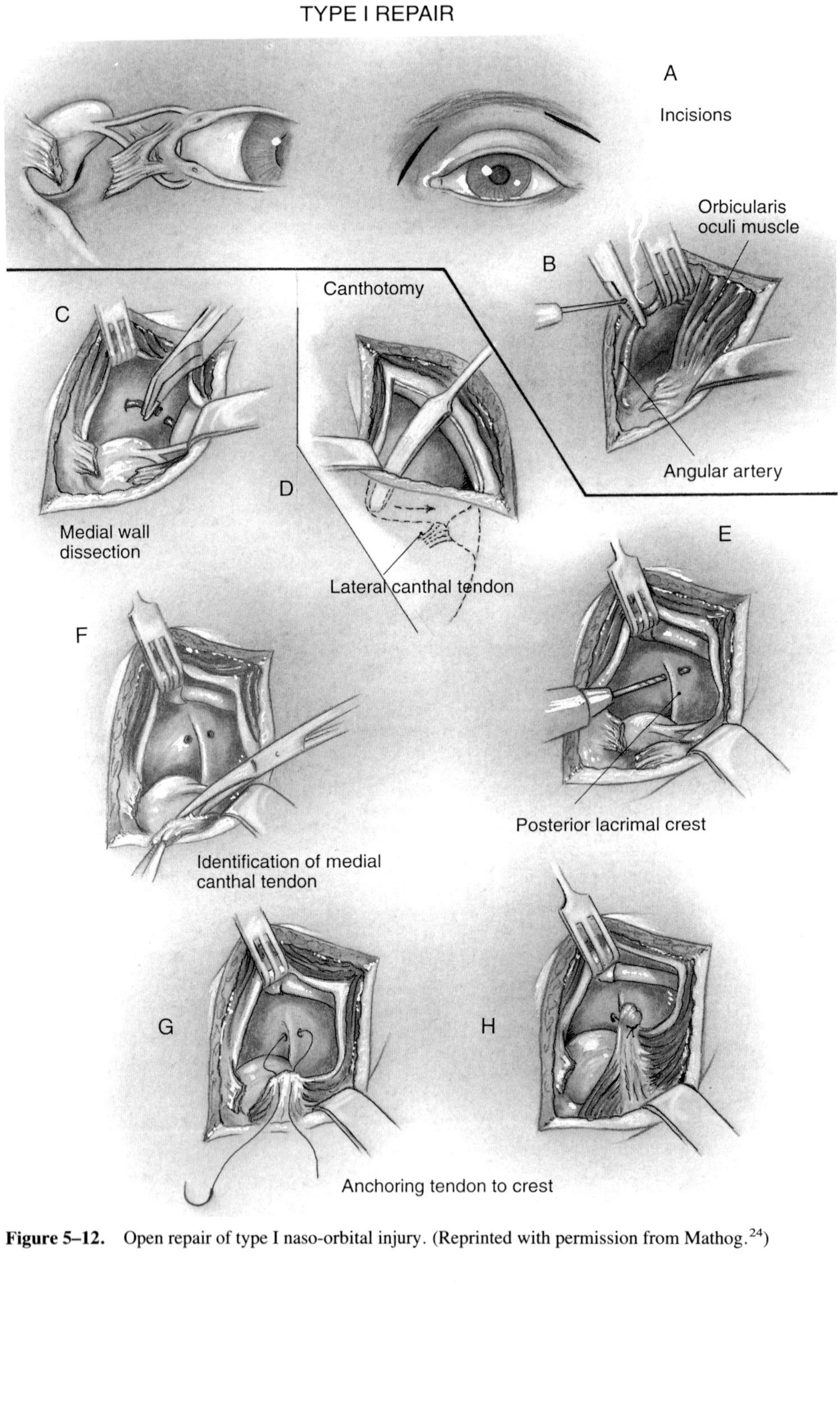

Figure 5–12. Open repair of type I naso-orbital injury. (Reprinted with permission from Mathog.[24])

severed from its insertion site, it should be reattached to the superior aspect of the posterior lacrimal crest using a strong, nonabsorbable suture. Better eyelid position and improved contact of the punctum with the surface of the globe is achieved by pulling the tendon in a superior and posterior direction. A minidriver and 0.035-in Kirschner wire can be used to make the hole through the posterior lacrimal crest (Fig. 5–12E–H). Forceps are used to grasp the firm, thickened medial canthal tendon and a cutting needle guides a 30-gauge stainless steel wire through the tendon. The wire is then placed through the hole in the posterior crest. Overcorrection of the tendon insertion is the ideal surgical outcome and eyelid laxity can be evaluated by repeating the eyelid tension test described earlier. The use of plates and buttons on the skin to hold the medial canthal tendon in position should be avoided as these materials tend to cause skin necrosis and scarring, and usually do not allow enough posteriorly directed pull of the tendon to maintain adequate alignment. A standard layered closure is performed and antibiotic ointment applied to the wound.

Postoperatively, the patient should be observed for 24 hours and undergo serial ophthalmologic examinations to evaluate for any increased intraorbital tension. The patient is discharged home on oral antibiotics for 5 days and sutures are removed in 5 to 7 days.

The more common complications associated with this procedure include persistent telecanthus or injury to the lacrimal collecting system. Persistent or recurrent telecanthus is a difficult management problem. Obviously, successful correction at the first operation is the ideal outcome. However, if this is not achieved as a result of undercorrection of the defect or detachment of the wire from the tissues, reexploration must be performed. Injury to the lacrimal collecting system can result in obstruction, epiphora, and dacryocystitis. Reexploration and repair (see "Repair of the Lacrimal Collecting System") should be performed for any suspected lacrimal collecting system injury. If dacryocystitis occurs owing to obstruction of the lacrimal collecting system, the patient should be placed on appropriate antibiotics and the collecting system evaluated for the degree and level of obstruction using the Jones dye test. If persistent dacryocystitis ensues, treatment should be conducted as described later in this chapter under "Repair of the Lacrimal Collecting System."

OPEN REPAIR OF TYPE II NASO-ORBITAL INJURY

Early repair of type II naso-orbital injuries is essential for good results. Patients with a type II naso-orbital injury have unilateral comminution of the medial wall of the orbit with displacement of the medial canthal tendon laterally. Like the type I injury the patient often presents with telecanthus, blunting of the inner angle, narrowing of the palpebral fissure, eyelid laxity, and epiphora. Additionally, the medial rectus and superior oblique muscles are often entrapped through bony defects in the medial orbital wall, causing diplopia. Because of the magnitude of force needed to cause such injuries, CSF leaks and optic nerve injury are sometimes seen. Repair of this type injury is difficult because there is inadequate bony support along the medial orbital wall for reattachment of the displaced tendon (Fig. 5–13). Wiring the tendon to the ipsilateral nasal or frontal bone will often result in anterior displacement of the tendon, failure of the puncta to contact the surface of the globe, and persistent epiphora. Therefore, the most effective repair usually includes transnasal wiring of the tendon to the opposite orbital wall.

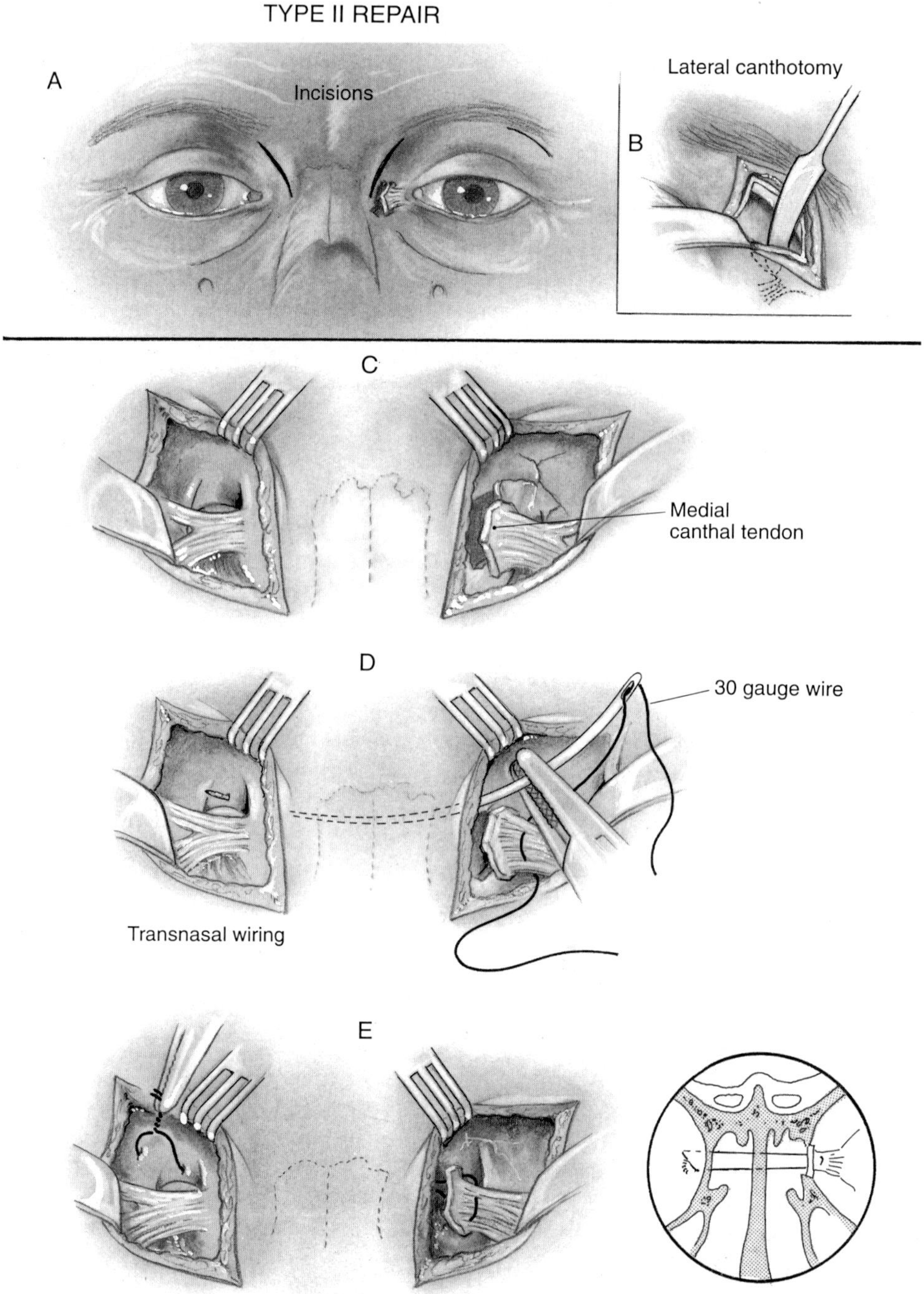

Figure 5–13. Open repair of type II naso-orbital injury with transnasal canthoplasty. (Reprinted with permission from Mathog.[24]

The patient is prepared as in the repair of type I injuries. The medial canthal and lateral brow incisions are outlined on the side ipsilateral to the injury, therefore providing exposure to the lacrimal crests and lateral canthal tendon, respectively (Fig. 5–13A). A third incision is outlined over the medial canthal region on the contralateral uninvolved side to provide exposure of the lacrimal crests for reattachment of the tendon to the intact orbital wall.

The interorbital dissection is conducted in a similar manner as described for the type I repair (Fig. 5–13B). Alternatively, the repair can be carried out through a bicoronal incision with a subperiosteal dissection of the orbital rims. If one chooses this technique care must be taken not to injure the supraorbital vessels and nerves. The lacrimal collecting system should be inspected for kinks, twists, or lacerations. Displaced fragments of bone should be replaced, herniated fat and entrapped muscle released, and the orbital wall, if necessary, reinforced with polyethylene mesh. Associated frontal, maxillary, and other orbital fractures should be repaired with appropriate fixation (ie, plates, wires) techniques. Once the lateral canthal tendon has been relaxed the medial canthal tendon is isolated and secured with a 30-gauge stainless steel wire (Fig. 5–13C–E). One end of the wire is attached to a large curved needle that is passed through the lacrimal bone defect, nasoseptum, and finally cut through the lacrimal bone just anterior to the posterior lacrimal crest on the opposite side. Care must be taken to pass the fixation wire superior to the lacrimal sac so that it is not obstructed by the wire. The other end of the wire is passed in a similar manner, except this time out through the lamina papyracea so that the wires exit on either side of the posterior lacrimal crest. If stability of the orbital wall is in question, the wire should be secured to a screw or hole placed along the edge of the frontal process. When passing wires, care must be taken to protect the globes with malleable retractors.

After the wires are passed they are secured to the opposite uninvolved lacrimal crest so that overcorrection of the displaced medial canthal tendon occurs. The ends of the wires are twisted flat against the orbital wall and the incisions are closed in a standard manner. Postoperatively, the patient should be observed for 24 hours for any signs of increased intraorbital tension, oral antibiotics should be prescribed for 5 days, and sutures should be removed in 5 to 7 days.

Complications associated with repair of type II naso-orbital injuries include persistent telecanthus, obstruction of the lacrimal collecting system with dacryocystitis, persistent or new onset CSF leaks, nasofrontal duct obstruction, and medial canthal scarring.

Persistent telecanthus and/or epiphora usually occurs when postoperative swelling pulls the soft tissues from the wire or the wire loosens from its bony attachment. Late repair of telecanthus (described later in this chapter) is difficult to perform because of increased scarring and tissue retraction.

Dacryocystitis can occur from obstruction of the lacrimal collecting system. The patient should be treated with appropriate antibiotics and evaluated for the degree and level of obstruction using the Jones dye test. Persistent dacryocystitis can be treated as described later.

Cerebrospinal fluid leaks after persist or present postoperatively. If this occurs appropriate antibiotics should be continued until the leak subsides, usually after a few days. If the leak continues beyond 2 to 3 weeks, despite a lumbar drainage procedure, the leakage site should be determined and preparation made for repair of the leak.

Nasofrontal duct obstruction can occur when the soft tissues attached to the transnasal wires are displaced into the ethmoid sinus. Postoperative complaints of periorbital pain and frontal headaches should alert the physician of frontal duct obstruction and an appropriate radiological evaluation should be initiated. Nasofrontal duct obstruction requires reconstruction of the nasofrontal duct or fat obliteration of the frontal sinus.

Scarring of the medial canthal region can result in web formation. This problem can be prevented by designing incisions with irregular patterns. Early treatment of postoperative web formation may include daily massage of the incision site in an attempt to relax the scar contracture and injection of triamcinolone (40 mg/mL) along the incision site. If this treatment fails, a zigzagplasty or Z-plasty may be performed to correct the deformity.

OPEN REPAIR OF TYPE III NASO-ORBITAL INJURY

The patient presenting with a type III naso-orbital injury has undoubtedly sustained severe upper midface trauma. As a result of bilateral comminution of the medial orbital walls, the patient may have bilateral telecanthus, displacement and blunting of the inner angles, narrowing of the palpebral fissures, eyelid laxity, and epiphora. Other associated problems include depressed nasal, frontal, and maxillary bones, orbital wall and ocular injuries, optic nerve damage, CSF leaks, and closed head injury. Because the medial orbital walls are unstable for reattachment of the medial canthal tendon, other techniques must be utilized; these include intercanthal tendon fixation or fixation to the frontal process of the maxilla (Fig. 5–14).

Early repair of naso-orbital injuries is essential for successful results, as long as the patient has been evaluated neurologically and cleared medically for a surgical procedure. The patient is prepared in a sterile fashion as described earlier. The surgeon has the choice of using bilateral medial canthal and eyebrow incisions or performing an open sky approach in which the bilateral medial canthal incisions are connected by a horizontal limb (Fig. 5–14A). An optional technique for exposure of the upper face may include a bicoronal incision.

Working on one side at a time, the dissection is performed similarly to that described for type I and II repairs except that additionally, the periosteum lining the glabellar region and brow prominence is incised and elevated superiorly. The medial wall of the orbit including the lacrimal fossa, crests, and collecting system are inspected, and displaced fragments of bone should be replaced, herniated fat and entrapped muscle released, and the orbital wall, if necessary, reinforced with polyethylene mesh. Interosseous wiring or bone miniplate techniques should be utilized for displaced nasal or anterior frontal bone wall fractures. Lateral canthotomies are performed to release tension on the medial canthal tendons as described earlier.

When bilateral dissections are complete, intercanthal medial canthal tendon fixation can be performed (Fig. 5–14B). As described previously, carefully placed malleable retractors should be used to protect the globes. Starting on one side, a 30-gauge wire attached to a large curved needle is passed through the medial canthal tendon. Both ends of the wire are attached to the needle, directed through the lacrimal bone region, superior portion of the cartilaginous nasoseptum, and then out the opposite lacrimal bone. One free end of the 30-gauge wire is then attached to a fine curved needle and the wire is passed through the medial canthal tendon. The wire is then tightened and the ends twisted flat against the orbital wall, pulling the tendons toward each other. As described for the type I and II repairs, the pull on the medial canthal tendon must be superior and posterior with

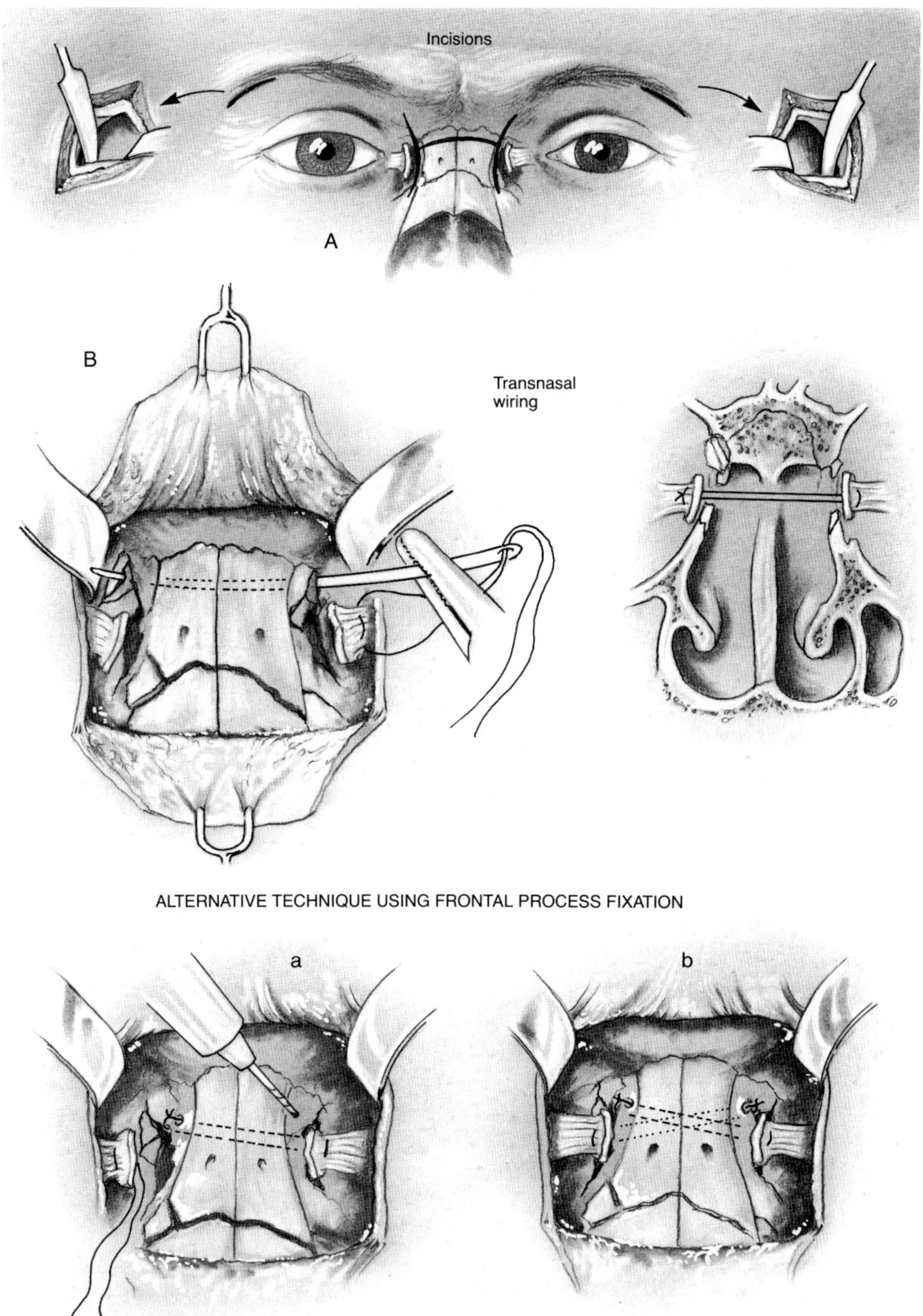

Figure 5–14. Open repair of type III naso-orbital injury with transnasal canthoplasty. (Reprinted with permission from Mathog.[24])

overcorrection toward the midline. To achieve proper tendon alignment the transnasal wire must be placed along the superior nasoseptum. A wire directed too far inferiorly through the septum will cause inferior displacement of the inner angle with resultant scleral show. The periosteum, subcutaneous tissue, and skin are closed with a standard layered technique.

An alternate technique using fixation to the frontal process of the maxilla can be performed if the medial canthal tendon and inner angle rotate inferiorly when performing a transnasal canthoplasty (Fig. 5–14a,b). The advantage of this technique over the transnasal canthoplasty is that the medial canthal tendons can be adjusted independently of each other. The incisions and exposure technique used are identical to those described above. Once the medial canthal dissection and lateral canthotomies have been performed, the medial canthal tendon is secured with a 30-gauge stainless steel wire. One end of the wire is attached to a large curved needle and passed through the lacrimal bone defect, cartilaginous nasoseptum, and out through the superior portion of the anterior lacrimal crest on the frontal process of the maxilla of the opposite side. The other end of the wire is passed in a similar manner, except this time out through a point several millimeters posterior to the initial hole. The ends of the wire are then tightened to bring the tendon into proper alignment. The opposite medial canthal tendon is required in a similar manner, therefore establishing a crossing of wires within the nasal vault. The wound closure and postoperative care are the same as those for earlier described techniques. Serial radiographs are obtained postoperatively to evaluate the frontal sinuses.

Complications associated with this technique are similar to those for type I or type II repairs, and include persistent telecanthus, lacrimal collecting system injury or obstruction, nasofrontal duct obstruction, CSF leaks, and webbing of the medial canthal incision site. Treatment of these complications has been discussed. Additionally, low placement of the transnasal wire can cause inferior displacement of the inner angle and scleral show. If only mild asymmetry persists, a V-Y or Z-plasty technique may be used to effect proper alignment of the medial canthal tendon. If there is pronounced asymmetry, reexploration should be performed, and the wire reattached high in the nasoseptum.

OPEN REDUCTION AND REPAIR OF TELESCOPING NASO-ORBITAL INJURY

Sometimes the naso-orbital complex is driven as a unit beneath the frontal bones. Forces directed posteriorly drive the nasal bones through their underlying vertical buttresses. Once these strong abutments are disrupted little further resistance is offered by the paper-thin structures of the ethmoid air cell system. As the nasal bones are pushed posteriorly, the septal cartilage and perpendicular plate of the ethmoid telescope backwards with subsequent dislodgment of the septum from the maxillary crest. A patient suffering this type of injury often presents with a characteristic pig-snout deformity in which the nasofrontal angle is accentuated. The medial walls of the orbit are often fractured with displacement of the lacrimal bones and splaying of the medial canthi laterally. This results in telecanthus, displacement and blunting of the inner angles, narrowing of the palpebral fissures, eyelid laxity, and epiphora. Forceful reduction of this type of fracture is necessary for successful repair (Fig. 5–15). Disruption of the optic canal with optic nerve compression can also occur from severe, posteriorly directed forces to the nasofrontal angle.

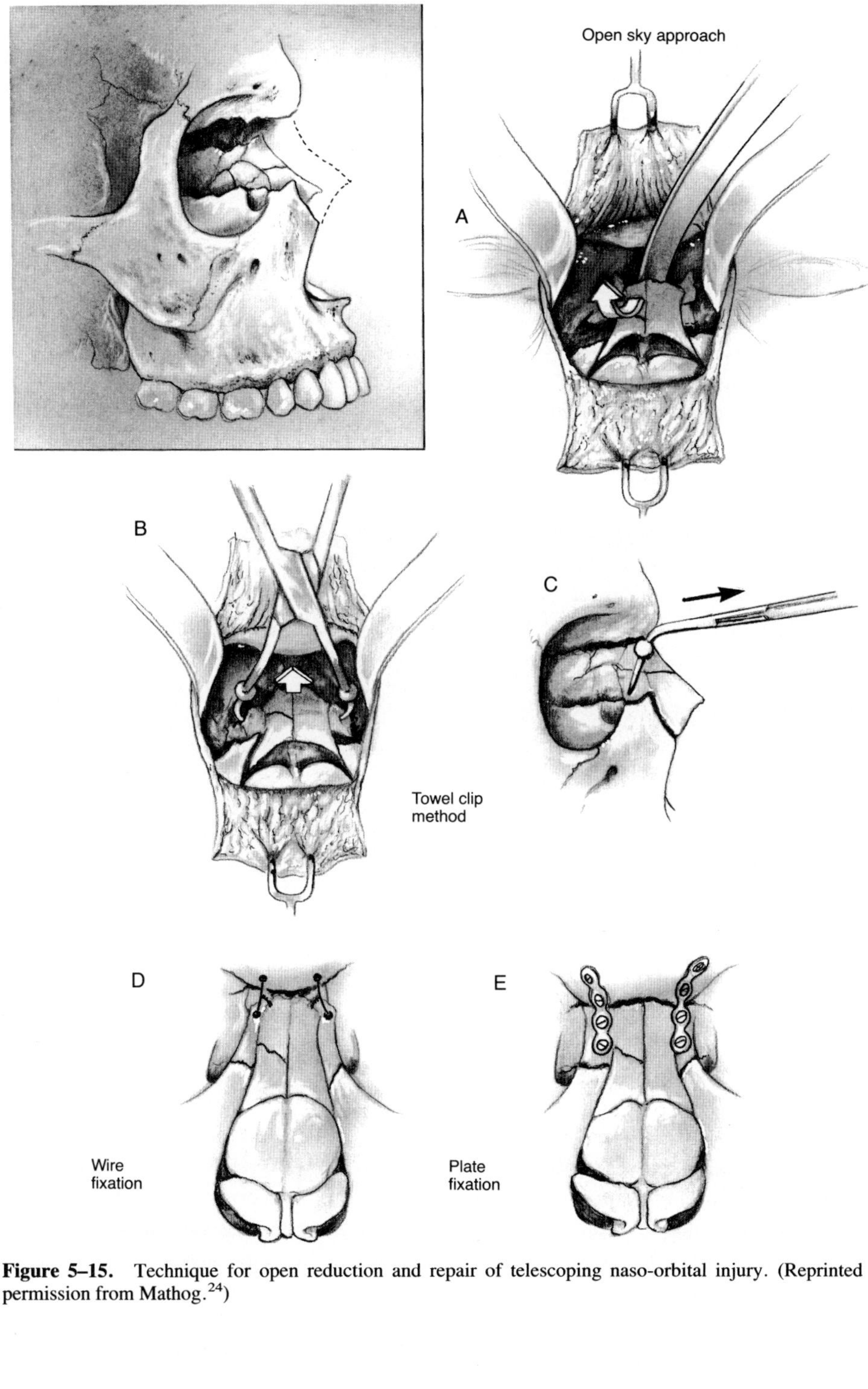

Figure 5–15. Technique for open reduction and repair of telescoping naso-orbital injury. (Reprinted with permission from Mathog.[24])

Commonly associated frontal bone, cribriform plate, and anterior cranial fossa fractures may cause dural tears, CSF leaks, and/or closed head injuries. A thorough evaluation for such injuries must be performed and treatment individualized to obtain acceptable results.

The patient is prepared in a standard sterile fashion and an open sky or bicoronal incision is outlined using marking solution followed by injection of the incision sites with 1% lidocaine containing 1:100,000 epinephrine to help provide hemostasis.

The periosteum is elevated from the nasal bones, anterior walls of the frontal bones, and medial orbital walls. Using a small curved osteotome, the nasoethmoid complex is reduced into proper alignment (Fig. 5–15A). This can be accomplished by placing the osteotome through the fracture line along the nasofrontal suture and using the frontal bone or superior orbital rim (if not fractured) as a lever point for reduction of the nasoethmoid complex. If the frontal bone and/or superior orbital rim is fractured and the nasoethmoid complex severely impacted beneath the frontal bone, reduction may be accomplished by applying a towel clip to the frontal processes of the maxillae and pulling anteriorly (Fig. 5–15B,C). Excessive outward force exerted on the complex can avulse bone from the craniofacial skeleton and possibly cause dural tears and/or CSF leaks, therefore care must be taken when performing this maneuver. Extraction of bone from the nasoethmoid complex can often be avoided by maintaining pressure over the dorsum of the nose and using a rocking motion as the lifting is performed. After reduction, the nasoethmoid complex is usually stable; however, if the complex remains unstable, miniplates or interosseous wires can be applied (Fig. 5–15D,E). Following bony reduction the medial canthal tendons are realigned as described for repair of type I, II, or III naso-orbital injuries. Nasoseptal injury should be managed by one of the closed or open techniques.

The incisions are closed with a standard layered technique and antibiotic ointment applied to the wounds. The postoperative treatment is similar to that described for repair of type I, II, or III injuries. Serial radiological exams of the frontal sinuses should be performed to evaluate nasofrontal duct patency.

Complications associated with repair of telescoping nasoethmoid injuries are similar to those described for type I, II, or III repairs. Additionally, depression of the nasofrontal angle may persist if adequate reduction is not accomplished with the initial repair. Correction of a nasofrontal angle deformity is best accomplished using cartilage and/or onlay bone grafts applied to the dorsum of the nose. Cantilevering techniques may be desirable. As described earlier, it is possible during reduction to extract all or part of the nasoethmoid complex. If this occurs, immediate replacement of the bone fragments and plating or interosseous wire fixation should be performed. Neurosurgical consultation should be obtained to evaluate any exposed or torn dura.

LATE REPAIR OF NASO-ORBITAL INJURY

Delayed treatment of type II or III naso-orbital injury results in malunion and new bone growth along the medial orbital walls, herniation of soft tissues through fracture lines with retraction, scarring and fixation of soft tissues around the orbit. These bony and soft tissue changes often cause twisting and kinking of the lacrimal collecting system, resulting in stasis of lacrimal secretions and eventually dacryocystitis. When the surgeon is faced with these problems, alternate repair techniques must be applied (Fig. 5–16).

The patient preparation, incisions, and approaches are similar to those used for acute

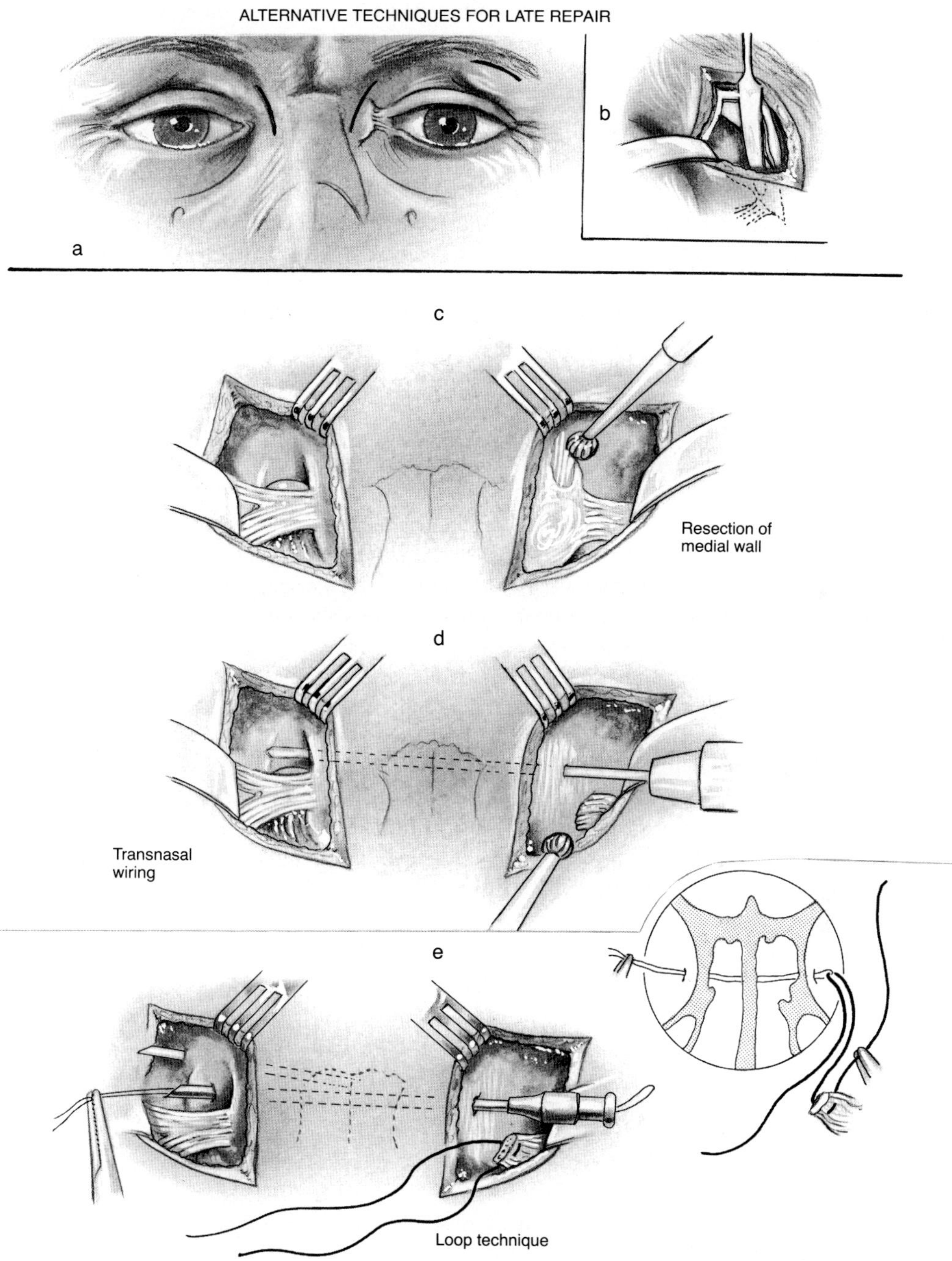

Figure 5–16. Technique for late repair of naso-orbital injury. (Reprinted with permission from Mathog.[24])

injury repair (Fig. 5–16a,b). Because of decreased elasticity of the soft tissues encountered with delayed repair, a larger area of periorbita must be elevated, including the superior orbital wall and orbital floor regions. New bone growth along the medial orbital wall, including bone along the planned tendon placement site, can be removed using a cutting bur or Kerrison rongeur (Fig. 5–16c). Passage of a large curved needle through the dense bone may be difficult and the use of a minidriver and 0.035-in K wire may be helpful (Fig. 5–16d). The drilled holes are cannulated with a 14-gauge needle and a 30-gauge loop of wire is passed through the needle (Fig. 5–16e). The needle is then removed leaving the 30-gauge loop in place. One end of the transnasal wire is attached to the loop and passed through the holes. Another cannulation is then performed with an exit point just beyond the first. A 30-gauge wire loop technique is used to pass the other end of the transnasal wire into place. Attachment of the transnasal medial canthal tendon wire to the opposite lacrimal crest, overcorrection of the medial canthal tendon, and incision closure are identical to those used for repair of acute injuries.

REPAIR OF THE LACRIMAL COLLECTING SYSTEM

Trauma to the naso-orbital region often results in injury to the lacrimal collecting system. The upper collecting system, including the puncta, and/or canaliculi may be damaged causing epiphora. The lower collecting system, including the sac, and/or nasolacrimal duct may be twisted or kinked resulting in stasis of secretions and subsequent dacryocystitis. It is important that early diagnosis and treatment of lacrimal collecting system injury be performed to avoid late complications such as scarring, chronic epiphora, and dacryocystitis. Obviously, a laceration through the medial upper or lower eyelid will suggest puncta or canaliculi damage. Lacerations of the canaliculi can be evaluated by cannulation and instillation of saline solutions. If no obvious soft tissue injury is noted and the patient has epiphora, it is important to use physiological testing to evaluate for obstruction of the collecting system. The primary and secondary fluorescein dye drainage tests, originally described by Jones in 1962,[25] will give accurate objective information of the level and degree of obstruction. The primary dye drainage test is performed by placing fluorescein dye into the lower conjunctival sulcus and allowing the natural Jones pump action to transmit the dye into the inferior meatus. Recovery of the dye in the nose signifies a positive test and a normal functioning collecting system. A negative dye test indicates that normal drainage from the eye to the nose is not occurring and the secondary dye drainage test should then be given. This test is performed by irrigating the puncta and canaliculi with saline. The appearance of dye in the inferior meatus indicates that there was retention of dye in the lacrimal sac (therefore normally functioning puncta and canaliculi) and that greater than normal physiological pressure was needed to advance the dye into the nose. Such findings suggest obstruction distal to the sac, called a functional block.

REPAIR OF CANALICULI

Early repair of lacrimal collecting system injury is important for successful restoration of normal anatomy and function. Lacerations through the medial portion of the upper or lower eyelid may sever the canaliculi causing epiphora. Failure to correct this problem early can result in chronic epiphora. Although the inferior canaliculus is responsible for collecting the majority of secretions, an attempt should be made to correct the superior canaliculus to ensure a more efficient excretion mechanism (Fig. 5–17).

Under general anesthesia the patient is prepared in a sterile fashion. One percent lidocaine with 1:100,000 epinephrine is injected over the medial canthal region to help provide vasoconstriction and therefore improved hemostasis. The procedure is performed using an operating microscope. The eyelid laceration is carefully irrigated and the edges of the wound examined for the ends of the severed canaliculi. By probing through the punctum, the proximal portion of the injured canaliculus is easily identified (Fig. 5–17A). If the distal end of the canaliculus is not visualized, the uninjured canaliculus can be irrigated with normal saline and the sac compressed allowing retrograde transport of fluid through the severed canaliculus. After identifying the ends of the injured canaliculus, a Silastic tube swaged on a flexible probe is passed through the uninjured punctum, canaliculus, and lacrimal sac, and out into the nose through the nasolacrimal duct (Fig. 5–17B-D). The opposite swaged end is passed in a similar manner through the injured canalicular system and out into the nose. The probes are then cut and the tubing is tied and placed along the floor of the nose. The tubing acts as a stent while the surgeon approximates the cut ends of the canaliculus with 8-0 nonabsorbable sutures.

The eyelid laceration is closed using a special suture technique (Fig. 5–17E-I). A buried 5-0 chromic suture is placed along the conjunctival edge of the distal tarsal plate. A 6-0 silk suture is placed at the level of the meibomian bland orifices. Care must be taken to place these sutures 1 to 2 mm from the wound margins. A second 6-0 silk suture is placed along the posterior eyelid at the junction of the skin and conjunctiva. A third 6-0 silk suture is placed in front of the first silk suture at the eyelash line. The sutures are then tied down and the ends brought out anteriorly to be held in position when the third, most anterior stitch is tied. Antibiotic ointment is applied to the wound for several days and the sutures are removed in 3 to 5 days. The stents exiting the nose are kept free of crusts by irrigating the nose regularly with normal saline and can be removed after 2 to 3 weeks.

Complications associated with canalicular repair include restenosis and recurrent epiphora, erosion with displacement of the tube, ectropion, or entropion. The most common complication of canalicular repair is restenosis of the lacrimal collecting system, resulting in recurrent epiphora. With the Silastic stent in place, function of the collecting system is difficult to evaluate. When the stent is removed, scarring with restenosis may develop and secondary procedures such as conjunctivorhinostomy or conjunctivodacryocystorhinostomy will need to be performed. Displacement of the Silastic tubing may occur because of loosening, breakage, or erosion through the canaliculi. To avoid these complications the patient should be instructed on the correct position of the tubing. If inflammation develops, appropriate antibiotic treatment should be initiated. Ectropion or entropion may develop secondary to problems with the canaliculus or eyelid repair. Correction of these complications should be conducted with the help of an ophthalmologist.

Conjunctivorhinostomy

Restenosis resulting in recurrent epiphora after initial canalicular repair should be treated with a bypass method. The degree and level of obstruction can be obtained by performing the Jones dye test. Conjunctivodacryocystorhinostomy, using a Jones tube, is generally an

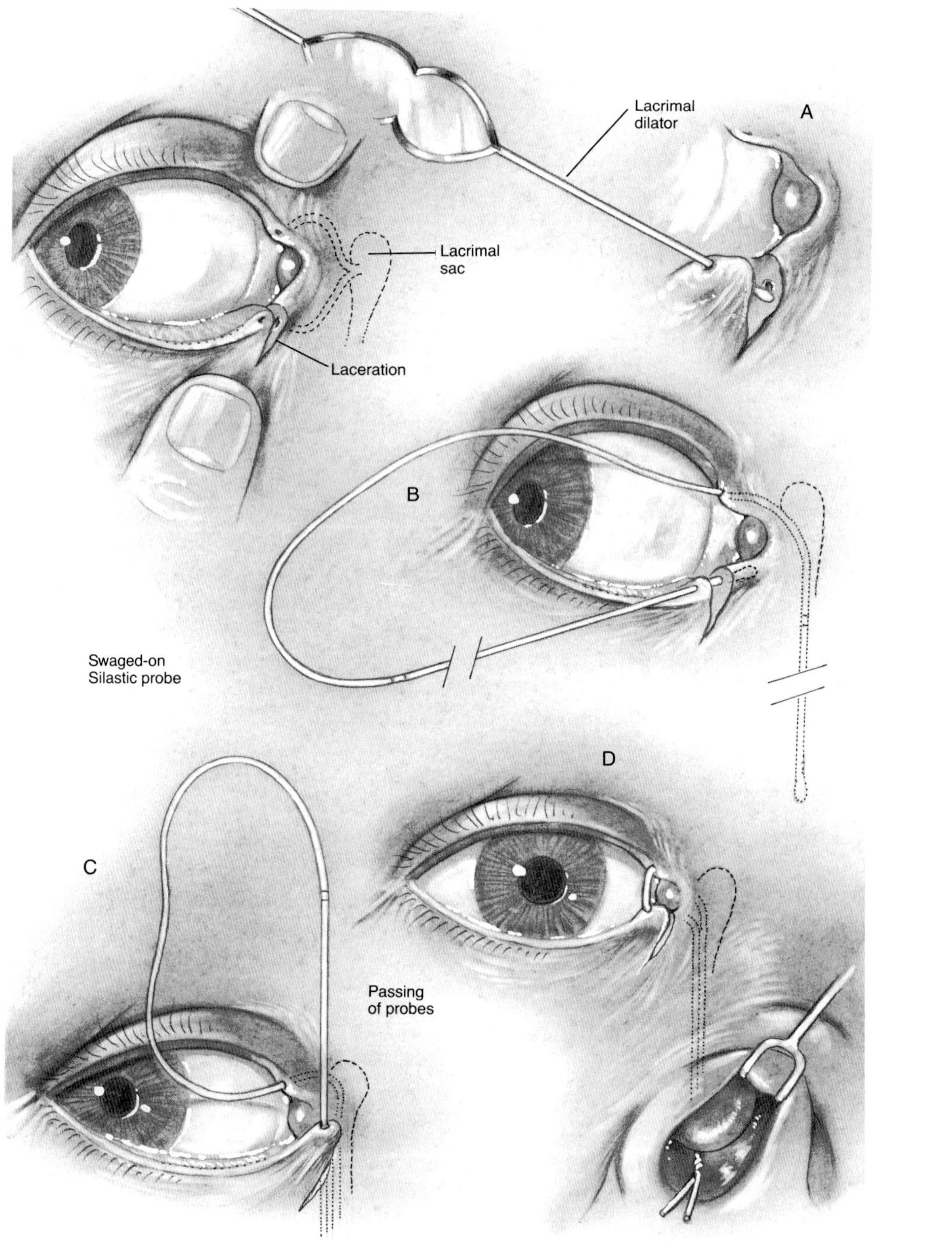

Figure 5–17. Technique for repair of canalicular injury. (Reprinted with permission from Mathog.[24])

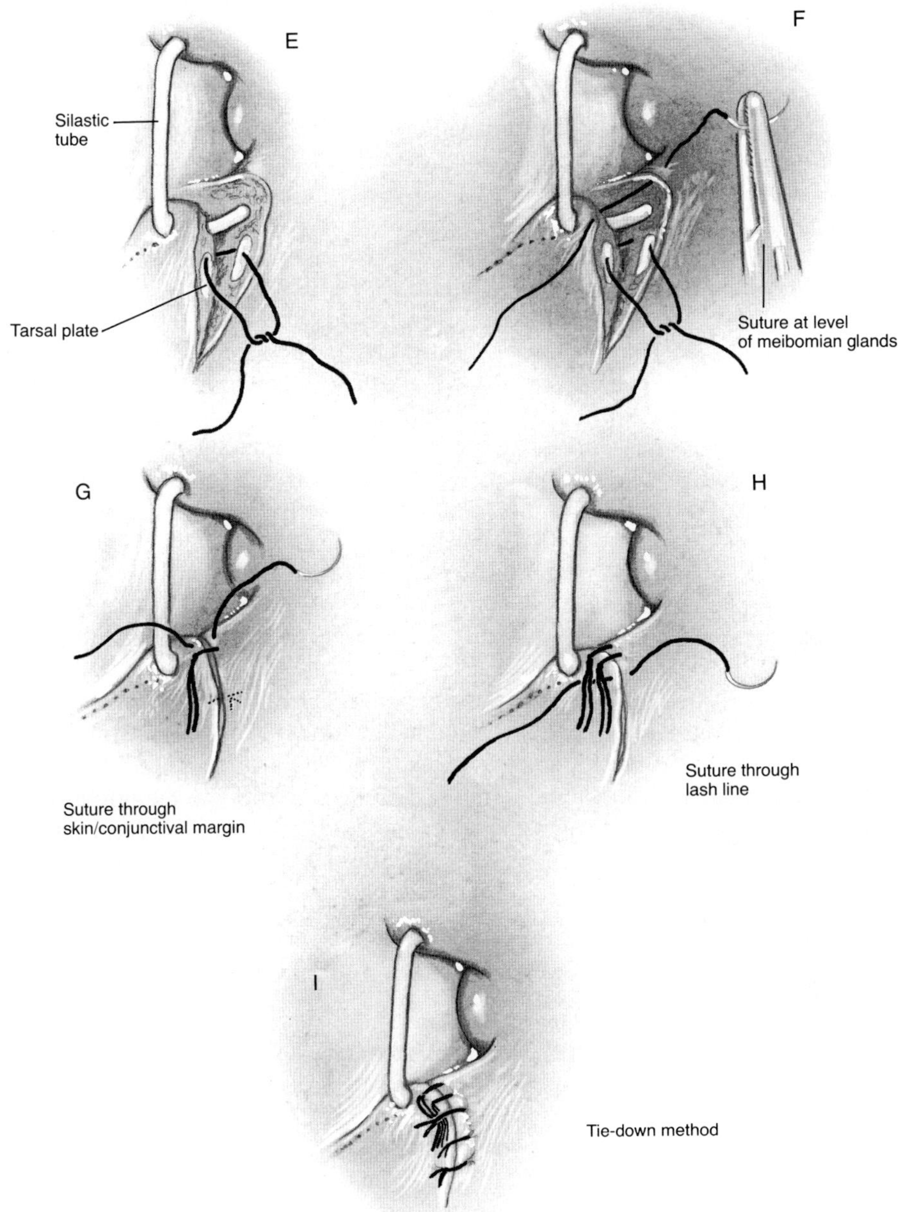

Figure 5–17. *Continued.*

effective procedure. However, because the technique involves the development of unopposed mucosal flaps there is a risk of increased granulation tissue and scarring as a result of healing from secondary intention, with restenosis and recurrent epiphora. Canaliculodacryocystorhinostomy offers physiological restoration of the lacrimal collecting system, but the procedure requires a lengthy tedious dissection under the operating microscope and often there is insufficient canaliculus remaining to perform this repair. A variant of the standard conjunctivorhinostomy technique can be performed, which offers a total lacrimal system bypass and has the advantages of bipedicled mucosal flaps, optimal temporary stenting, and improvement of epiphora (Fig. 5–18). Before attempting these procedures, the nose must be evaluated and treated for possible sinusitis, nasal masses, or polyps.

The patient is prepared in a standard sterile fashion. Using a medial canthal incision (Fig. 5–18a), with extension of the incision inferiorly along the inferior orbital rim, the angular vessels are visualized and ligated. The periosteum is incised and elevated off the nasal bones and medial orbital wall to expose the lacrimal crests and fossa.

If a telecanthus repair is to be performed in conjunction with a conjunctivorhinostomy, a medial canthal exploration with attachment of a 30-gauge wire to the tendon should be done first. The lacrimal repair is then performed, followed by placement and tightening of the medial canthal tendon. If the lacrimal repair is performed too early, there is a risk of pulling out the mucosal sutures with the transnasal wiring technique; exposure will be compromised if the lacrimal repair is performed too late.

Working medial to the lacrimal sac, the lacrimal fossa is fractured. Using a Kerrison rongeur, the opening is enlarged by removing the anterior and inferior portions of the anterior lacrimal cost and a portion of the frontal process of the maxilla. If dense thick bone is encountered, drilling with cutting burs may be performed (Fig. 5–18b). Moving intranasally, the middle turbinate is fractured medially and the mucoperiosteum of the nose is elevated, developing a flap along the anterolateral wall of the nose (Fig. 5–18c). Vertical and horizontal incisions are designed so that the flap is easily rotated through the rhinostomy defect.

On the orbital side, a 1 × 2-cm inferiorly based flap is developed from the medial aspect of the bulbar conjunctiva just lateral to the limbus (Fig. 5–18d,e). A tunnel is then formed, tracking from the eye to the rhinostomy defect, by making a horizontal incision medial to the conjunctival flap in the fornix and deepening it to join the original medial canthal incision. The conjunctiva is sutured end to end to the nasal mucosal flap using interrupted 5-0 chromic sutures. A Silastic tube stent is then placed through the fornix and into the nose, and the flaps sutured to surround the tube.

Dacryocystorhinostomy

Obstruction of the lacrimal collecting system distal to the lacrimal sac may be repaired by dacryocystorhinostomy (Fig. 5–19). If a telecanthus repair is to be performed in conjunction with a conjunctivorhinostomy, a medial canthal exploration with attachment of a 30-gauge wire to the tendon should be done first. The lacrimal repair is then performed, followed by placement and tightening of the medial canthal tendon (see conjunctivorhinostomy). Before attempting this procedure the nose must be evaluated and treated for sinusitis, nasal masses, or polyps.

The face is prepared in a standard sterile fashion. An incision is outlined with marking solution over the medial canthal region and extended inferiorly over the inferior orbital rim (Fig. 5–19A). The angular vessels are ligated and the periosteum incised and elevated over the frontal process of the maxilla, lacrimal fossa, and crests. Working medial to the lacrimal sac, the lacrimal fossa is fractured (Fig. 5–19B). Using a Kerrison rongeur, the opening is enlarged by removing the anterior and inferior portions of the anterior lacrimal crest and a portion of the frontal process of the maxilla (Fig. 5–19C,D). If dense thick bone

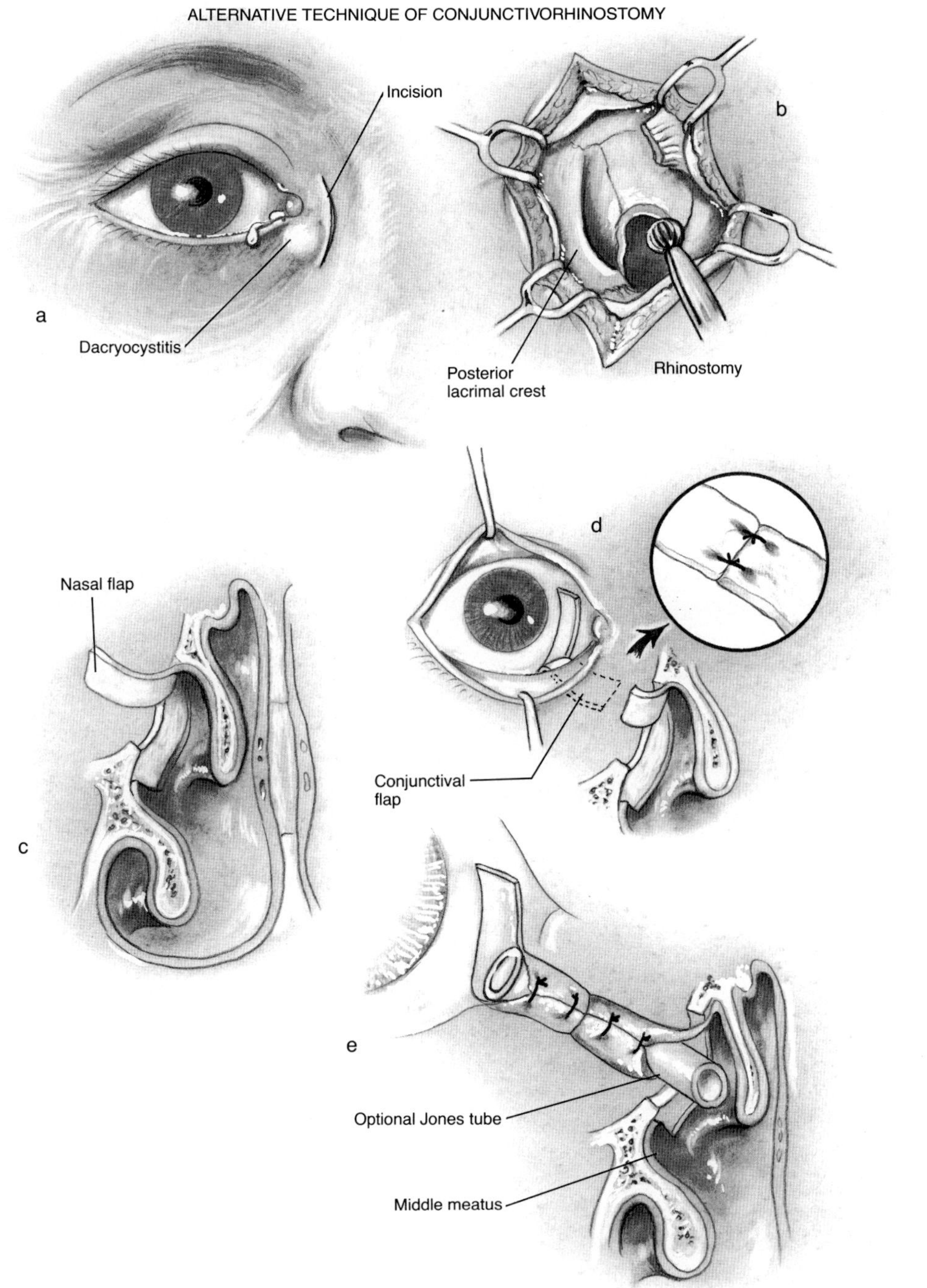

Figure 5–18. Shown above is a variation of the standard conjunctivorhinostomy technique for repair of lacrimal collecting system injury. (Reprinted with permission from Mathog.[24])

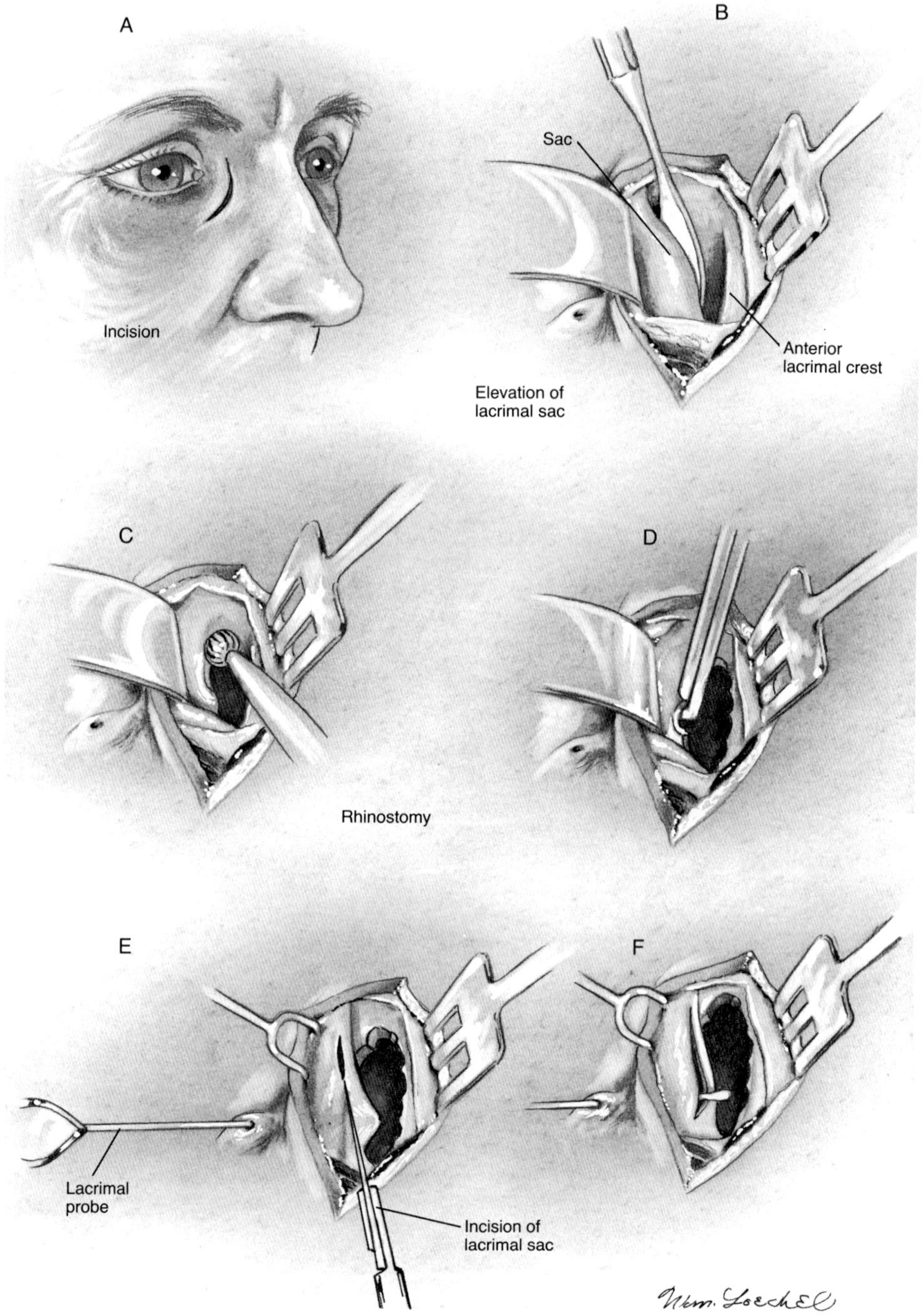

Figure 5–19. Obstruction of the lacrimal collecting system distal to the lacrimal sac may be repaired by dacryocystorhinostomy. (Reprinted with permission from Mathog.[24])

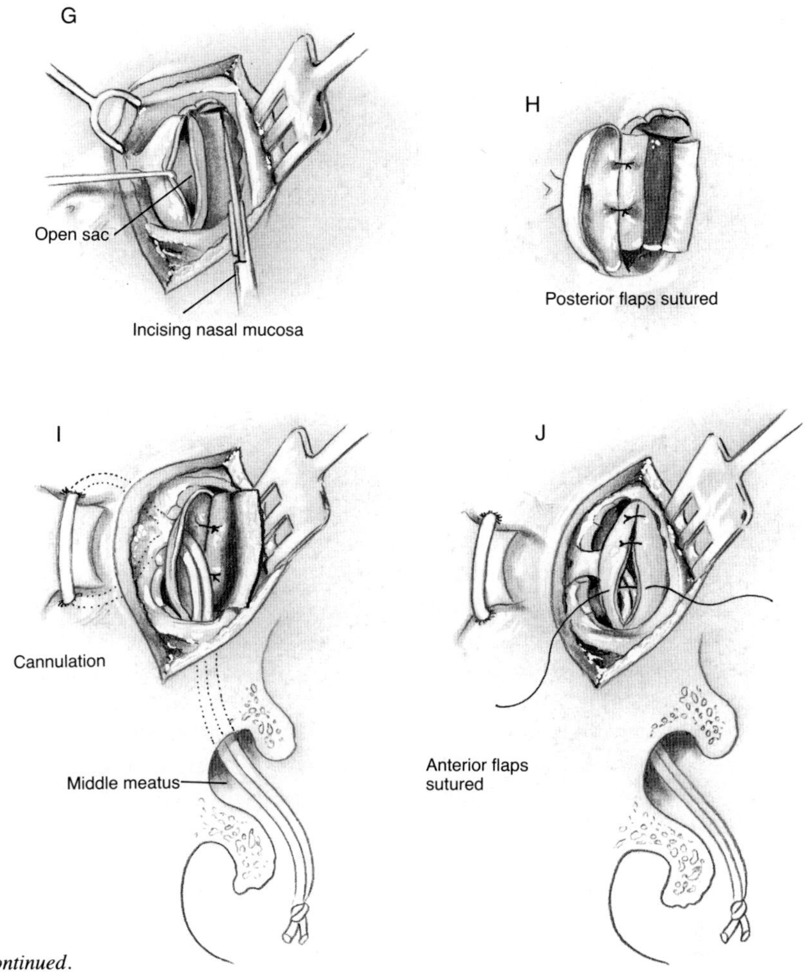

Figure 5–19. *Continued.*

is encountered, drilling with cutting burs may be performed. The mucosa of the nose should be left intact, and to avoid injury to the mucosa, elevation of the mucoperiosteum should be performed before removal of bone.

After the lacrimal sac and nasal mucosa are exposed, the lower canaliculus and puncta are dilated with a lacrimal probe and a no. 00 probe is then passed into the sac to help tent the sac wall (Fig. 5–19E,F). A vertical incision is made along the tented sac wall and two 4-0 chromic sutures are placed along the posterior flap of the sac for stabilization.

The nasal mucosa is now tented toward the lacrimal bone defect by placing a clamp intranasally against the lateral nasal wall (Fig. 5–19G,H). A vertical incision extending from superior to inferior is made over the mucosa, creating anterior and posterior mucosal flaps. The posterior nasal mucosal and lacrimal sac flaps are then sutured together using interrupted chromic sutures.

Silastic tubing is then placed through the superior and inferior canaliculi (see "Repair of Canaliculi," earlier in this chapter and into the nose (Fig. 5–19I,J). The tubing is tied and left in place along the nasal floor. The anterior nasal mucosal and lacrimal sac flaps are sutured together closing the newly formed drainage system over the Silastic tubing.

The periosteum, subcutaneous tissue, and skin are closed in a standard layered fashion, appropriate antibiotics are administered, the nose is cleared of crusts daily, and the stents are removed in 3 to 4 weeks.

Complications associated with lacrimal collecting system repair include restenosis with epiphora and dacryocystitis. If restenosis of the system occurs a repeat dacryocystorhinostomy should be performed. In elderly patients with diminished tearing a dacryocystectomy can be considered. Dacryocystitis must be treated with appropriate intravenous antibiotics until all signs of inflammation have subsided. After complete recovery from the infection, repeat dacryocystorhinostomy or dacryocystectomy should be performed.

REPAIR OF WIDENED SCARS, WEBS, AND DISPLACED ANGLES OF THE MEDIAL CANTHUS

Repair of posttraumatic telecanthus may result in cosmetic deformities such as widened scars, medial canthal webs, and displaced medial canthal angles. Widened scars and medial canthal webs can be repaired with the use of zigzagplasty or Z-plasty techniques (Fig. 5–20A,B). If there is pronounced displacement of the medial canthal angle, formal telecanthus repair is required. With minimal displacement of the inner angle (ie, 1 to 2 mm) advancement or rotational skin flaps can be used. Displacement of the inner angle upward or downward may be corrected with a transposition flap such as the Z-plasty.

Photographic documentation of the deformity should be obtained before any procedure. The palpebral fissure width and height should be measured and compared with the unaffected side, and recorded.

The medial canthal incision site usually heals with minimal scar formation. For those scars that become widened over time, or contract causing web formation, appropriate intervention should be initiated. If the problem is identified early, massage of the incision site and steroid injection with triamcinolone (40 mg/ML) may be helpful. Steroid injection should be used sparingly because this technique may cause atrophy and increased vascularity within the scar. If the scar has matured, surgical correction should be performed (Fig. 5–20A).

The face is prepared in a standard sterile fashion. Using local anesthetic with sedation the widened scar is outlined using a marking solution and then infiltrated with 2% lidocaine. Epinephrine should be avoided as small thin flaps will often not tolerate the reduced blood supply induced by this agent. If the inner angle is at the appropriate level, the widened scar is simply excised as a geometric broken line through the dermis. The tissues are undermined at the subcutaneous level around the entire wound, advanced, and closed in layers using 5-0 white nonabsorbable sutures to close the subcuticular tissues and interrupted 6-0 nylon sutures for the skin closure.

If the scar has contracted causing webbing of the inner angle, scar excision with a Z-plasty technique should be performed (Fig. 5–20B). The excised scar should correspond to the diagonal of the Z, and arms are created at 45 to 60° to the diagonal. Again, the flaps are undermined, transposed into position, and closed in layers using 5-0 white nonabsorb-

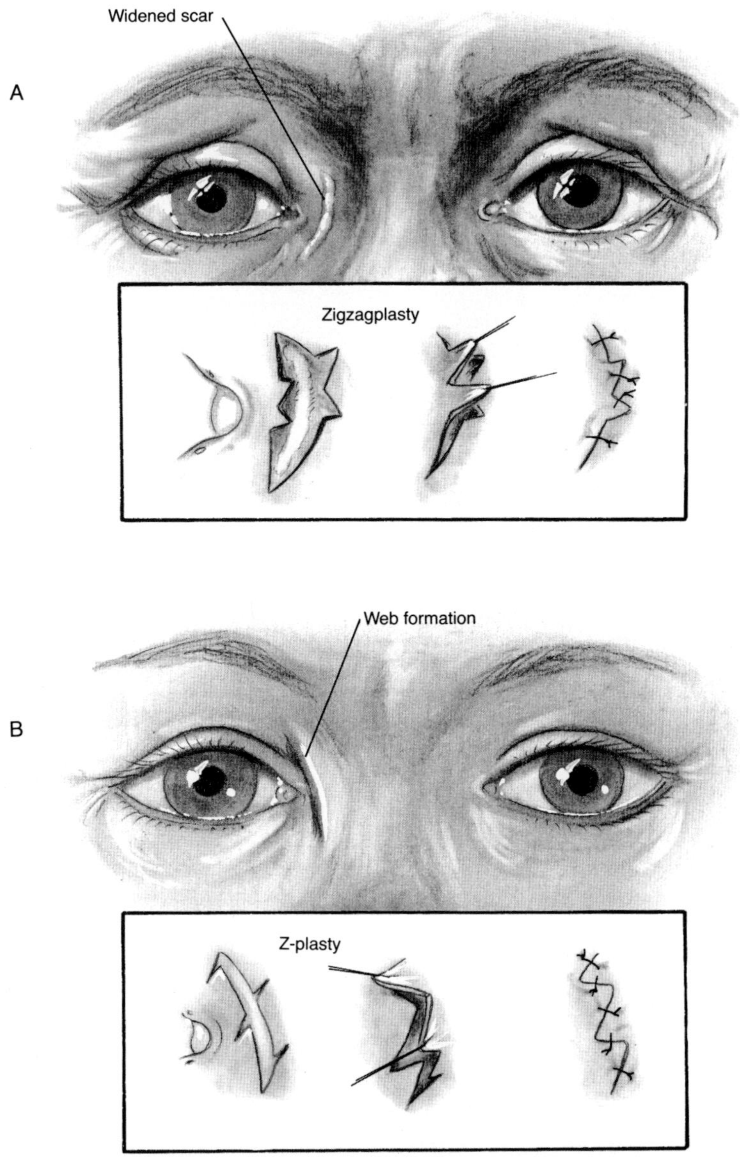

Figure 5–20. Techniques for repair of widened scars, webs, and displaced angles of the medical canthus. (Reprinted with permission from Mathog.[24]) (Figure continued on next page.)

C

D

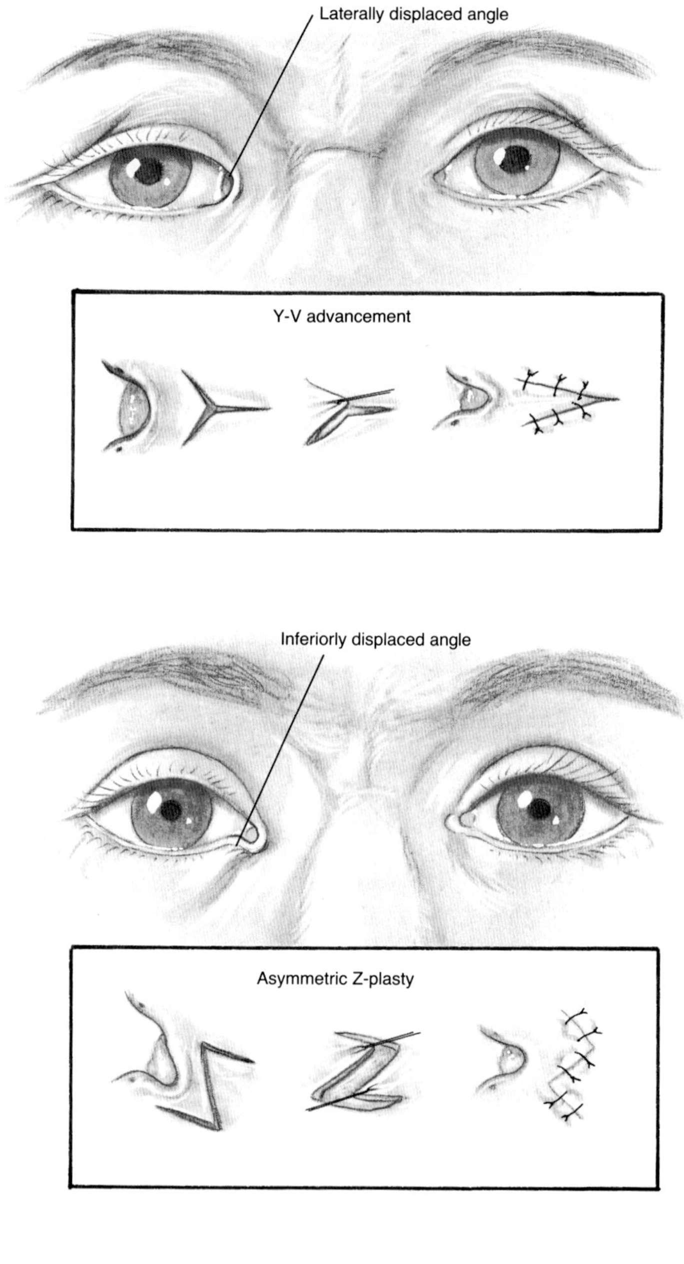

Figure 5–20. *Continued.*

able sutures to close the subcuticular tissues and interrupted 6-0 nylon sutures for the skin closure. Postoperatively, antibiotic ointment is applied to the wounds and sutures are removed in 4 to 5 days.

If the inner angle is displaced laterally, superiorly, or inferiorly it can often be corrected using an advancement and/or transposition technique (Fig. 5–20C,D). The patient is prepared as described above.

For lateral displacement of the inner angle a V-shaped incision is drawn with the lines of the V parallel to and 1 to 2 mm above and below the lid margins (Fig. 5–20C). The point of the V is then extended as a horizontal line in the medial direction to form a Y. The length of this horizontal line should approximate the distance the inner angle must be moved medially, plus an additional 1 to 2 mm to allow for overcorrection. The incisions are carried out through the dermis and subcutaneous undermining is performed for approximately 0.5 to 1 cm around the wound. The flap is then advanced medially to the end of the Y, forming a V-shaped incision. The wound is closed in layers using 5-0 white nonabsorbable sutures for the subcuticular tissues and interrupted 6-0 nylon sutures for the skin.

For upward or downward displacement of the inner angle, a Z-plasty technique should be utilized (Fig. 5–20D). One flap of the Z should contain the inner angle and the other flap should contain the space to which the inner angle will be transposed. Usually, one arm of the Z will parallel the eyelid margin; the second arm will be more acutely drawn to the diagonal. The tissues are conservatively undermined, transposed, and closed in layers using 5-0 white nonabsorbable sutures to close the subcuticular tissue and interrupted 6-0 nylon sutures for the skin closure. Postoperatively, antibiotic ointment is applied to the wounds and sutures are removed in 4 to 5 days.

SUMMARY

Fractures involving the naso-orbital complex pose considerable diagnostic and treatment challenges because of the complexity of the anatomy of the anatomy of this region, as well as its central location on the facial skeleton. Early diagnosis and treatment of naso-orbital injuries are essential for obtaining optimal results. Three general fracture patterns are described, and the physical findings, diagnostic workup, and corrective surgical techniques are outlined according to the degree of injury. Because of its anatomic association with the naso-orbital complex, the lacrimal collecting system may be injured. The clinical findings, diagnostic workup, and several repair techniques are presented. Last, a description for repair of widened scars, webs, and displaced angles of the medial canthus is delineated.

REFERENCES

1. Converse JM, ed. *Kazanjian and Converse's Surgical Treatment of Facial Injuries*. vols 1 and 2, 3rd ed. Baltimore, Md: Williams & Wilkins; 1974:337.
2. Foster CA, Sherman JE, eds. *Surgery of Facial Bone Fractures*. New York, Churchill Livingstone; 1987;39.
3. Habel MB, Ariyan S, eds. *Facial Fractures*. Philadelphia Pa: BC Decker; 1989.
4. Mathog RH, ed. *Textbook of Maxillofacial Trauma*. Baltimore, Md: Williams & Wilkins; 1984:303.
5. Leipziger LS, Manson PN. Nasoethmoid orbital fractures. *Clin Plast Surg*. 1992;19:167–193.

6. Jackson IT. Classification and treatment of orbitozygomatic and orbitoethmoid fractures. *Clin Plast Surg* 1989;16:77–91.
7. Gruss JS. Naso-ethmoid-orbital fractures: classification and role of primary bone grafting. *Plast Reconstr Surg*. 1985;75:303–314.
8. Paskert JP, Manson PN, Nicholas TI. Nasoethmoidal and orbital fractures. *Clin Plast Surg*. 1988;15:209–223.
9. Duvall AJ, Banovetz JD. Nasoethmoidal fractures. *Otolaryngol Clin North Am*. 1976;9:507–516.
10. Markowitz BL, Manson PN, Sargent L, et al. Management of the medial canthal tendon in nasoethmoid orbital fractures: the importance of the central fragment in classification and treatment. *Plast Reconstr Surg* 1991;87:843–853.
11. Gruss JS, Hurwitz JJ, Nik NA, et al. The pattern and incidence of nasolacrimal injury in naso-orbital-ethmoid fractures: the role of delayed assessment and dacryocystorhinostomy. *Br J Plast Surg*. 1985;38: 117–121.
12. Gruss JS. Fronto-naso-orbital trauma. *Clin Plast Surg*. 1982;9:577–589.
13. Peter H, Freihofer M. Experience with transnasal canthopexy. *J Maxillo fac Surg* 1980;8:119–124.
14. Duvall AJ, Foster CA, Lyons DP, et al. Medial canthoplasty: early and delayed repair. *Laryngoscope* 1981;91:173–183.
15. Stranc MF. Primary treatment of naso-ethmoid injuries with increased intercanthal distance. *Br J Plast Surg* 1970;23:8–25.
16. Converse JM, Hogan VM. Open-sky approach for reduction of naso-orbital fractures. *Plast Reconstr Surg*. 1970;46:396–398.
17. Beyer CK, Fabian RL, Smith B. Naso-orbital fractures, complications, and treatment. *Ophthalmology* 1982;89:456–463.
18. Heine RD, Catone GA, Bavitz JB, et al. Naso-orbital-ethmoid injury: Report of a case and review of the literature. *Oral Surg Oral Med Oral Pathol* 1990;69:542–549.
19. Calhoun KH, Rotzler WH, Stiernberg CM. Surgical anatomy of the lateral nasal wall. *Otolaryngol Head Neck Surg*. 1990;102:156–160.
20. Nixon J, Birchall IW, Virjee J. The role of dacryocystography in the management of patients with epiphora. *Br J Radiol*. 1990;63:337–339.
21. Benger R. Surgical management of the lacrimal drainage system. *Aust N Z J Ophthalmol*. 1988;16:281–290.
22. Fernandez-Valencia R, Pellico LG. Functional anatomy of the human saccus lacrimalis. *Acta Anat*. 1990;139: 54–59.
23. Della Rocca RC, Arthurs B, Silverstone P. Nasolacrimal disorders and their treatment. *Clin Plast Surg*. 1988;15:195–207.
24. Mathog RH, ed. *Atlas of Craniofacial Trauma*. Philadelphia, Pa: WB Saunders Co; 1992;316–348.
25. Jones LT. The cure of epiphora due to canalicular disorders, trauma, and surgical failures on the lacrimal passages. *Trans Am Acad Ophthalmol Otolaryngol*. 1962;66:506–524.
26. Mathog RH, Bauer W. Posttraumatic pseudohypertelorism (telecanthus). *Arch Otolaryngol*. 1979;105:81–85.
27. Rowe NL, Williams JL. Maxillofacial Injuries. Edenburgh: Churchill Livingstone; 1985.
28. Furnas DW, Bircoll MJ. Eyelash traction test to determine if the medial canthal ligament is detached. *Plast Reconstr Surg*. 1973;52:315–317.
29. Paskert JP, Manson PN. The bimanual examination for assessing instability in naso-orbitoethmoidal injuries. *Plast Reconstr Surg* 1989;83:165–167.
30. Kassel EE. Traumatic injuries of the paranasal sinuses. *Otolaryngol Clin North Am*. 1988;21:455–493.
31. Unger JM. Fractures of the nasolacrimal fossa and canal: a CT study of appearance, associated injuries, and significance in 25 patients. *AJR* 1992;158:1321–1324.
32. Koornneef L, Zonneveld FW. The role of direct multiplanar high resolution CT in the assessment and management of orbital trauma. *Radiol Clin North Am*. 1987;25:753–766.
33. Daly BD, Russell JL, Davidson ML, et al. Thin section computed tomography in the evaluation of naso-ethmoidal trauma. *Clin Radiol*. 1900;41:272–275.
34. Haeusler R. Facial injury to vehicle occupants associated with traffic crashes: maxillofacial injuries from vehicle accidents. *Clin Plast Surg*. 1975;2:47–51.
35. Mathog RH, Rosenberg Z. Complications in the treatment of facial fractures: symposium on maxillofacial trauma. *Otolaryngol Clin North Ann*. 1976;9:533–552.

6

Sphenoid Fractures

JEFFREY S. LEIDER, M.D.
ROBERT H. MATHOG, M.D.

Although the isolated sphenoid bone fracture is relatively rare, these injuries are commonly found with maxillary, zygomatic, ethmoid, frontal, and temporal bone fractures. Given its central location within the skull and proximity to major neural vascular structures, sphenoid bone fractures are associated with significant morbidity and mortality. Successful management depends on early diagnosis and appropriate surgical and medical management.

The purpose of this chapter is to review the anatomy, physiology, and classification of sphenoid fractures. Common etiologies along with current means of diagnosis are also discussed. Finally, treatment concepts, both medical and surgical, are addressed in conjunction with resultant central complications.

ANATOMY AND PHYSIOLOGY

The sphenoid bone is a complex structure lying in a central area of the craniofacial skeleton (Fig. 6–1). This large bone sits at the base of the skull between the occipital and ethmoid bones in front and the parietal and temporal lobes at the side. The wing-shaped sphenoid would appear to be protected by its central position, but it is particularly vulnerable to injury as fracture lines can extend through its multiple craniofacial attachments.

The sphenoid contributes walls to the orbit, nasal cavity, anterior middle cranial fossa, and the temporal, infratemporal, and pterygopalatine spaces.[1,2] It articulates anteriorly with the cribriform plate, perpendicular plate, and lamina papyracea of the ethmoid; posteriorly with the occiput; laterally with the temporal and parietal bones; inferiorly with the pyramidal process and horizontal plate of the palatine bone and vomer. The sphenoid bone is separated from the maxilla only by a small thin ledge of the ethmoid bone that lines that floor of the orbit and a narrow pterygoid process of the palatine bone. The sphenomandibular ligament, extending from the spine of the sphenoid bone to the lingula of the mandible, attaches to the mandible and to the sphenoid.

Numerous muscles either insert or take origin from the sphenoid. Consequently, interference with these muscular attachments may result in dysfunction and may be

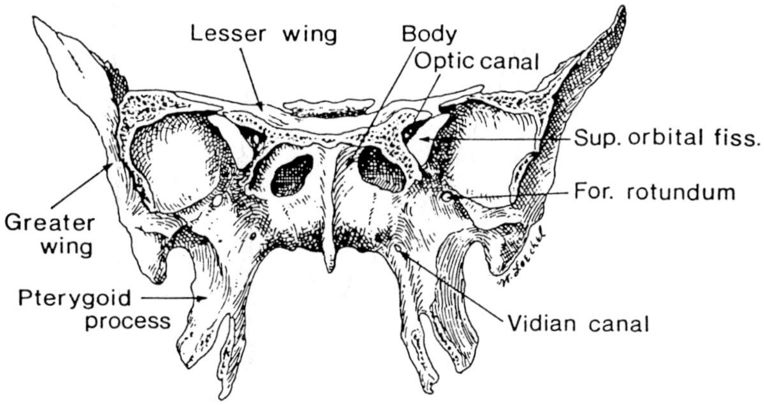

Figure 6–1. Anatomy of the sphenoid bone. (Reprinted with permission from Ghobrial et al.[3])

important sequelae of sphenoid injury. The lateral and medial pterygoid muscle originate from the lateral pterygoid plate and insert into the mandible. The levator palpebrae superioris and the four rectus muscles join in the annulus tendinous that surrounds the optic canal in the medial part of the superior orbital fissure. The superior pharyngeal constrictor takes origin from the medial pterygoid plate. The tensor velli palatini is associated with the hamulus, which serves as a pulley, as an extension of the medial pterygoid plate. Consequently, any change in the musculature attachment secondary to sphenoid trauma may result in alterations in ocular motility, mastication, speech, swallowing, or eustachian tube function.

Neurovascular structures are also at risk as they traverse the foramina associated with the sphenoid (Fig. 6–2). The superior orbital fissure transmits the recurrent meningeal branch of lacrimal artery, the superior and inferior ophthalmic veins, the oculomotor (III),

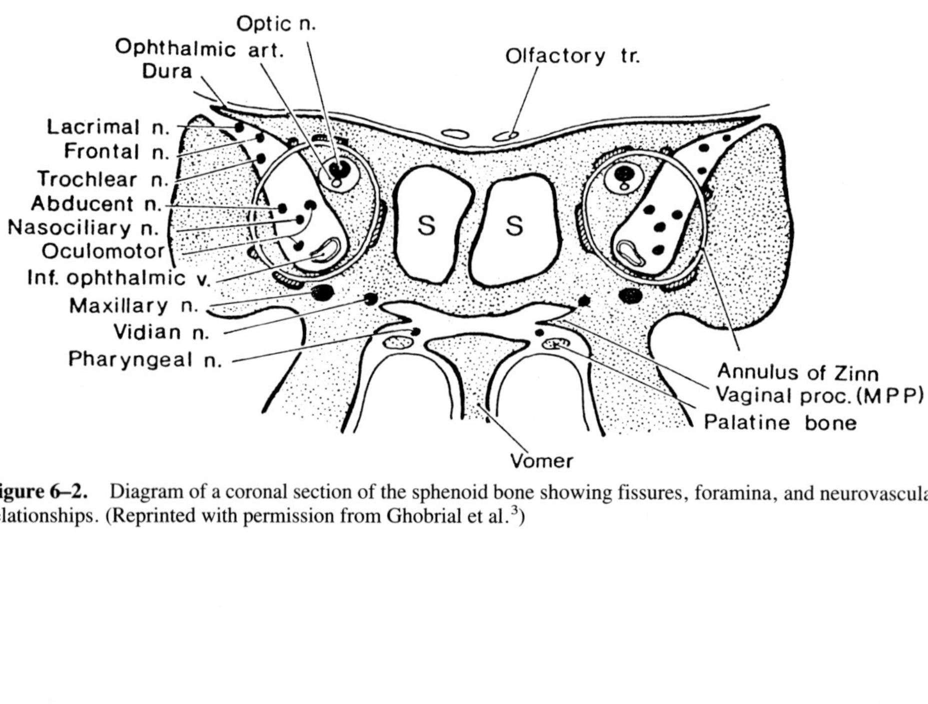

Figure 6–2. Diagram of a coronal section of the sphenoid bone showing fissures, foramina, and neurovascular relationships. (Reprinted with permission from Ghobrial et al.[3])

trochlear (IV), lacrimal, frontal, and nasal ciliary branches of the ophthalmic (V_1) and the abducens (VI) nerves and the sympathetic fibers to the globe. The foramen ovale, rotundum, and spinosum transmit the mandibular and maxillary nerves, the middle meningeal artery, and lesser petrosal nerve, respectively. The optic canal houses the optic nerve and ophthalmic artery and the pterygopalatine fissure transmits the maxillary nerve, branches of the sphenopalatine ganglion, and the terminal part of the maxillary artery. Injury to any of these structures may cause serious sensory and/or motor dysfunction.

ETIOLOGY

Sphenoid fractures are the result of severe blunt trauma to the head and facial region. Falls from excessive heights, sports accidents, assault with a blunt weapon, gunshot injuries, and motor vehicle accidents are all associated with sphenoid fractures. Frontal impact would be expected to cause combined sphenoid and frontal or maxillary fractures. More laterally directed blows would be expected to result in zygomatic and sphenoid wing fractures.

Ghobrial et al[3] presented a retrospective analysis of sphenoid fractures in 112 patients with a diagnosis of skull base fractures. Of this group, 17 patients (15%) had radiological evidence of sphenoid fractures (Table 6–1). The sphenoid fractures were commonly associated (in order of decreasing frequency) with maxillary, zygomatic, ethmoid, frontal, and temporal bone injuries. Nasal, mandibular, occipital, and parietal injuries were also noted. All anatomic areas of the sphenoid bone were found to be fractured in the series (Fig. 6–3). Pterygoid plate fractures were most commonly seen and observed to be associated with maxillary fractures, which also predominated in this series. Greater and lesser wing, body, and sinus fractures were also noted but could not be related to any facial bone injury.

DIAGNOSIS

The diagnosis of sphenoid bone fractures can almost always be made by the evaluation of historical and physical findings. The physician must correlate the mode of injury with

Table 6–1. Craniofacial and Sphenoid Fractures

TYPE OF FRACTURE	NUMBER*
Sphenoid	17
Maxillary	13
Zygomatic	10
Ethmoid	9
Frontal	5
Temporal	4
Nasal	3
Parietal	2
Mandibular	2
Occipital	1

From Ghobrial et al.[3]
*Each patient may have more than one fracture.

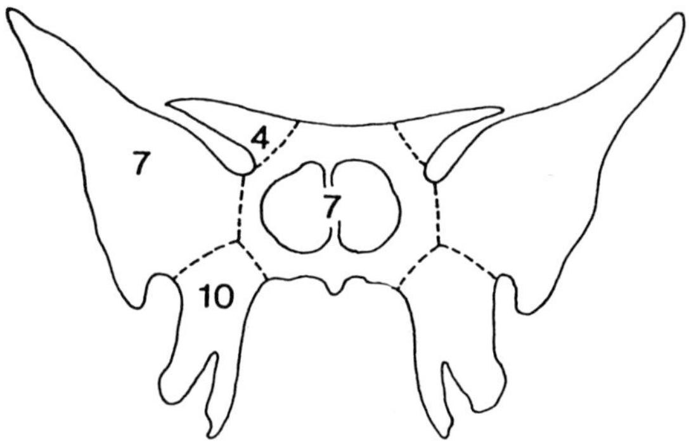

Figure 6–3. Number of fractures occurring in different anatomic areas of the sphenoid bone. (Reprinted with permission from Ghobrial et al.[3])

physical findings. Certain clinical syndromes can be expected depending on the site of the fracture. Specific signs and symptoms may develop as a result of injury to the body, sphenoid sinus, lesser and greater wings, and pterygoid plates. Various combinations of ocular injury, visual disturbances, extraocular movement dysfunction, hypoesthesia, malocclusion, and cerebrospinal fluid (CSF) leaks can be related to fractures in various anatomic areas. Confirmation of the fracture, however, should take place with appropriate imaging studies.

Greater and lesser wing fractures of the sphenoid can result in combinations of motor and sensory deficits. Hypoesthesia of the middle and lower face can occur from injury to the foramen ovale. Superior orbital fissure fractures can cause injury to cranial nerves III, IV, and VI. This results in a superior orbital fissure syndrome: dilated pupil, ptosis, and extraocular movement dysfunction. When the optic nerve is involved this syndrome is then designated orbital apex syndrome.

Pterygoid plate fractures can cause occlusion and mastication problems. Protrusion and lateral movement of the mandible can be limited as a result of pterygoid muscle dysfunction. As stated, maxillary fractures are commonly associated with pterygoid plate fractures and further aggravate occlusal relationships secondary to maxillary displacement. Pterygoid plate fractures can also cause dysphagia, middle ear fluid, and hypoesthesia. Compromise of the tensor velli palatini and superior constrictors can result in a poor pharyngeal phase of swallowing and eustachian tube dysfunction. Hypoesthesia secondary to ipsilateral infraorbital nerve and sphenopalatine ganglion injury can also occur.

Sphenoid body injuries can result in CSF leaks into the sinus and/or damage to the optic nerve within the optic canal. Cerebrospinal fluid leaks are determined by the presence of clear rhinorrhea after injury. The degree of optic nerve injury within the canal can range from edema, infarction, and hemorrhage to shearing and transection injuries.[4,5] Outside of the canal, visual loss can be caused by other factors such as increased central retinal artery compression and direct ocular damage.[6–8] As demonstrated by the Ghobrial et al[3] series, sphenoid fractures overall are associated with a 76% incidence of orbital injuries. Direct globe injuries occurred in 18% of patients with sphenoid fractures. No tendency, however, has been observed for ocular injury to occur more commonly with any specific type of sphenoid fracture. In 29% of patients a decrease in vision was observed secondary to direct ocular injury or optic nerve damage. Impaired extraocular muscle function, due to entrapment and neurological injuries, was found in 53% of patients.

The diagnosis of optic nerve injury within the canal can manifest with sudden or delayed-progressive visual loss. The nerve can be injured mildly as in a physiological block or severely as with severance or degeneration. The early determination of sudden versus delayed-progressive loss time is critical regarding treatment decisions. An afferent pupillary defect (Marcus Gunn pupil) will result when optic nerve injury has occurred. The involved pupil will react consensually, but not to direct light stimulation. It may actually appear as a relative dilation of the involved pupil as the clinician moves the light from the uninvolved to the involved eye. Associated third nerve injuries result in variable degrees of pupillary dilation.

The site and extent of a sphenoid bone fracture should be determined by radiological evaluation. The best studies are obtained several days after injury when the sinuses have become reaerated and the soft tissue swelling of the face has diminished. Computed tomographic (CT) scans are particularly suited to evaluate specific details of the injury whereas the posteroanterior and lateral skull, submental vertex, orbital apex, and sinus views are generally useful for initial screening.

The Waters view provides a general appraisal of the base of skull and details of certain areas of the sphenoid bone. The orbital oblique line, which continues as an outline of the pterygoid plate, can be well visualized as it extends into the middle of the maxillary sinus. The foramen rotundum can also be observed as a small opening inferiorly and laterally to the superior and orbital fissure. The body of the sphenoid and sphenoid sinus itself can also be visualized, especially when the view is obtained in an open mouth position.

The Caldwell projection is important in identifying, through the orbit, the greater and lesser wings of the sphenoid and superior orbital fissure. The optic canal is usually not seen. The planum sphenoidale is visualized as a horizontal line above the nasal cavity. Not uncommonly, air in the tissues secondary to ethmoid injury will obscure fine bony detail.

On lateral views of the face, the sphenoid sinus and anterior projections of the greater wings and planum sphenoidale are well seen. The pterygoid plates can be visualized as they form an oval-shaped pterygomaxillary fissure between them and the posterior wall of the maxilla. This view may also demonstrate an air-fluid level in the sphenoid sinus.[9] (Fig. 6–4).

Post-traumatic sphenoid sinus effusions (air-fluid levels) seen on plain films are of great clinical concern. In a review by Quinn and Smothers,[10] 93% of patients with a posttraumatic sphenoid effusion had abnormal CT scans. Of these patients, 31% had intracerebral hematomas, 24% had extracerebral hematomas, 13% had pneumocephalos, and 13% had cerebral edema. Thus it appears that posttraumatic sphenoid sinus effusions on skull radiograph are a useful and sensitive sign for intracranial damage, suggesting an immediate head CT to rule out associated central nervous system injury.

The Waters, Caldwell, and lateral views are informative but the submento vertex is the most important skull radiograph for evaluating sphenoid injury. This view best shows the outline of the sphenoid sinus and the Y-shaped divergence of the pterygoid plates and the wings of the sphenoid bone. The foramen ovale and foramen spinosum can also be observed. Patient cooperation and extension of the neck however are essential for obtaining satisfactory images.

Although helpful, conventional radiographs poorly demonstrate bony and optic canal injuries. Axial CT scans are quite accurate in these areas and are the best imaging techniques for sphenoid fractures.[11] Not only do CT scans give excellent bony detail, they also demonstrate the globe, extraocular muscle, optic nerve, and brain.

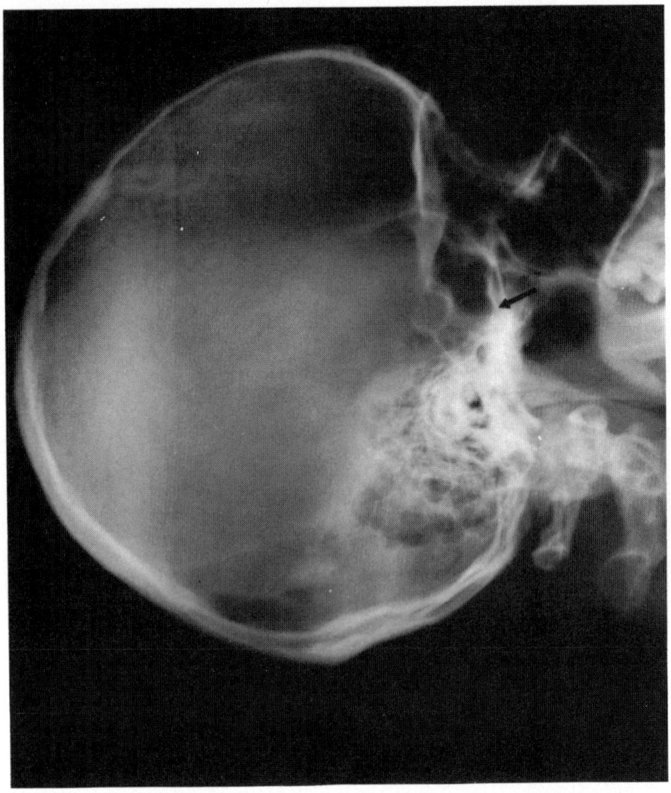

Figure 6–4. Lateral skull film demonstrating a sphenoid sinus air-fluid level. (Reprinted with permission from Jacobs.[9])

Sudden traumatic blindness is best evaluated with high resolution CT scans. The incidence of optic canal fractures varies but it is increased when CT is used over plain film examination.[12] Seif et al[12] had three of nine patients with sudden traumatic blindness present without CT scan documented evidence of optic canal fractures. On the other hand, cases of visual loss not directly explained by fracture noted on CT or magnetic resonance image of the orbit have been well documented, and optic nerve injury should be suspected. Edema, nerve contusion, stretching of the nerve, hematoma within the nerve sheath, shock wave effect, compression of the nerve, and neuroproxia have all been proposed as mechanisms of optic nerve injury[5] (Fig. 6–5). The history in such cases is critical to management and if immediate loss of vision occurs after head injury, the prognosis for visual return is quite poor.[13,14] In cases of delayed visual loss there is a reasonable chance for visual improvement. It is therefore essential to diagnose optic nerve injury as early as possible so that appropriate treatment can be undertaken.

Early and accurate diagnosis of CSF leaks is also critical in the management of patients with sphenoid bone fractures. The CSF leak can result in retrograde contamination and untoward sequelae such as meningitis and brain abscess. The leak can occur secondary to several pathologic processes. If the dura is torn, pressure differences will force the fluid into the upper respiratory/digestive tract. If the dura is partially torn, constant intracranial

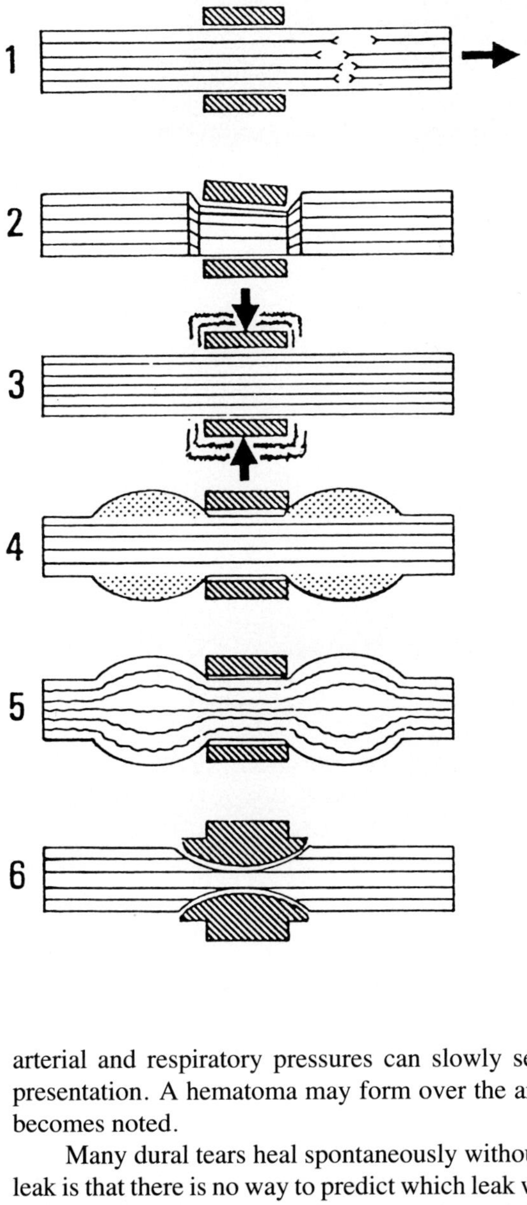

Figure 6–5. Schematic representation of common mechanisms of optic nerve injury: (1) stretching or torsion causing axonotmesis; (2) optic canal and/or anterior clinoid fracture; (3) shock wave; (4) hemorrhage; (5) edema; (6) callus formation. (Reprinted with permission from Osguthorpe and Sufferman.[5])

arterial and respiratory pressures can slowly separate dural fibers and cause a delayed presentation. A hematoma may form over the area of injury and as it dissolves, the fluid becomes noted.

Many dural tears heal spontaneously without sequela. The main problem with a CSF leak is that there is no way to predict which leak will stop and which will be associated with intracranial infection. Thus for most patients, it is important to localize the site and nature of the injury and, if the leak does not stop, to prepare for surgical exploration and repair. The leak of the cribriform plate must be distinguished from other leaks of the frontal sinus, sphenoid sinus, roof of the orbit, and temporal bone.

The history and physical examination are helpful in localizing the site of the leak (Fig. 6–6A). Gushing clear fluid from the nose associated with a change in head position suggests a fluid collection in one or several paranasal sinuses. Anosmia is often associated with leaks through the cribriform plate. Visual problems suggest injury to the tuberculum sella, sphenoid sinus, and posterior ethmoid sinus. Loss of cochlear, vestibular, or facial

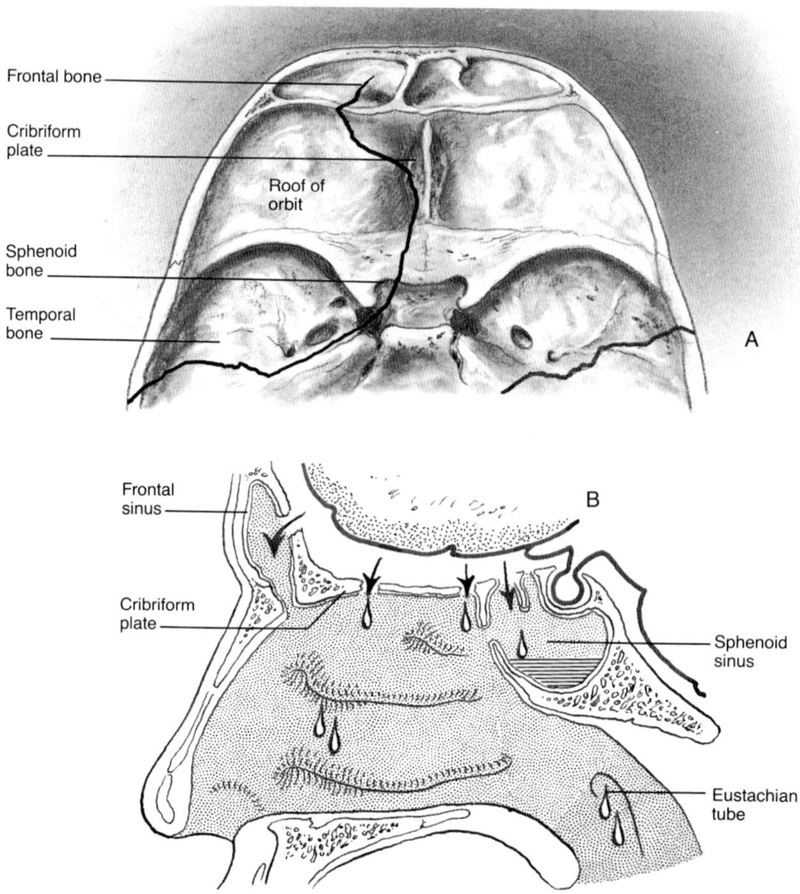

Figure 6–6. Sites and signs of CSF leak. (Reprinted with permission form Mathog.[19(p425)])

nerve function indicates a temporal bone injury. Paraesthesia or anesthesia of the face and forehead suggest damage to one or several branches of the trigeminal nerve.

On physical examination of the nose, the surgeon should shrink the mucus membranes with phenylephrine hydrochloride (Neo-Senephrine) and observe for clear fluid discharge (Fig. 6–6B). Leakage superiorly from the vault and/or from the superior meatus is indicative of cribriform plate, ethmoid, or sphenoid injury. Leakage from the middle meatus is often associated with a flow of fluid from the frontal sinus by way of the nasofrontal duct. Fluid coming from behind the inferior turbinate may indicate eustachian tube transmittal of fluid from a dural tear of the temporal bone. In most patients, the CSF can be increased by placing the patient in a head-down position; a stream or drops of fluid may be observed at the tip of the nose. In some patients, fluid may be seen behind the tympanic membrane.

With small leaks, CSF fluid may be difficult to collect and analyze. However, if the fluid can be collected, it should be evaluated in the laboratory and compared chemically and physically to the known properties of the spinal fluid. Glucose-sensitive sticks are usually not diagnostic as glucose can vary in CSF and in lacrimal and nasal secretions. A handkerchief test in which the surgeon observes different rings can be suggestive; bloody mucus will separate from CSF and generally cause rings. A cloth soaked with spinal fluid the handkerchief will not stiffen with drying.

The site and size of the defect must be obtained by special imaging and/or dye studies. Plain radiographs of the facial bones and coronal and horizontal CT scans are useful in demonstrating fracture sites. The studies may also show the accumulation of fluid in adjoining sinuses. Computed tomographic scans with metrizamide are very helpful in defining larger leaks. Fluorescein dye is also a useful method, but the surgeon must be aware of potential reactions to the intrathecally placed substance.

TREATMENT AND MANAGEMENT

Patients with life-threatening subdural hematomas, intracerebral hemorrhage, etc will require immediate neurosurgical evaluation and treatment. Ophthalmologic consultation is essential for determining the site and extent of ocular and orbital damage. Any treatment that can be delayed should be delayed until the patient is stable and suitable for further evaluation.

In most cases, expectant waiting with appropriate prophylactic antibiotic therapy is indicated. In others there is a need for immediate, aggressive medical and/or surgical decompression of one or several nerves. This is most noticeable in patients with visual loss secondary to blunt trauma who require immediate medical or surgical decompression of the optic nerve. In addition, persistent CSF leaks, masticatory dysfunction, and diplopia may also require surgical treatment but generally on a more elective basis.

The treatment of optic nerve damage following head injury is controversial and numerous treatment strategies have been proposed. In cases where vision has been affected and an optic nerve injury is suspected one must decide whether a surgical and/or medical decompression is indicated. As noted earlier, immediate and complete visual loss implies direct optic nerve trauma and a poor prognosis. In some cases especially where visual loss is delayed, early surgical intervention (less than 7 days) can be effective.[5] A review of these surgical series is seen in Table 6–2.

Table 6–2. Results of Transethmoid Optic Nerve Decompression

AUTHOR(S)	NO. OF PATIENTS	AMELIORATION (%)
Fukado	400	55
Hadjean	30	60
Sugita et al.	29	72
Niho et al	25	80
Hager et al	25	48
Baumann	23	52
Strohm and Jahnke	15	40
Matsuzaki et al	11	43
Karnik et al	10	20
Beuthner	9	56

From Osguthorpe and Sufferman.[5]

Most protocols prescribe a trial of medical management, and if this is not successful, surgical intervention should be considered. Management consists of high-dose intravenous steroids (Solumedrol 30 mg/kg four times per day for the first 48 hours). Patients should be informed of the potential side effects of this megadose therapy including ulcer disease and bony necrosis. Patients should also be placed on H2 blockers. If the patient responds, the steroids are tapered. If the patient does not respond or there is a relapse after the initial treatment then the steroids are stopped and surgical decompression is considered.

Several surgical approaches are available for decompression of the optic nerve. A transfrontal craniotomy (Fig. 6–7D) is particularly useful in patients with coexisting intracranial injuries. This approach is also useful when there is damage to the dura, frontal sinus, and orbital roof. It has the advantage over the frontoethmoid approach when important craniofacial landmarks along the skull base are lost or distorted by injury. The surgery is carried out under general anesthesia. Coronal skin flaps are marked behind the hairline, and about 2 to 3 cm of hair is shaved along the incision line (Fig. 6–7A). The incision is carried to a subperiosteal plane. Hemostasis is achieved with electric cautery and/or hemostatic clips. The scalp flap is then rotated forward and held in place with fish hooks or self-retaining retractors.

The craniotomy is best performed through a frontotemporal (Frontopterional) approach (Fig. 6–7B). One bur hole is made just behind the frontal process of the zygoma, another 2 to 3 cm laterally and posteriorly in the temporal bone, and a third just above the frontal sinus, 3 or 4 cm lateral to the midline. The dura is then elevated around the bur holes and from the deep surface of the bone with special malleable dissectors. Injury to the middle meningeal artery may occur, particularly at the transition from the bony portion to the epidural part. Electrocautery and bone wax are used for control. A craniotome or Gigli saw is used to divide the bone and remove the flap.

The dura is elevated from the floor of the frontal fossa (Fig. 6–7C). Medially the surgeon should avoid injury to the dura over the area of the cribriform plate, as the olfactory fibers cannot be adequately elevated without tearing the fibers and entering the dura. Often it is not even necessary to dissect this area.

On exposure of the roof of the orbit, the dural elevation should be carried medially and posteriorly to the edge of the lesser wing of the sphenoid. The orbital roof is then opened with a small osteotome or high-speed drill, and a portion of the roof is removed (Fig. 6–7D). The dissection is directed toward the optic canal. All bone fragments and splinters should be carefully removed and the dura of the optic canal should probably be opened. When the anatomy is obscure, it may be safe to open the anterior fossa dura and visualize the optic nerve before a decompression is carried out.

Bleeding should be controlled with electric cautery and bone wax. Dural openings and tears should be carefully repaired and openings into the sinuses closed with muscle, fat, or periosteum.

The bone flap is held in place with four or five 3-0 nonabsorbable sutures, and the scalp flap is closed with interrupted and inverting galeal 3-0 chromic sutures. Staples or nonabsorbable sutures can be used for the skin. Antibiotics (ie, nafcillin and gentamicin or cefazolin) are administered for 5 to 7 days. The head dressing can be removed at 48 hours and sutures/staples can be removed at 7 to 10 days.

If there is no associated intracranial surgical problems, several extracranial approaches have been developed to decompress the optic nerve. The transethmoid approach

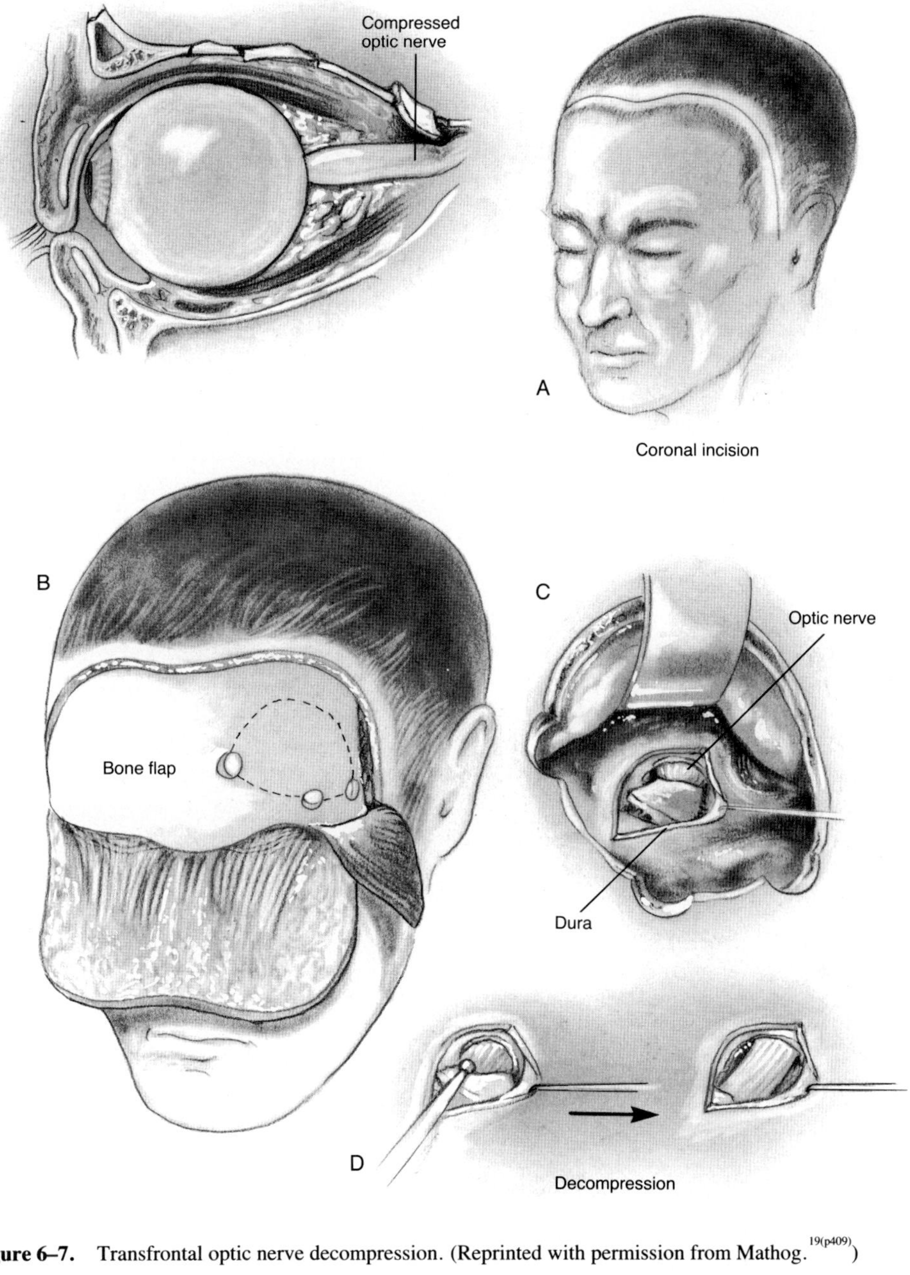

Figure 6–7. Transfrontal optic nerve decompression. (Reprinted with permission from Mathog.[19(p409)])

is the most commonly employed. Since the first described by Niho et al[15] in 1970 numerous studies have reported on this technique.[16–18] The transethmoid approach both obviates the need for a frontal craniotomy and is easily mastered by the maxillofacial surgeon who is well versed in sphenoethmoid anatomy (Fig. 6–8). With the surgeon sitting

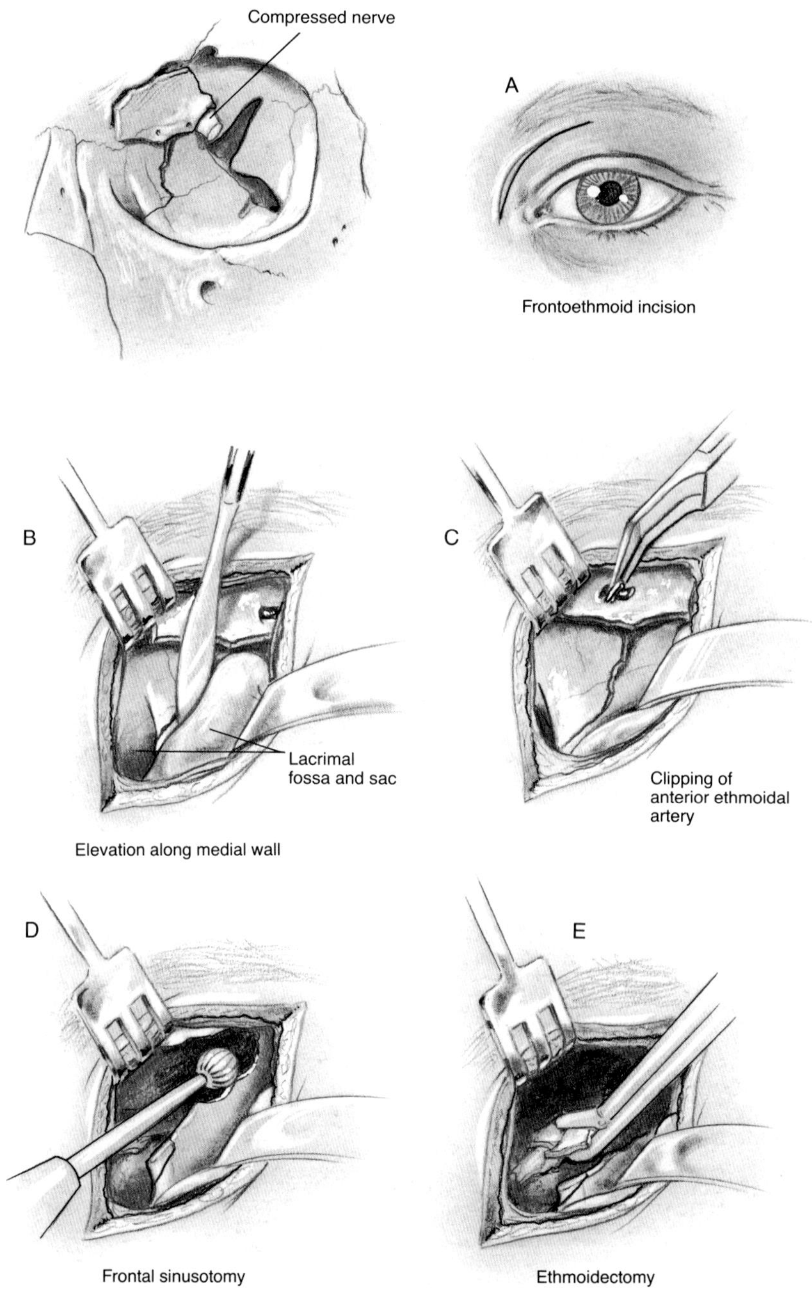

Figure 6–8. Transethmoidal decompression of the optic nerve. (Reprinted with permission from Mathog.[19(pp405,406)])

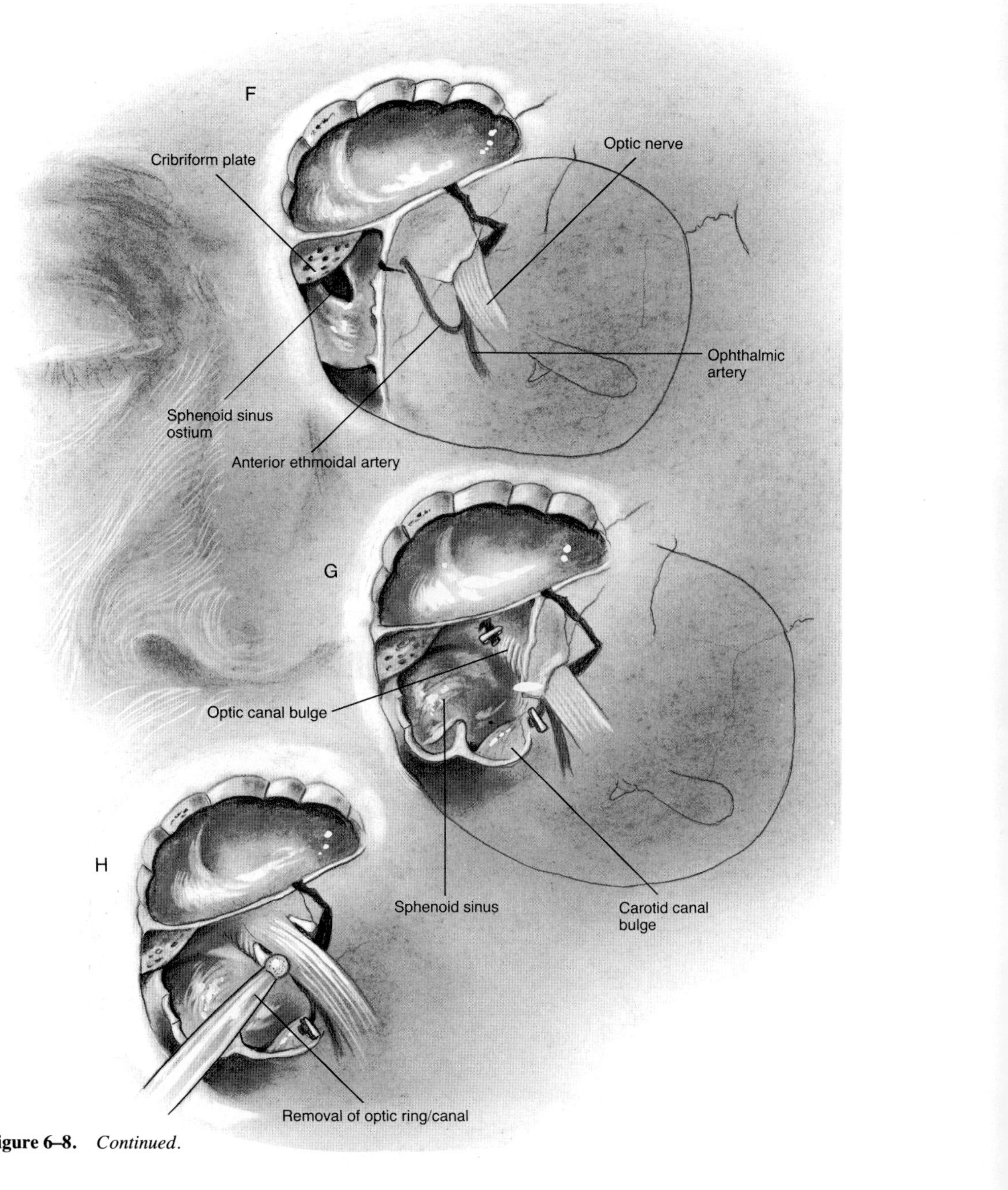

Figure 6–8. *Continued.*

at the head of the table, a curvilinear incision is made one half the distance between the inner caruncle of the eye and the dorsum of the nose (Fig. 6–8A). The incision is carried through the subcutaneous tissues; the angular vessels are ligated and bleeding is stopped with cautery. The incision can also be extended to the shadow area beneath the brow.

The periosteum is elevated off the nasal bones and the frontal process of the maxilla (Fig. 6–8B). The lamina papyracea and the lacrimal bones are exposed and the lacrimal sac is retracted laterally. The trochlea is released from its attachment. The periosteum is elevated off the medial wall of the orbit with a Freer elevator. The anterior ethmoidal artery is clipped or avulsed and bleeding is controlled by gentle pressure (Fig. 6–8C). Posteriorly the dissection should expose, but not injure, the posterior ethmoidal artery.

A frontoethmoidectomy is then performed by removing portions of the floor of the frontal sinus, the nasal bone, and the frontal process of the maxilla (Fig. 6–8F-H). The frontal sinus is opened by a small drill hole and enlarged with Kerrison rongeurs. The inferiorly located ethmoid cells are then removed with Takahashi rongeurs. The curved posterior wall of the frontal bone should be visualized and followed inferiorly and posteriorly along the base of the skull. The undersurface of the cribriform plate is exposed.

The operating microscope with a 300-mm lens is used for the remainder of the procedure (Fig. 6–8F,H). Self-retaining retractors are helpful in holding the soft tissues of the orbit from the sinus cavity. We prefer to open the sphenoid sinus with Hajek rongeurs, which in turn exposes the intersinus septum and those landmarks that identify the optic nerve and carotid artery. The transverse bulge superiorly shows the course of the optic nerve; a wider bulge laterally and posteriorly represents the carotid artery canal.

With the optic nerve bulge identified within the sphenoid sinus and the posterior ethmoidal artery visualized within the orbit, the posterior ethmoidal artery is clipped or treated with a bipolar cautery. The bone along the posteromedial wall of the orbit is then removed, exposing more of the sphenoid sinus. The periorbita is elevated 1 or 2 mm at a time, and immediately posterior to the posterior ethmoidal artery the surgeon will see the optic nerve sheath entering the optic canal. The entrance to the canal (ring) is quite thick and diamond burs on a long drill handle should be used to open this area. The canal is thinned with burs and extracted with small elevators. Approximately one half to three fourths of the canal is opened. Any displaced bone spicules are removed.

Bleeding should be minimal and nasal packing should not be needed. The periosteum is closed with 3-0 chromic sutures and the trochlea should be returned to its anatomic position. The subcutaneous tissues and skin are closed in layers.

The patient should be treated with prophylactic antibiotics (ie, cefazolin or ampicillin) and the eye checked periodically for visual function and for changes in pressure on the globe. The patient can be discharged in 24 to 48 hours.

With regard to CSF leaks, early reduction of any associated facial fractures is often successful, stopping most within 2 to 3 weeks. A lumbar drain may be helpful. The efficacy of the prophylactic antibiotics is still unclear in today's literature. If a leak persists despite these measures, then site localization and surgical repair must be considered. Three approaches for repair of a sphenoid bone CSF leak are the transseptal, frontoethmoid, and frontal craniotomy. The transseptal dissection is reliable and does not have the potential problems of diplopia and enophthalmos found with the frontoethmoid procedure or the morbidity associated with the craniotomy and exploration of the anterior fossa. Repair via functional endoscopic sinus surgery techniques is also possible.

The transseptal procedure is initiated by a sublabial degloving incision from the molar-to-molar region (Fig. 6–9). The periosteum is elevated off the premaxilla to expose the anterior nasal spine and piriform apertures (Fig. 6–9A,B). A septal/columella incision with extension along the nostril skills provides for additional elevation of tissues and wider entry into the vestibule of the nose (Fig. 6–9C).

The septal cartilage and bone are exposed by a subperichondrial and subperiosteal dissection (Fig. 6–9D,E). First, the mucoperichondrium is elevated off the quadrilateral plate; the mucoperiosteum is subsequently lifted off the perpendicular plate of the ethmoid and vomer. The dissection is continued along the maxillary crest, and after cutting the decussating fibers, the mucosal flaps are elevated off the floor region. Cottle elevators and speculae may be helpful. An identical procedure is carried out on the opposite side of the nose.

With the septum completely exposed, the quadrilateral plate is separated from the maxillary crest and ethmoid and swung to the side as a "swinging-door" flap (Fig. 6–9F). The perpendicular plates of the ethmoid and vomer are removed by to-and-fro rotation and fracture with Takahashi rongeurs. Additional exposure is obtained by excising portions of the maxillary crest, anterior nasal spine, and piriform aperture with sharp osteotomes.

At this stage, a large self-retaining speculum is inserted and the patient placed into Trendelenburg's position (Fig. 6–9G–I). With the surgeon sitting at the patient's head, the microscope is positioned and the sphenoid sinus is inspected. The rostrum and ostia of the sphenoid are identified, and after the mucosa is elevated laterally along the basisphenoid, the anterior wall is removed with Hajek and Takahashi rongeurs. The remainder of the midline septum of the sphenoid is removed, and the mucosa is stripped from the walls of the sphenoid sinus with elevators and a Takahashi rongeur.

The CSF leak should then be identified (Fig. 6–9J). The surgeon can, if necessary, inject fluorescein into the spinal fluid to distinguish the spinal fluid from other tissue fluids. Fascia lata and muscle from the leg (approximately 3 × 3 cm) are harvested. A small piece of fascia is then cut and pushed into the hole to plug the intracranial side of the defect. Additional muscle and fascia are then placed on the sinus side against the defect. The sphenoid sinus is filled with additional tissue (muscle and fascia). The speculum is removed and the mucosal flaps are placed back into original position.

The septal/columella incision is closed with interrupted 4-0 chromic sutures. The mucosa of the sublabial incision is approximated with additional chromic sutures. The nose is then packed bilaterally with nasal tampons or 1/2-in gauze treated with bacitracin ointment.

Postoperatively the patient is placed in the head-up position and told to avoid any straining, sneezing, and coughing, or blowing of the nose. The patient is given a stool softener and placed on antibiotics (ie, cefazolin or ampicillin) for approximately 2 weeks. The nasal packing is removed at about 5 days and the nose is treated with saline mists at least three times daily.

In summary the management of sphenoid fractures will depend on the problems created by the injury. In most cases expected waiting with appropriate prophylactic antibiotics is indicated. In others there is a need for immediate aggressive medical and/or surgical decompression of the optic nerve. Other conditions such as CSF leaks can be treated on a more elective basis after thorough evaluation and stabilization of the patient. The prognosis and response to treatment will be governed by the degree and complexity of the injury, the accuracy of the diagnosis, and the timeliness of competent medical and surgical interventions.

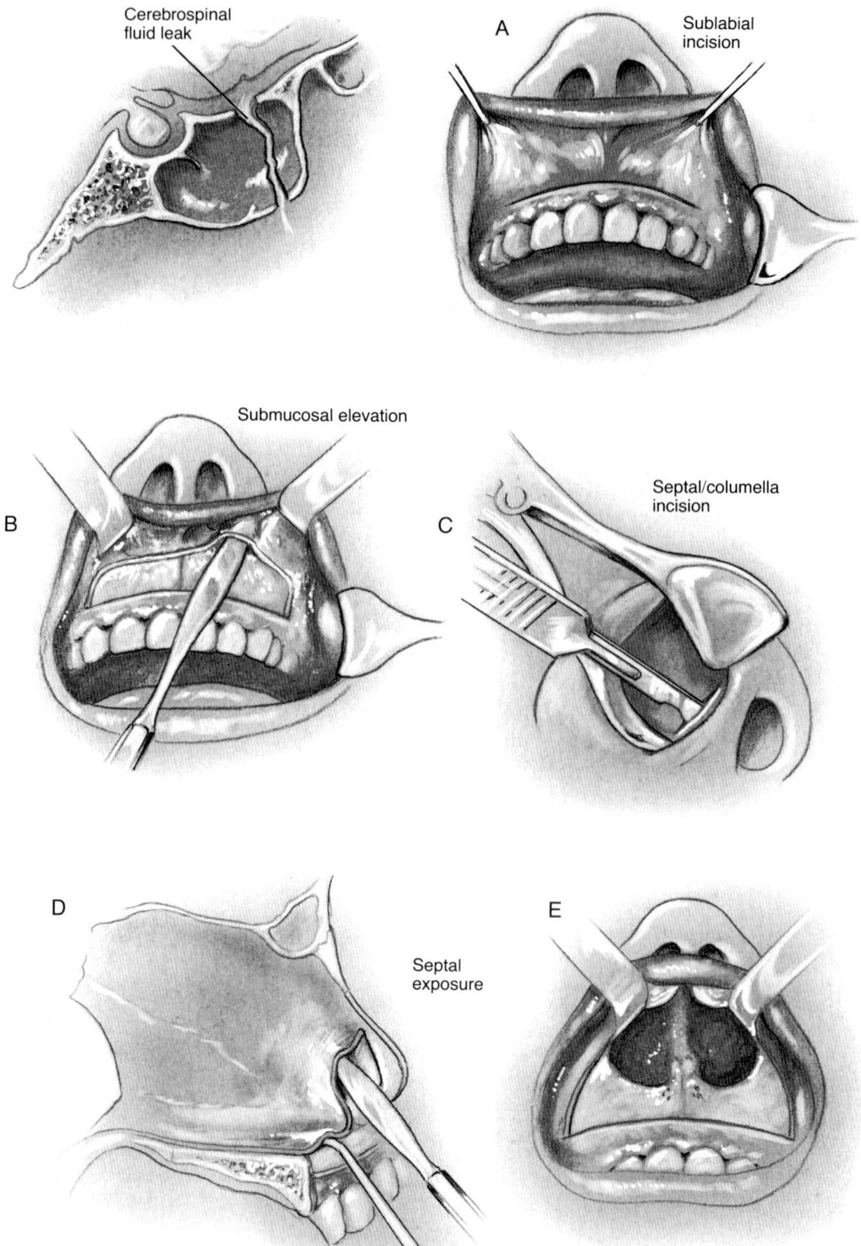

Figure 6–9. Transsphenoidal repair of CSF leak (Reprinted with permission from Mathog.[19(pp417,418)])

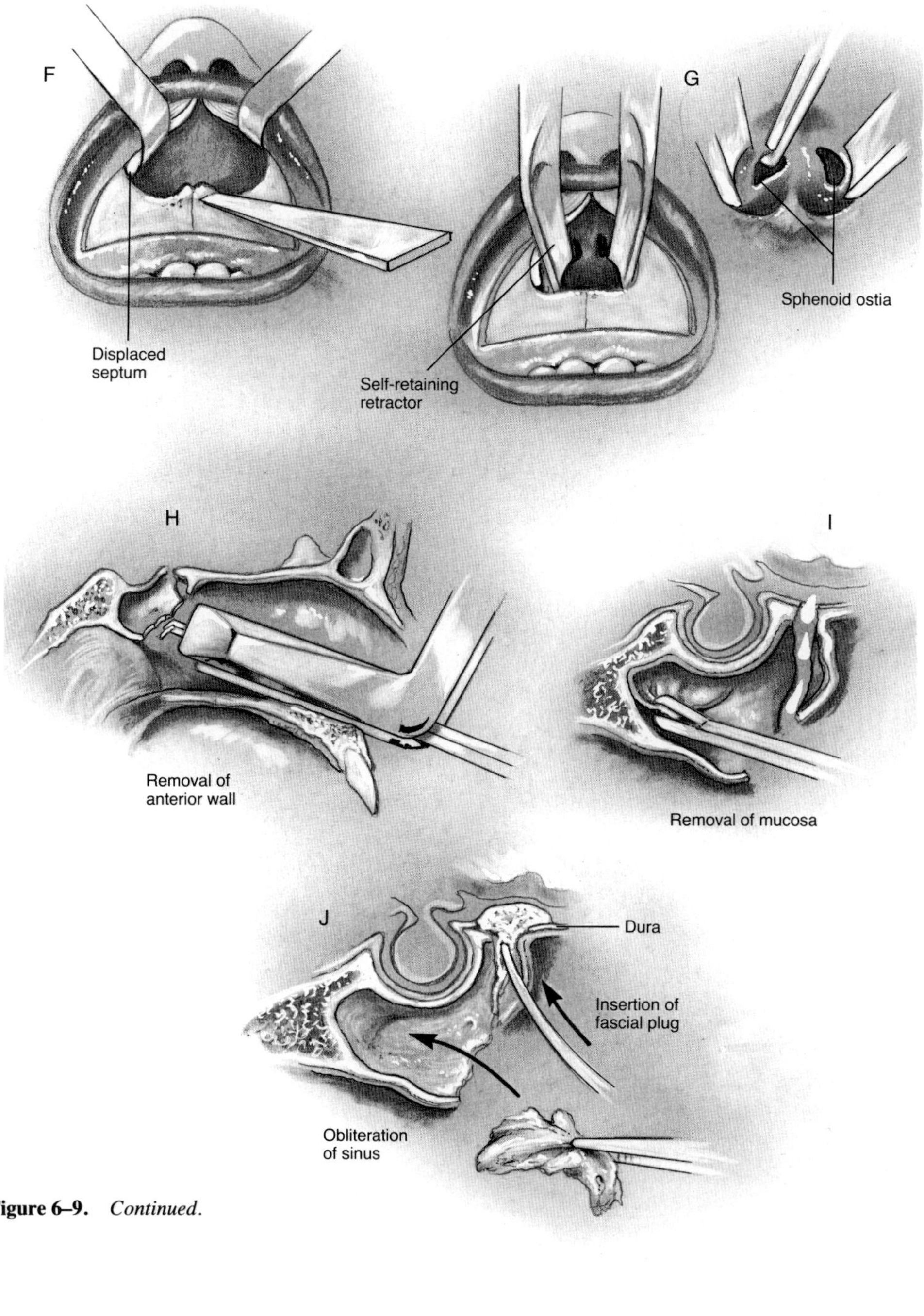

Figure 6–9. *Continued.*

REFERENCES

1. Maisel H. Postnatal growth and anatomy of the face. In: Mathog RH, ed. *Maxillofacial Trauma*. Baltimore, Md: Williams & Wilkins; 1984:21–38.
2. Katton KR, Potter GD. Lateral extension of the sphenoid sinuses. *Med Radiogr Photogr*. 1983;59:9–12.
3. Ghobrial W, Amstuz S, Mathog R. Fractures of the sphenoid bone. *Head and Neck*. July/August 1986:447–455.
4. Ramsay JH. Optic nerve injuries in fractures of the canal. *Br J Ophthalmol*. 1979;63:607–610.
5. Osguthorpe JD, Sufferman RA. Optic nerve decompression. *Otolaryngol Clin North Am*. 1988;21:155–169.
6. Nicholson DH, Guzak SV. Visual loss complicating repair of orbital floor fractures. *Arch Ophthalmol*. 1971;86:369–375.
7. Gelman HK, Janzen WR, Skolnik EM. Ocular hypertension following the use of an antral balloon. *Arch Otolaryngol*. 1974;99:449, 450.
8. Ketchum LD, Ferris B, Maskers FW. Blindness without direct injury to the globe: a complication of facial fractures. *Plast Reconstr Surg*. 1976;58:187–191.
9. Jacobs JR. Cerebrospinal fluid fistula. In: Mathog RH, ed. *Maxillofacial Trauma*. Baltimore, Md: Williams & Wilkins; 1984:297–302.
10. Quinn S, Smothers R. The diagnostic significance of post-traumatic sphenoid sinus effusions: correlation with land computed tomography CT. *J Comput Tomogr*. 1984;8:61–64.
11. Manfred SJ, Raji MR, Sprinkle PM, Weinstein CW, Minardi LM, Swamson TJ. Computerized tomographic findings in facial fractures associated with blindness. *Plast Reconstr Surg*. 1981;68:479–490.
12. Seiff S, Mitchel S, Guyon J, Pitts L. Computed tomographic evaluation of the optic nerve canal in sudden traumatic blindness. *Am J Ophthalmol*. 1984;98:751–755.
13. Bodrussion EH. Evaluation of orbital injuries. *Adv Ophthalmol Plast Reconstr Surg*. 1987;6:37–49.
14. Joundeph BC. Blunt ocular trauma, *Emerg Med Clin North Am*. 1988;6:147–167.
15. Niho S, Niho M, Niho K. Decompression of the optic canal by the transethmoidal route and decompression of the superior orbital fissure. *Can J Ophthalmol*. 1970;5:22–40.
16. Fukado Y. Results in 350 cases of surgical decompression of the optic nerve. *Trans Assoc Pacific Acad Ophthalmol*. 1972;4:96–99.
17. Sufferman RA. Sphenoethmoid approach to the optic nerve. *Laryngoscope*. 1981;91:184–196.
18. Kennerdell JS, Amsbaugh GA, Meyers EN. Transantralethmoidal decompression of the optic canal fracture. *Arch Ophthalmol*. 1976;94:1040–1043.
19. Mathog RH. *Atlas of Craniofacial Trauma*. Philadelphia, Pa: WB Saunders Co; 1992.

7

Mucoceles and Sinusitis

JORGE D. LATONI, M.D.
STEVEN C. MARKS, M.D.

Inflammatory conditions of the nose and the paranasal sinuses are a natural result of maxillofacial trauma. There are a number of factors that contribute to this association beginning with the initial trauma itself, which can lead to mucosal edema with a resultant decrease in ciliary function. Hemorrhage into the sinuses creates a clot within the sinus, which liquifies over time and finally clears through the natural ostium due to the ciliary activity of the mucosa. During this process, however, bacterial contamination of the sinus either through direct inoculation from trauma or by any iatrogenic means, can progress to an infectious process. Trauma may also directly impair mucociliary clearance by the obstruction of the sinus ostia or the mucosal drainage pathway.

Despite these incumbent risks, the actual incidence of inflammatory complications of nasal and sinus trauma appears to be quite low. Although acute infection in this setting is uncommon, the true incidence of inflammatory complications following sinonasal trauma is still not known. In 1987, Chole[1] studied the role of antibiotic prophylaxis in maxillofacial trauma. In this prospective randomized trial, there were no infections in any Le Fort, zygomatic, or subcondylar fractures even when associated with other infected mandibular fractures. They found no statistical advantage to using prophylactic antibiotics in nonmandibular maxillofacial fractures, a finding that may be related to the overall low incidence of infection in these patients.

The incidence of chronic sinus disease after maxillofacial trauma is also low but it is even less well understood. Chronic sinusitis can occur owing to alterations in anatomy such as a deviated nasoseptum or a medial orbital wall fracture. The resulting conditions are typical of chronic sinusitis, the diagnosis and management of which are beyond the scope of this chapter. More important to this discussion is the association between mucoceles and sinonasal trauma.

MUCOCELES

Mucoceles are benign, locally expansile masses filled with mucus and lined by the mucoperiosteum of the involved sinus.[2–5] Mucoceles occur equally between sexes[5,6] and have a peak incidence in the third or fourth decade of life.[5] They are believed to be formed secondary to obstruction of the sinus ostium, with the accumulation of fluid within a mucoperiostally lined cyst.[4] As the mucosal lining secretes fluid, the mucocele slowly enlarges, resulting in erosion and resorption of the sinus walls.[4,7] Secondary bacterial infection of this fluid can lead to a period of rapid expansion and bony wall destruction, also known as a pyocele.

The two most common causes of sinus obstruction that lead to mucocele formation are chronic infections and allergic nasal disease.[8,9] In a large number of cases, however, the etiology is not known.[10] Rarely, a fracture through a sinus ostium, with or without entrapment of mucosa along the fracture line, can lead to the formation of a mucocele.[9] Iatrogenic mucoceles can also occur, particularly in the maxillary sinus. It has been estimated that 50% of all maxillary sinus mucoceles are, in fact, related to antral operations.[9] Typically, this postoperative mucocele occupies only a portion of the antral cavity[9] and commonly follows a Caldwell-Luc approach.[10–12]

Mucoceles are most commonly found in the frontoethmoidal region.[3,6,13–19] The ethmoid, sphenoid, and maxillary sinuses then follow in decreasing order of frequency.[10,20] Approximately 10% of mucoceles occur in the maxillary sinus.[9,21] Frontal and frontoethmoidal mucoceles are typically the most dangerous, as they may extend superiorly and posteriorly to encroach on the anterior cranial fossae, or alternatively, extend inferomedially to invade the orbit. Because of their close proximity to the intracranial structures sphenoid sinus mucoceles can also be dangerous. They can erode into the sella turcica or into the middle cranial fossae and present with hormonal or neurological abnormalities.[22–28]

Palubinskas and Davis noted that mucoceles do not always contain mucus or mucoid material. In fact, mucocele content can vary from a light serous fluid[29] to a thick greenish fluid[30] or a mucoid material that may or may not contain pus.[31]

DIAGNOSIS

Mucoceles are diagnosed by correlation of a careful history and physical examination with radiographic findings. Patients with advanced frontoethmoidal mucoceles typically present with proptosis, frontal pain, and headaches.[5,6,20] Earlier findings include diplopia, frontal tenderness, swelling over the medial canthal area, or a small degree of lateral globe displacement.[20] Intranasal exam may show a mucopurulent discharge, nasal polyps, or in some cases no pathologic findings are found.[5] If a mucocele is complicated by osteomyelitis of the frontal bone, the patient may present with a boggy or fluctuant swelling of the forehead (Pott's puffy tumor).[6] The differential diagnosis in these patients includes primary or metastatic neoplasms, meningiomas, fibro-osseous dysplasia, and encephaloceles.[4,20]

Sphenoethmoid mucoceles may present with headaches referred to the occipital or vertex regions and ophthalmologic complaints such as diplopia and globe displacement.[3,6] Rarely, they may present with signs of pituitary gland involvement such as galactorrhea and amenorrhea.[24] The differential diagnosis of sphenoethmoidal mucoceles must include pituitary tumors, craniopharyngiomas, meningiomas, gliomas, dermoids, metastatic lesions, and vascular aneurysms.[4,24]

When a mucocele is suspected, radiographs are obtained to help define the nature and extent of the disease process. Early on, a mucocele will not show any characteristic findings on plain radiographs. At this time, nonspecific opacification of the sinus may be the only significant finding.[7,9] As the mucocele enlarges, however, a loss of the marginal scalloping of the sinus, an enlarged sinus size, and the presence of marginal bone porosis and sclerosis can usually be identified with plain films.[7] The information gained from these studies is quite limited, as it does not sharply define soft tissue margins or the presence or absence of intracranial and intraorbital invasion.

Computed tomography (CT) is the diagnostic method of choice because it shows the extent of the mucocele as well as orbital or intracranial extension.[22,32] Unlike neoplastic processes, mucoceles will not enhance on CT scan[10,23] whereas the periphery of a pyocele does, however, enhance with intravenous contrast administration.[9,21] Also, although neoplastic processes show irregular patterns of bone erosion and mottling, mucoceles usually demonstrate bone expansion and concentric erosion (Fig. 7–1).[33]

Magnetic resonance imaging can be of benefit in the differentation of neoplastic processes from mucoceles.[6,10,34] Typically, a mucocele will appear bland on T1 weighted images and will enhance on T2 weighted images. However, this will vary with the content of the mucocele thus limiting the usefulness of this modality.[33]

Maxillary mucoceles often present with painless bulging of the cheek, diplopia, and dental complaints.[9] Nasal obstruction due to medial displacement of the medial antral wall and the inferior turbinates can also occur.[35] The differential diagnosis of maxillary sinus mucoceles includes sinusitis, retention cysts, and antrochoanal polyps.[20]

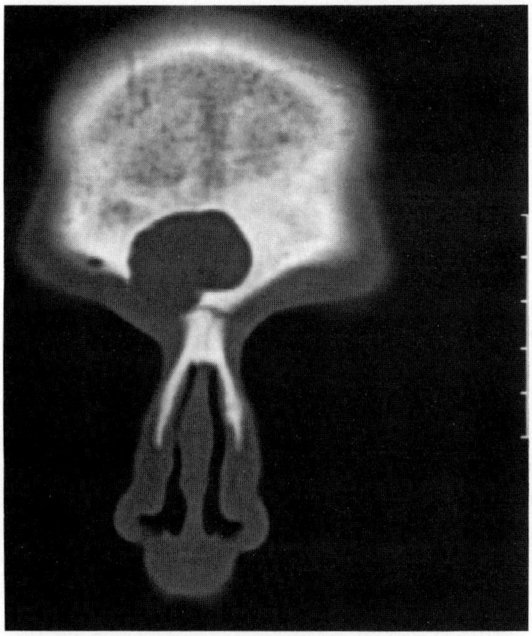

Figure 7–1. Frontal sinus mucocele demonstrating concentric expansion and bone erosion.

TREATMENT

The management of paranasal sinus mucoceles depends on a number of factors including the location and extent of disease as well as the skill and experience of the surgeon. In each case the surgeon must choose between intranasal and external approaches. If possible, the least invasive intranasal approach should be utilized. A number of factors, however, may be present that would favor an open surgical technique. Posttraumatic mucoceles are usually related to obstruction of sinus ostium or to mucosal entrapment along the fracture line. These conditions predispose many of these mucoceles to early complications and, possibly, to inaccessibility by intranasal surgical techniques. Also, large mucoceles with significant extension beyond the sinus walls may contain recesses that would inadequately drain through the natural ostium.

The experience of the surgeon should also not be discounted. Techniques such as frontoethmoidectomy, osteoplastic flaps with obliteration, and endoscopic drainage are technically difficult and challenging procedures. Most surgeons will tend to favor that technique with which they are most comfortable. In the remainder of this chapter the basic approaches to paranasal sinus mucoceles will be outlined with the criteria in which these procedures can be utilized.

ENDOSCOPIC DRAINAGE

Intranasal drainage of mucoceles has been performed for many years. Many surgeons had, however, abandoned this approach because of a high rate of stenosis of the opening and subsequent recurrence of the mucocele. Since the advent of endoscopic sinus surgery, enlargement of the natural sinus ostium has become possible. Also, the ability to effectively follow the patient postoperatively and assure long-term patency have been improved by the use of intranasal endoscopic techniques. Other advantages to the endoscopic drainage of paranasal sinus mucoceles include the ability to perform it under local anesthesia with sedation, thus avoiding the risks of general anesthesia, and a shorter hospital stay. These factors have led to a tremendous increase in the popularity of intranasal drainage of mucoceles.

Although long-term follow-up data is lacking, the early results of endoscopic drainage of paranasal sinus mucoceles have shown uniformity of success when the mucoceles themselves can be endoscopically opened.[6,36] Accessibility of the mucocele remains the principal criterion for endoscopic drainage. A relative contraindication to endoscopic sinus mucocele drainage is extension of the mucocele outside the sinus walls. Generally, significant extension into the orbit or soft tissues of the face may require open surgical techniques for complete removal of the mucocele and to prevent future complications.

Specific locations amenable to this approach include frontal mucoceles extending into the frontal recess, any ethmoid or sphenoid mucocele, and maxillary sinus mucoceles that abut the natural ostium or that extend into the nose. Sphenoethmoid mucoceles are especially good candidates for endoscopic management. When compared with other techniques, this approach provides superior exposure and visualization for either simple drainage or complete excision.

The endoscopic management of mucoceles first involves an endoscopic ethmoidectomy as previously described.[37–39] The procedure is then modified according to mucocele location. For frontal mucoceles, a detailed and careful dissection of the frontal recess is required. The agger nasi cells should be widely opened and the root of the middle turbinate removed to increase exposure (Fig. 7–2a). The skull base is skeletonized forward from the attachment of the bulla while identifying the anterior ethmoidal artery (Fig. 7–2b). The opening of the frontal sinus is usually found posterior to the agger nasi cells and anterior to the anterior ethmoidal artery (Fig. 7–2c). Often the 70 or 90° giraffe forceps are used to take down the posterior wall of the agger nasi cells. Visualization is best achieved with either the 30 or 70° telescope. The mucocele is opened widely but care should be taken to minimize trauma to the mucosal lining beyond the limits of the bony opening. Stripping or abraiding the mucosa in this location can lead to synechia formation and permanent obstruction of the nasofrontal drainage system.

Sphenoid sinus mucoceles require wide opening of the sinus. Again, the initial step is a complete endoscopic ethmoidectomy. The sphenoid is then entered either through the natural ostium or at the medial and inferior extent within the ethmoidectomy cavity. The anterior wall of the sinus is completely removed using the rotating sphenoid punch. Complete resection of sphenoid mucoceles is possible via the endoscopic approach; however, this appears to carry no advantage over wide marsupialization. Although it is possible to perform this technique without prior ethmoidectomy by removing only the posterior aspect of the middle turbinate, experience has shown that postoperative care and monitoring of the sphenoid sinus are optimized by the wide exposure gained by a complete ethmoidectomy.

Maxillary sinus mucoceles are dealt with by wide opening of the natural ostium. Care must be taken to avoid excessive anterior enlargement to avoid injuring the nasolacrimal duct. Usually an antrostomy alone will suffice to achieve adequate drainage; however, if the mucocele is only partially filling the sinus, it will be necessary to enter the sinus itself to approach these mucoceles. This is done endoscopically by using the 30 and 70° telescopes and giraffe forceps. In this instance, complete resection of the mucocele may be possible.

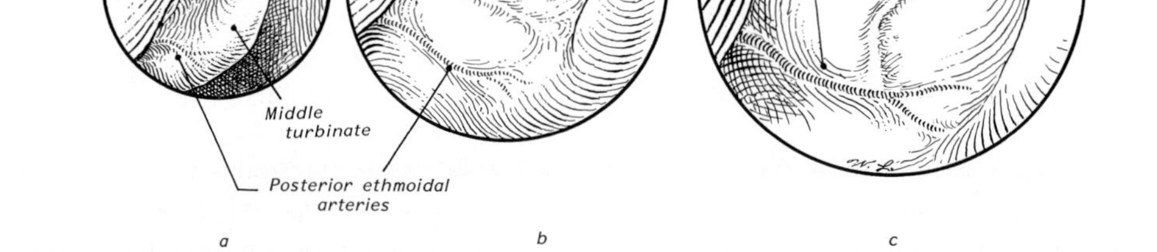

Figure 7–2. Endoscopic approach to the frontal sinus. (a). Endoscopic view following ethmoidectomy. The root of the middle turbinate has been removed to increase exposure. (b). Thirty-degree view after removal of the agger nasi cells. The anterior ethmoidal artery is identified. The ostium lies anterior and medial to the artery. (c). Seventy-degree view with enlargement of the ostium.

EXTERNAL APPROACH

Frontoethmoidectomy

There are two procedures that have gained wide acceptance for open surgical treatment of frontal sinus mucoceles, the frontoethmoidectomy and the osteoplastic sinusectomy with obliteration. The principle of the frontoethmoidectomy technique is that the sinus is preserved and the nasofrontal drainage pathway is reconstructed. An advantage of this procedure is that is a shorter, less invasive procedure that can usually be performed through a small incision. The external frontoethmoidectomy, however, requires long-term postoperative stenting and in the best hands has a 20 to 30% incidence of stenosis, which can often lead to mucocele recurrence.[2,40–43] It is well recognized that closure of the nasofrontal communication is the most common cause of failure of this procedure, and creation of a large nasofrontal opening does not guarantee a patent passageway.[40–44]

These factors make the external frontoethmoidectomy a reasonable alternative for an older patient or for patients less tolerant of major surgery. The frontoethmoidectomy has also been advocated as a method to avoid a longer surgery with the knowledge that close follow-up will be needed and the potential for reoperation is significant.

The frontoethmoidectomy is performed through a medial canthal incision with extension into the medial brow. Often, a notch is placed in the center to help camouflage the scar (Fig. 7–3a). Important landmarks to identify include the lacrimal crest and fossa, the anterior ethmoidal artery, and the supraorbital nerve (Fig. 7–3b). After the anterior ethmoidal artery is identified and ligated (or cauterized) a complete external ethmoidectomy is performed. This is usually accomplished with a headlight, forceps, and curettes. The frontal sinus is entered in its medial extent using a drill with a cutting bur (Fig. 7–3c). The floor of the frontal sinus is generally removed laterally only as far as the supraorbital nerve. If more exposure is required, the nerve can be mobilized out of its bony canal and the exposure then extended laterally as far as is necessary. The frontoethmoid sinuses are then connected using either a rongeur or a cutting bur (Fig. 7–3d).

The contents of the sinus are removed at this point and if desired, local mucosal flaps can be rotated to reconstruct a nasofrontal duct. A carefully sized stent is then placed through the nasofrontal connection and sutured to the lateral nasal wall or septum with an intranasal stitch. After surgery, the stent is regularly cleaned and can also be used to irrigate the sinus. The stent is usually left in place for a minimum of 4 to 6 weeks, although a longer period is sometimes desirable and is usually well tolerated.[44] Frontoethmoidectomy patients should be monitored closely postoperatively for several years with interval radiographs or CT scans to assure aeration of the frontal sinus.

Osteoplastic Frontosinusectomy

As mentioned earlier, definitive management of frontal sinus mucoceles can usually be obtained with an osteoplastic frontal sinusectomy with obliteration. When properly performed, this technique provides excellent success rates with minimal postoperative complications.[45] It relies on complete exenteration of the sinus mucosa, permanent obstruction of the nasofrontal connection, and obliteration of the frontal sinus. Advocates of this procedure prefer it for management of most chronic inflammatory conditions of the frontal sinus, including mucoceles.

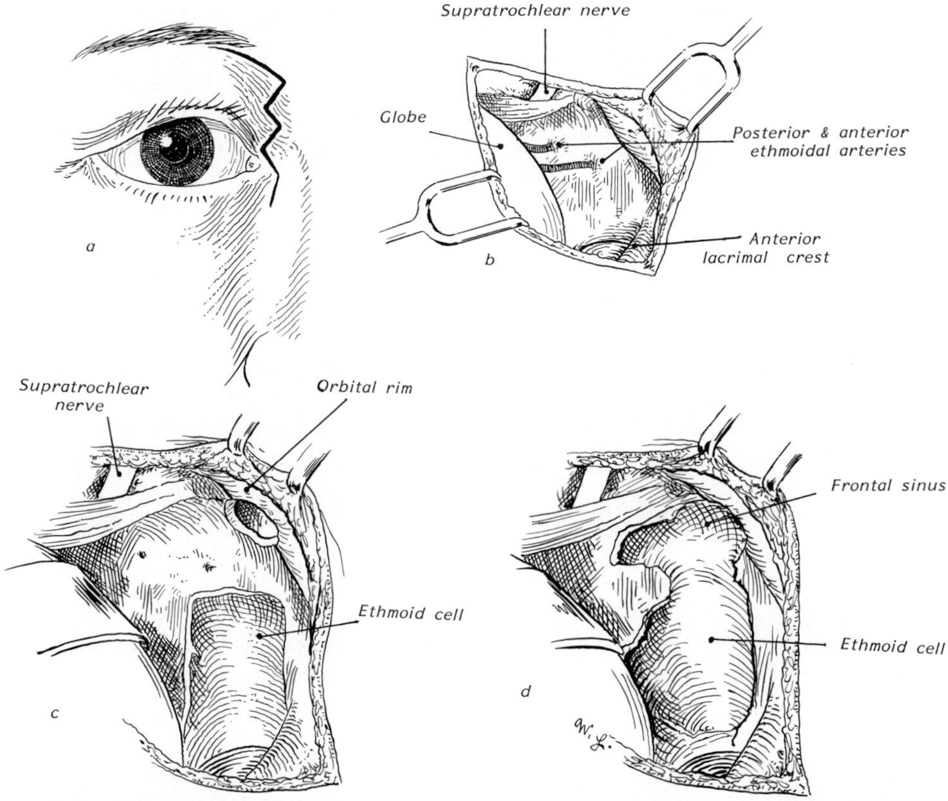

Figure 7–3. External frontoethmoidectomy. (a). Preferred incision incorporating W- plasty. (b). After elevation of the orbit showing positions of the anterior and posterior ethmoidal arteries and supratrochlear nerve. (c). After completion of the ethmoidectomy and frontal sinus trephination. (d). Completed operation before reconstruction of the nasofrontal duct.

There are however, several drawbacks to this technique. First, it requires a large incision that carries an increased risk of cosmetic and neurosensory complications. Also, a frontal bone flap must be created and this may lead to intracranial penetration with possible cerebrospinal fluid leaks and/or intracranial hemorrhage. Furthermore, the obliterated sinus is difficult to assess radiographically, making late complications more dangerous, though rare. Finally, postsurgical hospitalization for several days is necessary after this technique.

For the above-mentioned reasons, we perform the osteoplastic obliteration technique only in those patients who are either ineligible or fail endoscopic management.

SPHENOETHMOID SINUS MUCOCELES

Isolated sphenoid or ethmoid mucoceles are rare. When they do occur, however, they are usually adequately treated by intranasal excision or drainage. Removal can also sometimes be accomplished through an external or transantral approach if the mucocele is limited to its respective sinus cavity. These latter approaches offer no definitive advantages over

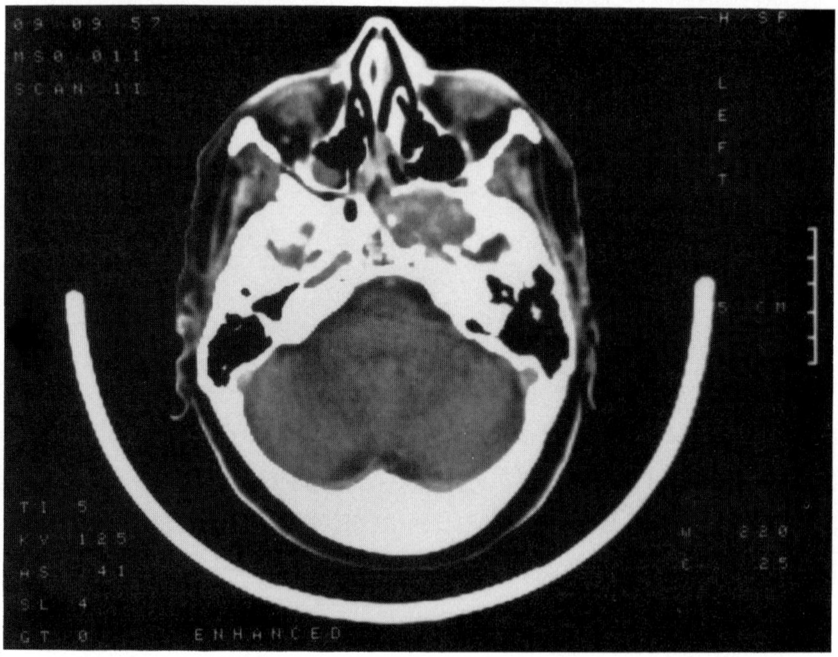

Figure 7–4. Sphenoid sinus mucocele before treatment by endoscopic decompression.

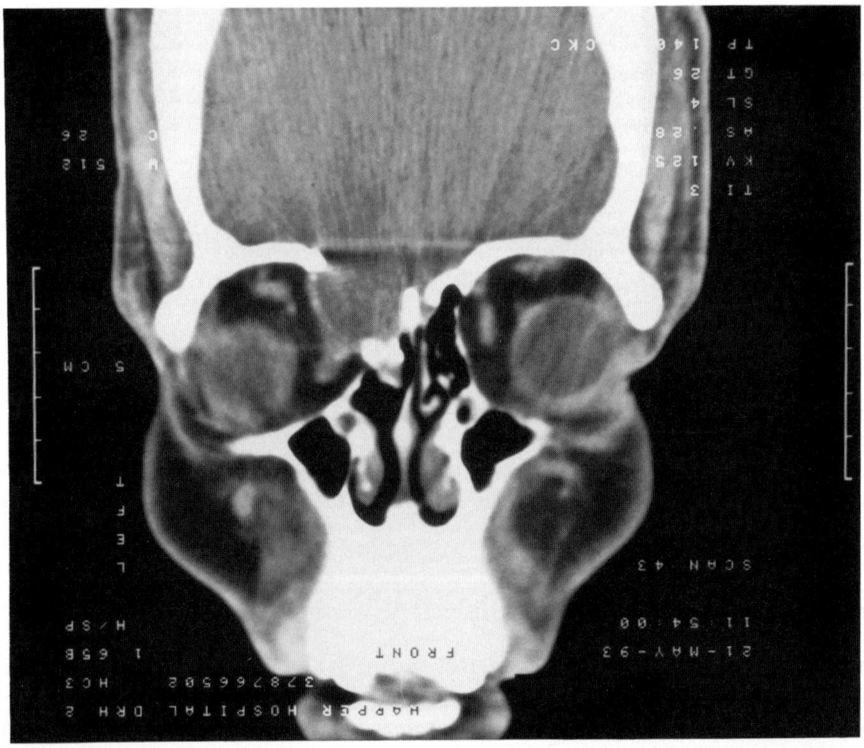

Figure 7–5. Ethmoid sinus mucocele before endoscopic drainage.

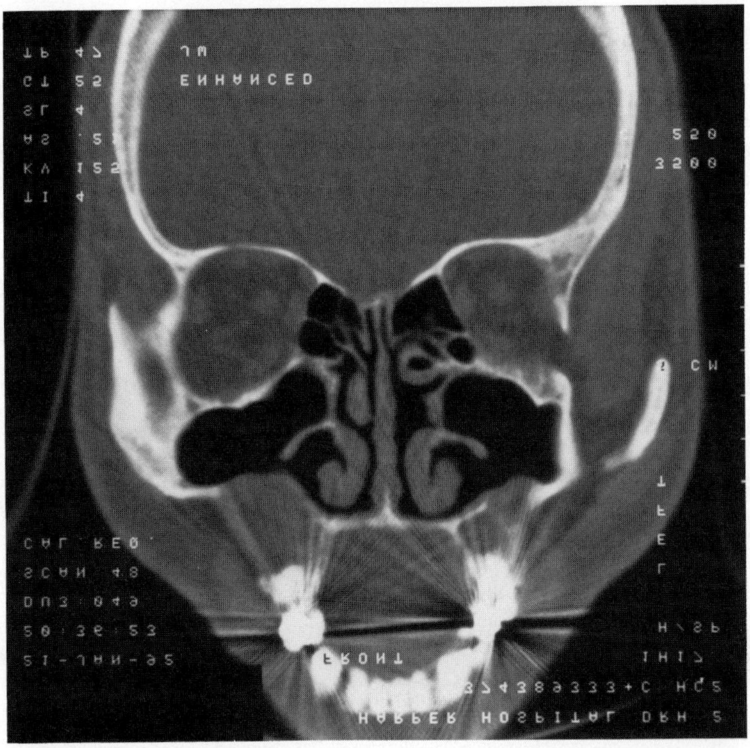

Figure 7–6. Maxillary sinus mucocele extending into the face before resection by the Caldwell-Luc procedure.

intranasal approaches and have the disadvantages of external incisions and the inability to follow the postoperative course of the patient with intranasal endoscopic examinations. These techniques are primarily advocated by surgeons who lack adequate training in endoscopic sinus surgery.

Ethmoid and sphenoid sinus mucoceles extending through the bony sinus walls into the anterior or the middle cranial fossa create difficult management decisions. Removal usually requires a craniotomy with significant brain retraction and an increased risk of serious neurological morbidity and mortality. Intranasal drainage is also an alternative in these cases. We have managed two such patients recently. The first patient was a 55-year-old woman, 10 years after a frontoparietal approach for a pituitary adenoma. She had a large sphenoid sinus mucocele with extension into the middle cranial fossa (Fig. 7–4). The second patient was a 25-year-old man 6 years after a gunshot wound to the head. He had a large ethmoid sinus mucocele with extension into the orbit and the anterior cranial fossa (Fig. 7–5). Both patients were managed with endoscopic drainage of the mucoceles. The patients have not developed any complications and are doing well 2 years and 6 months, respectively, after surgery.

MAXILLARY SINUS MUCOCELES

These entities are rare and more commonly associated with trauma or previous sinus surgery. Endoscopic management with a large middle meatus antrostomy has proven successful in the management of mucoceles limited to the sinus cavity. Alternatively, a Caldwell-Luc with mucocele resection and inferior nasal antral window for drainage would be equally successful but carries the risk of long-term complications.[46]

For larger mucoceles extending into the orbit, face, or infratemporal fossa, excision using a Caldwell-Luc or a Weber- Ferguson incision is usually necessary. These lesions tend to have recesses that do not usually drain adequately through an endoscopic middle meatus antrostomy (Fig. 7–6).

SUMMARY

Mucoceles are an uncommon but important complication of maxillofacial trauma. They can be successfully managed in most cases by endoscopic drainage through the natural sinus ostia, however, the surgeon must be well versed in all forms of sinus surgery to be able to adequately manage all variations of this important and difficult clinical entity.

REFERENCES

1. Chole RA, Yee J. Antibiotic prophylaxis for facial fractures. *Arch Otolaryngol Head Neck Surg*. 1987;113: 1055–1057.
2. Canalis RF, Zajtchuk JT, Jenkins HA. Ethmoidal mucoceles, *Arch Otolaryngol Head Neck Surg*. 1978;104: 286–291.
3. DeSanto LW, Garrity JA. In: Paparella MM, Shumrick, DA, Meyerhoff, WL, Gluckman JL, eds. Exophthalmos for the Otolaryngologist. *Otolaryngology. Vol. IV*. Philadelphia, Pa: WB Saunders Co; 1991:3057–3083.
4. Close LG, O'Connor WE. Sphenoethmoidal mucoceles with intrcranial extension. *Otolaryngol Head Neck Surg*. 1983;9:350–357.
5. Steinberg CM, Bailey BJ, Calhoun KJ, Quinn FB. Management of invasive frontoethmoidal sinus mucoceles. *Arch Otolaryngol Head Neck Surg*. 1986;112:1060–1063.
6. Kennedy DW, Josephson JS, Zinreich SJ, Mattox DE, Goldsmith MM. Endoscopic sinus surgery for mucoceles: a viable alternative. *Laryngoscope*. 1989;99:885–895.
7. Palubinskas AJ, Davies H. Roentgen features of nasal accessory sinus mucoceles. *Radiology*. 1959;72:576–584.
8. Schenck NL, Rauchback E, Ogura JH. Frontal sinus disease: II. Development of the frontal sinus model: occlusion of the nasofrontal duct. *Laryngoscope*. 1974;84:1233–1247.
9. Som PM, Shugar JMA. Antral mucoceles: a new look. *J Comput Assist Tomogr*. 1980;4:484–488.
10. Weber AL. Inflammatory diseases of the paranasal sinuses and mucoceles. *Otolaryngol Clin North Am*. 1988;21:421–437.
11. Hawegawa M, Saito Y, Weinake I, Kern EB. Postoperative mucoceles of the maxillary sinuses. *Rhinology*. 1979;17:253–256.
12. Kaneshiro S, Nakajima T, Yoshikawa Y, Iwasari H, Tokiwa N. The postoperative maxillary cyst: report of 71 cases. *J Oral Surg* 1958;16:251–253.
13. Bordley JE, Bosley WR. Mucoceles of the frontal sinus: causes and treatment. *Ann Otol Rhinol Laryngol*. 1973;82:696–702.
14. DeWilde R, Fossion E, Raas P, Ostyn F. Mucoceles of the paranasal sinuses. *Acta Stomatol Belg*. 1984;81:91–106.
15. Mortada A. Pulsating frontocele and exophthalmos. *Am J Ophthalmol*. 1968;65:425–427.
16. Natvig K, Larsen TE. Mucoceles of the paranasal sinus. *J Laryngol Otol*. 1982;92:1075–1082.
17. Van Alyea OE. *Nasal sinuses: An Anatomic and Clinical Consideration*. 2nd ed. Baltimore, Md: Williams & Wilkins Co; 1951.
18. Wolfowitz BL, SolomanA. Mucoceles of the frontal and ethmoid sinuses. *J Laryngol Otol*. 1972;86:79–82.
19. Zizmour J, Noyek AM. Cysts and benign tumours of the paranasal sinuses. *Semin Roentgenol*. 1968;3:172–185.
20. Evans C. Aetiology and treatment of fronto-ethmoidal mucocele. *J Laryngol Otol*. 1981;95:361–375.

21. Rothberg R, Goldfinger M, Noyek AM, Wortzman G. Diagnostic Imaging of the Head and Neck. Paparella MM, Schumrick DA, Gluckman JL, Meyerhoff WL, eds. *Otolaryngology*. Vol. IV. Philadelphia, Pa: WB Saunders Co; 1991:3103–3160.
22. Diaz F, Latchow R, Duvall AJ, Quick CA, Erickson DL. Mucoceles with intracranial and extracranial extension: report of two cases. *J Neurosurg*. 1978;48:443–451.
23. Gore RM, Weinberg PE, Kim KS, Ramsey RG. Sphenoid sinus mucoceles presenting as intracranial masses on computed tomography. *Surg Neurol*. 1980;13:375–379.
24. Green DC, Calcaterra TC. Sphenoethmoid sinus mucocele presenting with amenorrhea and galactorrhea. *Otolaryngol Head Neck Surg*. 1991;104:856–857.
25. Hukuba A, Katsuyama J, Matsuoka V, Shim JH, Nishimura S. Sphenoid sinus mucocele: report of two cases. *J Neurosurg*. 1975;43:368–373.
26. Nugent GR, Sprinkle P, Bloor BM. Sphenoid sinus mucoceles. *J Neurosug*. 1970;32:443–451.
27. Roberson GH, Price AK, Deeb ME, et al. Sphenoethmoidal mucoceles: radiographic diagnosis. *AJR*. 1976;127:595–599.
28. Simms NM, Brown WE, French LA. Mucocele of the sphenoid sinus presenting as an intrasellar mass: case report. *J Neurosurg*. 1979;32:708–710.
29. Turner AL. Mucocele of the accessory nasal sinuses. Edinburgh Med J. 1907;64:369–410.
30. Howarth WG. Mucocele of the frontal sinus caused by a large osteoma. *J Laryngol Otol*. 1924;39:265–267.
31. Linthicum FH, Rand CW, Reeves DL. Mucocele of the sphenoid sinus: report of case with autopsy findings. *J Neurosurg*. 1946;3:444–453.
32. Hesselink JR, Weber AL, New PF, et al. Evaluation of mucoceles of the paranasal sinuses with computed tomography. *Radiology*. 1979;133:397–400.
33. Som PM. Sinonasal cavity. In: Som PM, Bergeron RT, eds. *Head and Neck Imaging*. 2nd ed. St Louis, Mo: CV Mosby; 1991:114–168.
34. Lanzieri CF, Shah M, Krass D, Lavertu P. Use of gadolinium enhanced MR imaging for differentiating mucoceles from neoplasms in the paranasal sinuses. *Radiology*. 1991;178:425–428.
35. Zizmor J, Noyek AM, Chapnik JS. Mucocele of the paranasal sinuses. *Can J Otolaryngol*. 1974;3(suppl 1): 1.
36. Stankiewicz JA. Sphenoid sinus mucocele. *Arch Otolaryngol Head Neck Surg*. 1989;115:735–740.
37. Kennedy DW, Zinreich SJ, Rosenbaum AE, Johns ME. Functional endoscopic sinus surgery: theory and diagnostic evaluation. *Arch Otolaryngol Head Neck Surg*. 1985;111:576–582.
38. Kennedy DW. Functional endoscopic sinus surgery: technique *Arch Otolaryngol Head Neck Surg*. 1985;94: 643–649.
39. Stammberger H. Endoscopic endonasal surgery-concepts in treatment of recurring rhinosinusitis. Part II. Surgical technique. *Otolaryngol Head Neck Surg*. 1986;94:142–156.
40. Lillie HI, Williams HL. The external frontoethmo-sphenoid operation: a critical review of the literature and details of the technique in use at the mayo clinic. *Minn Med*. 1935;18:786–789.
41. Rubin JS, Lund VJ, Salmon B. Frontoethmoidectomy in the treatment of mucoceles. *Arch Otolaryngol*. 1986;112:434–436.
42. Schenck NL. Frontal sinus disease: III. Experimental and clinical factors in failure of the frontal osteoplastic operation. *Laryngoscope*. 1975;85:76–92.
43. Williams HL, Holman CB. The causes and avoidance of failure in surgery for chronic suppuration of the frontoethmo-sphenoid complex of sinuses: with a previously unreported anomaly which produces chronicity and recurrence, and the description of a surgical technique usually producing a cure of the disease. *Laryngoscope*. 1962;72:1179–1227.
44. Neel HB, McDonald TJ, Facer GW. Modified lynch procedure for chronic frontal sinus diseases: rationale, technique, and long-term results. *Laryngoscope*. 1987;97:1274–1279.
45. Hardy JM, Montgomery WW. Osteoplastic frontal sinusotomy: an analysis of 250 operations. *Ann Otol Rhinol Laryngol*. 1976;85:523–532.
46. DeFreitas J, Lucente FE. The Caldwell-Luc procedure: institutional review of 670 cases: 1975–1985. *Laryngoscope*. 1988;98:1297–1300.

8

Cosmetic Complications of Sinus Fractures

BEN GOLDWYN, M.D.
RICHARD L. ARDEN, M.D.

Fractures of the paranasal sinuses remain a common occurrence. Whether these are from a motor vehicle accident, interpersonal altercation, or from penetrating trauma, the end result may be a functional or cosmetic deformity or a combination of both. The first priority in fracture management is to stabilize and evaluate the patient for potential life-threatening injuries. The next priority is to reduce and stabilize fractures after clinical and radiological evaluation. Only after these details have been attended to can attention be turned to the cosmetic defects. The overall surface topography of the face is the result of the interaction between the facial skeleton and the overlying soft tissue structures. Interruption of either the skeletal or soft tissue components resulting from trauma to the paranasal sinuses can lead to the perception of facial disharmony or cosmetic defect. It is hoped that by restoring adequate function acceptable cosmesis will follow; unfortunately, this is not always possible at the time of acute injury.

The type of cosmetic deformities commonly associated with trauma is dependent on the site and mechanism of injury. Also important are the actual surgical reduction and fixation of the fracture(s). Occasionally, if the fracture reduction is good, there still may be cosmetically unsatisfactory soft tissue defects. Large conspicuous scars from the trauma itself, or from the skin incision related to the surgical approach, may be aesthetically unappealing. The trauma may interfere with important facial landmarks such as that seen in traumatic telecanthus. Even after adequate occlusion has been restored in a complex maxillary fracture there can remain a defect in the facial profile. Despite seemingly adequate reduction there may be malunion or non union resulting in a facial contour defect. Less than optimal results follow when conditions preclude definitive intervention, or when there is unrecognized injury, misdiagnosis, or unsuccessful initial management. Clearly, the most important point in the treatment of cosmetic deformities is their prevention. Careful diagnosis and treatment planning in the acute or semiacute situation may avert future deformity.

SOFT TISSUE INJURIES

Injuries to the soft tissues often accompany paranasal sinus fractures. Unfortunately for the patient, contour deformities and scars on the face and neck often remain conspicuous and may be a source of focused attention in normal interpersonal relations. The scars associated with paranasal sinus fractures can be divided into three groups: (1) scars that are the result of laceration which accompany the trauma; (2) scars that are the result of soft tissue loss related to the traumatic event; and (3) iatrogenic scars resulting from the surgical repair of the original fracture. Whatever the cause, these soft tissue lesions can be a difficult problem to correct secondarily. Consequently, facial surgeons should be prepared not only to repair the original fracture and associated soft tissue injury but they should be knowledgeable in the techniques of scar revision to make these scars less conspicuous.

Proper closure of wounds at the time of acute injury may obviate the need for future revision. When the dermis is violated it heals by forming a scar. There are many factors that influence this healing process such as timing of the wound repair and location of the injury. The optimum time for repair is within the first 8 hours after initial injury. Delay of more than 24 hours usually means that the wound will heal by secondary intent, or delayed primary closure, dependent on the patient's condition, location of the wound, and other factors. If the wound is the result of blunt trauma, the underlying edema and inflammatory reaction can have a negative impact on wound healing and lead to a potentially unfavorable result. An unfavorable scar can also be expected when a laceration crosses the mandible or involves the lower half of the nose.

The most significant factors relate to wound location and orientation relative to the relaxed skin tension lines (RSTLs). The closer a laceration is to being parallel to these favorable lines (Fig. 8–1), the more favorable the prognosis is for less conspicuous scarring.[1] By lying in the RSTL, and therefore at right angles to the lines of maximum extensibility (LME), closure tension is minimized. Tension provides a fibroblastic stimulus favoring widening and hypertrophy. Unfortunately, traumatic lacerations often do not orient themselves in the RSTLs, typically necessitating a need for secondary revision to optimize scar camouflage. In general, the goals of primary closure should not be focused on reorientation of the closure line but rather on creation of an environment that favors wound-healing conditions and minimizes tissue loss. Atraumatic handling of the tissue, meticulous hemostasis, aseptic technique, and careful closure of dead space are all critically important factors.

PRIMARY CLOSURE

The facial skin is a well-vascularized structure. An attempt should therefore be made to save all facial skin whenever possible for primary repair as it is likely to survive. This makes extensive debridement of tissues unnecessary and lessens the likelihood of tissue distortion. The wound should be well cleansed by copious irrigation and closely inspected for foreign objects. Blood and debris should be carefully removed. Automobile glass, teeth, grease, tar, asphalt, and gunpowder may all be found. Meticulous attention should be paid to removing these as they may cause permanent skin tattooing. These can be removed by scrubbing with a small toothbrush. In case of extensive soft tissue infiltration with glass or other more particulate matter, it may be necessary to use a small curette.

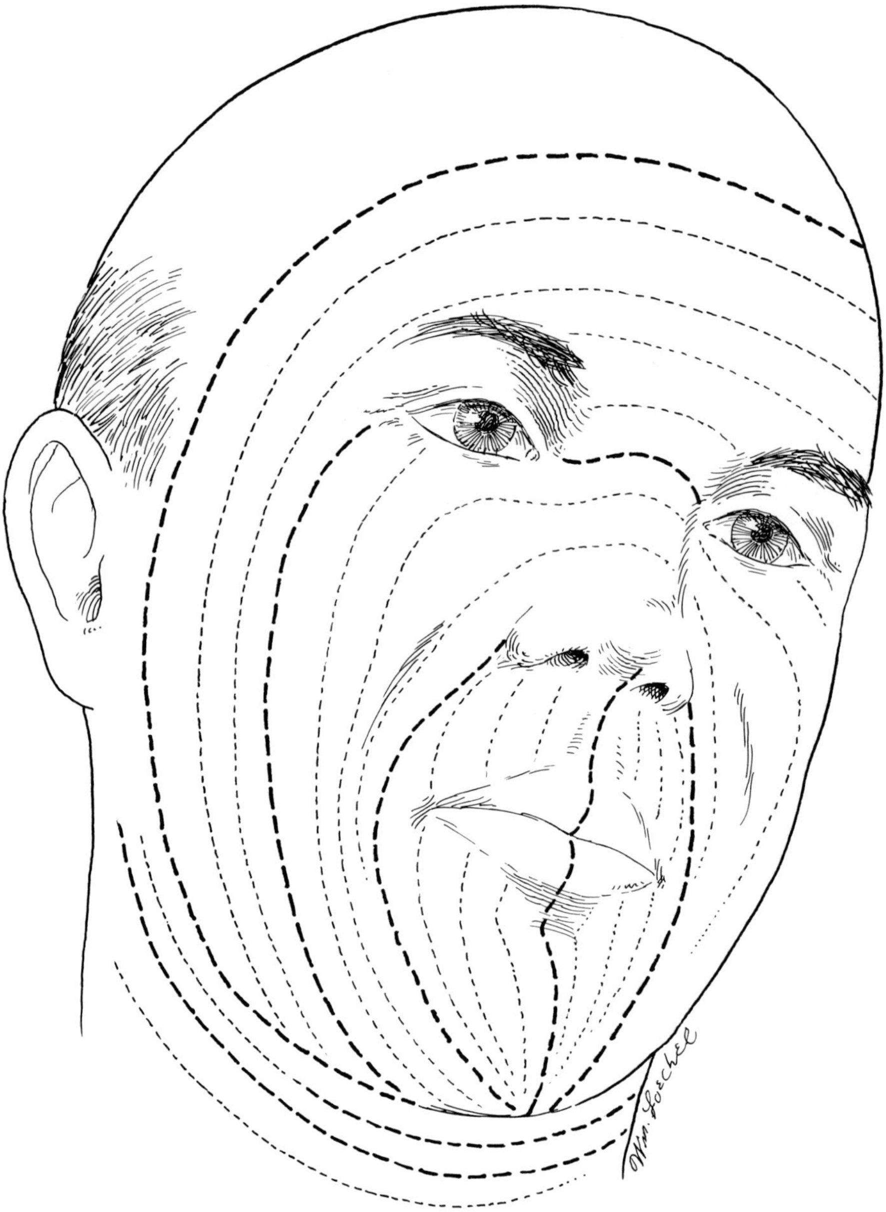

Figure 8–1. Relaxed skin tension lines (RSTLs) of the face.

After the wound has been cleansed and anesthetized, a mild antiseptic paint such as povidone-iodine (Betadine) can be utilized. Most wounds lend themselves to primary closure in two layers as previously described. However, when there is significant contusion associated with the trauma, and the wound margins are irregular, it may be best to conservatively excise these and convert the wound margins to straight surgical lines that will heal less conspicuously. Large stellate or irregular lacerations should be repaired primarily. These scars will contract and may be revised at a later time. Avulsion injuries, or soft tissue loss from penetrating trauma, can be handled in a number of ways. The wound may be left open to granulate and heal by secondary intent if it is believed that the wound is contaminated and there is significant risk of infection. Alternately, if the wound cannot be closed primarily without tension, a local flap may be advanced or rotated for coverage. Split-thickness skin grafts should ideally be avoided in the face as they do not provide optimal aesthetic results, except in secondary repair of eyelid trauma and ectropion.

There are certain areas of the face that are functionally as well as aesthetically important. Areas of the face associated with sinus fractures are the forehead, nasoethmoid area, and maxilla. The eyelids and nasal ala are particular areas where methodical closure at the time of injury will often obviate the need for future procedures.

In eyelid lacerations the first priority is the status of vision. Only after the globe has been cleared by the ophthalmologist and the wound carefully inspected for foreign bodies can closure begin. Horizontal superficial lacerations paralleling the eyelid margin can be closed in a single layer with 6-0 monofilament suture. Full-thickness lacerations should be closed in two layers, with the appropriate underlying structures such as the levator and orbicularis oculi muscles aligned to ensure adequate function of the lid apparatus. An absorbable 3-0 or 4-0 suture deep and a 5-0 or 6-0 cutaneous suture are typically used in closure.[2]

Vertical lacerations present a more difficult management problem. The eyelid margin needs to be carefully approximated or notching can occur. First, the wound edges should be carefully and conservatively debrided to provide linear closure. Next, the eyelid margins are approximated by utilizing a 6-0 silk suture passed through the orifice of the meibomian gland on one side of the laceration and brought through the gland orifice on the other side (gray line). The margin must be absolutely aligned at this point. A similar suture is then placed posteriorly but far enough away from the conjunctiva that the suture will not abrade the cornea. Before tying these sutures a 5-0 polyglactin 910 (Vicryl) may be used to close the tarsal layer if necessary. These sutures are then tied and left long. A third anterior marginal suture is then placed. These long strands are then tied together to minimize contact with the cornea. The remainder of the laceration is closed as a single layer with 6-0 monofilament including the orbicularis muscle in the closure.[2] Defects with loss of up to 25% of the eyelid margin can be closed primarily.[3] Defects larger than this will need flap repair and will be covered in the section on flap reconstruction.

The nasal ala presents another area where there is a potential for cosmetic and functional deformity. Lacerations involving the nasal rim, if not reapproximated adequately, may notch or even stenose. Again, aggressive debridement is to be avoided, but trimming the wound margins to obtain a straight, more "surgical" scar may lead to a better result. In through and through lacerations the closure is started deep through the wound. The nasal vestibular skin is closed with an absorbable suture. Next, the nasal rim is carefully lined up and approximated with a 6-0 monofilament suture. Torn cartilage can be seen through the wound and reapproximated by reduction into anatomic alignment. Closure of the perichondrium is usually sufficient to hold it into place. This stitch can be accomplished with a 6-0 monofilament suture encompassing the skin. Subcutaneous sutures are often unnecessary.[4] Stenosis can be further minimized by intranasal placement of a soft sponge or Silastic roll to stent the nostril open.

CONCEPTS IN SCAR REVISION

Facial trauma often results in scars that are not aesthetically pleasing to the patient, despite the best efforts on the part of the operating surgeon. Unfortunately, the scar cannot be removed. The goal in scar revision, therefore, is to adequately camouflage the scar to deceive the observer's eye into not seeing it. This is a realistic goal and the patient needs to know that the scar will still always be there.

The timing of scar revision is controversial. The standard teaching has been to let the scar mature for 6 to 12 months before attempting revision. However, several authors, notably Borges,[5] advocate revision as early as 2 months postinjury. This is especially true of scars that are uneven and lie perpendicular to the RSTL. Thomas and Ehlert[6] state that if it is possible to tell that a scar will not diminish with maturation there is no compelling reason to wait. Borges[5] believes that the patient who has scar revision after the scar has matured is not as happy with the result because the change is not as obvious.

The type of scar revision will depend on the scar itself and its location. The scar direction with respect to the RSTL, the width of the scar, its levelness (depression/hypertrophy), the length of the scar, its shape, pigment qualities, and relationship to anatomic landmarks all must be factored into the equation before undertaking a revision.

Objectives

The goal of scar revision is to make the scar as inconspicuous as possible. To do this, the ideal scar needs to be defined. An ideal scar should be flat and level, of good color match with the surrounding skin, narrow, and follow the RSTLs. Optimally, it should also be without straight unbroken lines that may be easily followed by the eye. Not all of these tenets of the ideal scar can always be met. Scar revision should be undertaken with specific goals in the surgeon's and patient's mind, and this should ultimately determine the type of revision procedure that is chosen. Techniques may be broken down into those of excision, irregularization, abrasion, and flap repair. It is not the purpose of this chapter to detail a complete methodology of scar revision techniques. What follows is a select list of techniques that are useful adjuncts to the armamentarium of the surgeon who treats fractures that involve the paranasal sinuses.

Fusiform Excision

Scars that lay parallel to the RSTLs and are less than 2 cm in length are ideal candidates for fusiform excision.[1] This is a simple technique that is perhaps the oldest and most common type of scar revision undertaken. The wound is marked and an ellipse drawn around it. This is done so that the opposed angles of the ends of the ellipse are less than 30°. Angles greater than 30° can result in dog ears at the closure margins. This can be overcome by incorporating Burrows triangles to correct this problem after the wound is closed. Another method for correcting this problem, if the angle is greater than 30° but less than 60°, is the use of the M-plasty. This minimizes the sacrifice of normal tissue otherwise required for an elliptic excision, but creates a nonlinear closure with two divergent limbs at each end.

Serial Partial Excision

Large lesions, or those in which surrounding skin needed for closure is relatively inelastic and poorly mobile, may not be able to be closed without gross distortion of normal anatomic landmarks. These types of scars may be revised by serial partial excision.[7] This technique entails partial excision of the scar with reapproximation of the normal tissue to the remaining scar. This is usually done from the center, and not the margins of the scar, so as not to necessitate repeated excisions of normal bordering skin. After a number of procedures the entire scar can usually be totally excised. This is done after wide undermining to facilitate advancement of the normal skin. The number of times this procedure needs to be performed is a function of the elasticity and redundancy of the patient's skin. Diminishing returns with successive attempts is the general rule, such that a plateau response is often reached following two or three excision cycles.

A useful adjunct to this procedure is tissue expansion. Conventional tissue expansion involves strategic placement of a subcutaneous prefabricated balloon-injection port system that is slowly expanded with saline over a period of time, typically one to two times per week over 4 to 6 weeks. This expands the overlying soft tissues, providing additional tissue for repair and obviating the need for serial excisions. Although tissue expansion works well in the forehead, it is associated with a high number of complications in the cheek area, most notably extrusion.[8] Rapid intraoperative tissue expansion, although not a true tissue expansion, does facilitate tissue mobilization to assist in closure after sequential cyclic loading in one operative procedure.[9] This technique is probably best applied over bony prominences such as the frontal and zygomatic regions. Caution must be exercised with either of these procedures to not expand the scar tissue itself.

REPOSITIONING TECHNIQUES

Horner[10] first described Z-plasty for release of ectropion in 1837 and it is still used for that procedure today. Z-plasty is a transposition flap in which two triangles are transposed about two pivot points. This procedure can be utilized for scar lengthening, changing the direction of a scar, releasing a scar, irregularization of existing scar lines, and shifting anatomic areas. Also, Z-plasty is the most powerful leveling technique in scar revision. The classic Z-plasty is designed with a central member and two parallel limbs, all equal in length (Fig. 8–2). Traditionally, the angles of the limbs with respect to the central portion are 60°; however Z-plasty can have angles designed from 30 to 90°. Angles less than 30° may contribute to compromised blood supply and tip necrosis whereas angles greater than 60° may lead to undesirable dog ear formation on closure. Therefore, angles of 30 to 60° are most commonly used. The angle of the Z-plasty will determine the amount of scar lengthening that will take place. An angle of 30° will theoretically increase scar length by 25%, 45° will increase it by 50%, and a 60° angle will lengthen the scar by 75%. Actual gain may be more owing to the elasticity of the skin. After rotation of the triangles this increase in length is seen along the direction of the original central member. This has the added benefit of distributing the forces that lead to wound contracture in several directions. The final direction of the central limb will be in the direction of a line connecting the ends of the two arms. Owing to the length of curvature of the scar, it is often necessary to utilize

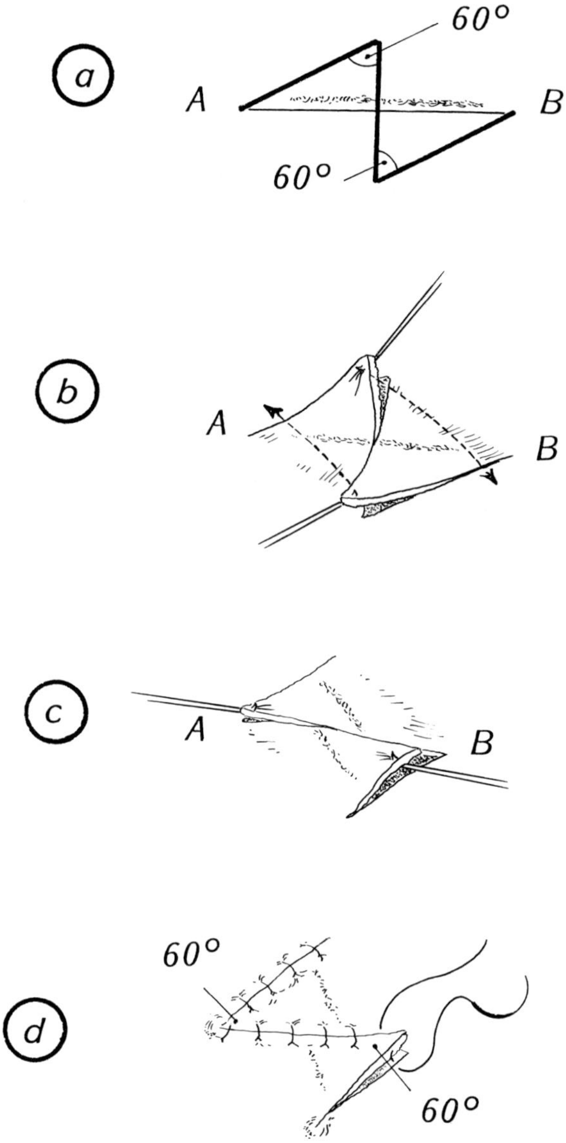

Figure 8–2. Classic Z-plasty. (a). Z- plasty outlined with 60° angles around central member. (b,c). Flaps are undermined and transposed. (d). Flaps are sutured, resulting in change in direction of scar as well as scar lengthening.

multiple Z-plasties. This enables a long scar to be broken up into multiple smaller scars, with some of the limbs in the RSTLs. Z-plasties are also useful in the revision of small flaps that have a pin-cushioned appearance such as the trap-door deformity. The placement of multiple Z-plasties allows the smaller triangles to interdigitate permitting the scar to lay down better. It should be noted that although Z-plasty is a technique that can fulfill many roles, it should not be used in situations where the anatomic area cannot tolerate the elongation or tension vectors. To its advantage, no additional tissue loss is imposed through its use.[11]

Scars over 2 cm long and not parallel to the RSTLs are easily noticed. W-plasty[5,12] is the simplest of the irregularization techniques for antitension line (ATL) scars and is more correctly called a running W-plasty because a single W formation is never utilized. W-plasty is often used with scars oriented greater than 35° from the RSTL. When a scar is greater than 2 cm, a Z-plasty revision will create a large scar with large amounts of tissue transposition. Multiple smaller Z-plasties have the disadvantage of giving rise to depressions and ridges making the scar more visible, which does not occur with W-plasty. Because the W-plasty is a form of advancement flap, dog ears are eliminated. Additionally, it tends to eliminate bowstringing on the wound as the scar heals and contracts. In contrast to Z-plasty, there is no gain in scar length, but excision of some normal tissue is inherent in its design. Also, W-plasty entails actual excision and advancement, not just transposition of tissue.

The W-plasty (Fig. 8–3) is constructed with the angles in the small flaps of 55 to 60°. The length of the triangles should be between 5 and 7 mm depending on the size and location of the scar. Longer segments will excise to much normal skin and tend to place more tension on the incision. The base of the triangle at the ends of the incision should be oriented at 90° to the scar to minimize dog ears at the ends. Incisions should be perpendicular to the skin surface and can easily be made with a no. 11 blade. The wound should be extensively undermined for several centimeters to decrease closing tension. The wound is then closed in layers, first with several loose horizontal mattress sutures to aid in bringing the skin edges together. Next, an absorbable suture can be placed intradermally to eliminate dead space and relieve tension. The wound margins are then approximated with interrupted monofilament 6-0 sutures.

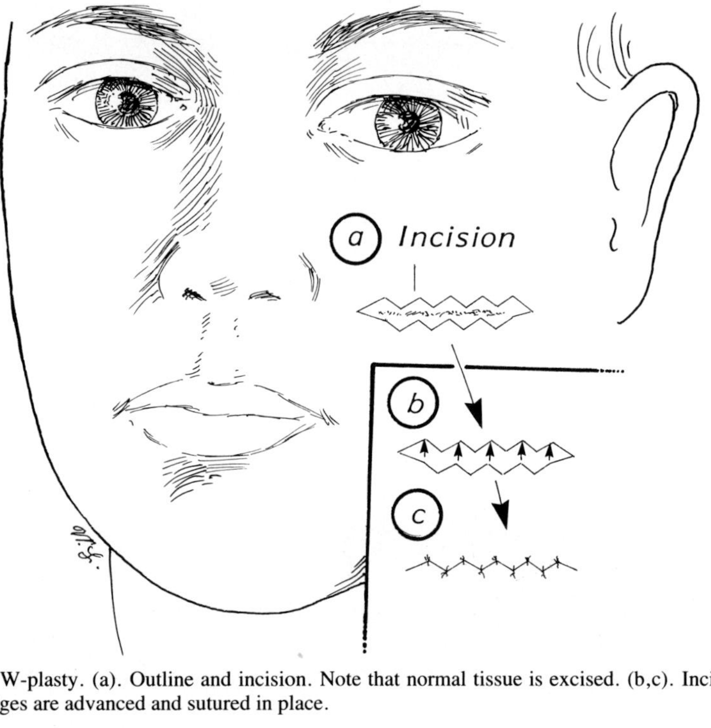

Figure 8–3. W-plasty. (a). Outline and incision. Note that normal tissue is excised. (b,c). Incision is undermined, skin edges are advanced and sutured in place.

There are several modifications of the W-plasty worth noting. The angles of the flaps can be adjusted when the incline of the scar is between 35 to 60°. As the angle of inclination of the scar decreases, the angles of the W-plasty should be increased so that they more closely run in the RSTL. When the inclination is 50°, the angles of the flaps need to be increased to 70°. From 35 to 45°, the angles need to be opened up to 90°. W-plasty is not indicated in revision of long straight scars. Although this technique does result in the irregularization of the scar, this is a regularly irregular result that can be picked up by the eye after a certain point. Borges[5] states that W-plasty is best used on the forehead, eyebrows, temples, cheeks, and chin. The inner aspect of the face (ie, the eyelids, nose, nasolabial folds, and lips) is better revised with Z-plasty.

Geometric Broken Line Closure

As the W-plasty increases in length it becomes more perceptible to the eye. The geometric broken line closure (GBLC) overcomes this problem. Although still a form of scar irregularization, this technique is somewhat more sophisticated than W-plasty. The GBLC (Fig. 8–4) changes the configuration of the scar by first excising the scar and then creating interposition flaps that are a series of irregular random geometric shapes. These shapes include triangles, rectangles, squares, and half circles that are excised and interposed with their mirror image on the opposite side of the scar margin. This procedure is generally

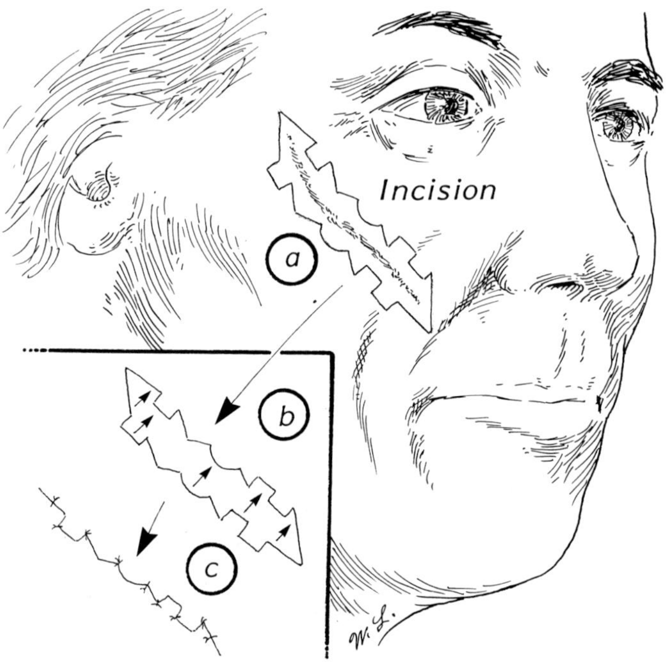

Figure 8–4. Geometric broken line closure. (a). A variety of geometric shapes are used when the incision is planned. (b). Undermining and advancement of flaps. Great care is exercised when handling these small flaps as their viability can be compromised easily. (c). The wound is sutured resulting in an irregular scar.

more time-consuming, technically more difficult, but results in improved scar camouflage by breaking up the linear scar into smaller, less predictable, randomly placed scars closer to the RSTL.

The procedure is initiated by delineating the scar with a fusiform outline. Lines are then drawn across the scar and parallel to the RSTL, spaced approximately 2 to 6 mm apart. The longest segment of these "mini" flaps should not exceed 6 mm and these should preferably be placed in the center. Webster et al[12] advocates the addition of smaller 1 to 2 mm zigzags at the end of the flaps to further aid in camouflage. Once the scar and flaps are outlined, a no. 11 blade is used to incise the skin at right angles and the scar and the outlined components are taken out en toto. The scar should be excised back to normal tissue. If the underlying scar is not tethering the skin, then some may remain behind as bulk if needed. The wound is then undermined and closed in layers. Interrupted intradermal 4-0 or 5-0 sutures are used to bring the margins into approximation. Caution should be used in closure as these flaps are tiny and unnecessary or indiscreet handling of the flap margins can affect their viability. The skin edges are then approximated with a 6-0 suture. Some authors use 6-0 monofilament whereas others prefer to use a 6-0 fast absorbing gut suture. This suture dissolves quickly so that suture removal is not necessary and further manipulation of the flaps can be avoided. This skin closure is actually treated as two suture lines because of the complicated nature of the new scar. The suture is passed on one side in a loose running interlocking fashion catching all the flap tips with small 1-mm bites. The other side of the wound margin is then closed in a similar fashion. The wound is then overlaid with steri-strips for added protection and support.

Scar Leveling Using Injectables

Physicians have long sought an injectable filler that could raise a superficial skin deformity without surgery. Many substances have been tried, often with spectacular success initially, followed by adverse side effects in the long run. The perfect injectable implant still does not exist but several good alternatives are available.

Fat that has been harvested during liposuction has been injected locally on the face to improve soft tissue deformities.[13] This procedure has several theoretical advantages in that donor material is virtually limitless and there is minimal morbidity to both donor and recipient sites. However, success has been mixed at best, with many noting a marked but incomplete resorption in 3 to 6 months.[14]

Silicone has been used in an injectable microdroplet form to augment soft tissue, however, initial enthusiasm has been tempered secondary to problems with availability, potential for autoimmune responses, and soft tissue irregularities. At this time, silicone is not approved by the Federal Drug Administration (FDA) for soft tissue augmentation, and it is illegal to transport across state lines for this purpose.[15]

Bovine collagen, listed by the FDA as a device and not a drug, has become the most widely used injectable filler for soft tissue augmentation.[14] It is available in three forms: (1) Zyderm I is 3.5% collagen and appears to be rapidly broken down by tissue collagenases; (2) Zyderm II is 6.5% collagen and appears to last longer than Zyderm I; however, it is ultimately resorbed; and (3) Zyplast is injectable collagen that is cross-linked with glutaraldehyde to provide longer-term stability, although it too disappears with time. All come with 0.3% lidocaine for anesthesia and are easily injectable through a 30-gauge needle.

Zyplast I and II are injected at the level of the lower papillary dermis so as to raise a skin wheal. Zyplast needs to be implanted deeper at the junction of the dermis and subcutaneous tissue. When placed too superficially, Zyplast can cause visible beading that can take months to resolve. Injectable collagen is not without its drawbacks also. There is a 1 to 2% chance of local or systemic hypersensitivity, therefore, any patient in whom collagen implantation is contemplated needs to be injected with a small test dose 1 month before the beginning of the therapy. Regardless of the material utilized, optimal correction rarely lasts longer than 6 to 9 months.[15] Patients need to be made aware of the need for repeated injections until the desired effect is reached. For improvement in scar profile, the correction is optimally undertaken at 2 to 3 months postevent (surgery or trauma), although good results can be obtained in older more mature scars over a longer period of time.[16] Both Zyderm I and Zyplast are efficacious in these cases. Some authors do not use Zyderm II[17,18] as it is more difficult to use.

Fibrel is a recently introduced gelatin matrix implant that incorporates porcine collagen, epsilon aminocaproic acid, and the patient's own serum before implantation. This combination of ingredients is thought to simulate the normal wound healing process, with the ultimate deposition of the patient's own collagen. In a large series using this implant, more than half the scars corrected had maintained at least moderate to better correction over 5 years.[19] The apparent advantages include longer duration of correction and fewer treatments than injectable collagen.

Dermabrasion

Dermabrasion is a useful adjunct to surgical scar revision. Although dermabrasion does not remove scars per se, it is a mechanical abrasive process that removes superficial epidermis and dermis, which can smooth contour irregularities.[20] By "blending" the scarred area with the surrounding skin, overall appearance is enhanced. Patient selection is important. Although people with dark pigmented skin can be dermabraded, there is a significant chance of hypopigmented areas particularly if the dermabrasion is carried too deeply. Thick oily sebaceous skin predisposes the patient to increased risk for hypertrophic scar formation. The ideal patient is fair haired with light skin. Patients that are pregnant or taking birth control pills are also at higher risk for permanent pigmentary changes.

Before dermabrasion the skin may be painted with gentian violet, which provides a dual advantage. It serves as an antiseptic and it also aids in delineation of the skin topography. The procedure is usually performed under local anesthesia that is supplemented with intravenous sedation. Regional anesthesia, blocking the cutaneous sensory nerves, is preferable to local infiltration of the skin because this can distort the anatomy and tissue planes. Further anesthesia is obtained by application of a topical skin refrigerant. This not only aids in anesthesia but it keeps the skin in a temporary rigid state that facilitates planing of the skin. Segments of the skin between 2.5 and 7.5 cm^2 are typically frozen and planed one at a time. Larger areas may thaw before they can be planed. Dermabrasion can be accomplished with either of two types of wheels. The diamond wheel or the wire brush both come in a variety of sizes. The diamond wheel comes as regular or coarse, with the coarse usually preferred. It is more forgiving as it abrades slower. The wire brush cuts deeper and faster and carries a higher risk of catching the skin. The dermabrader should be applied at right angles to the direction of wheel rotation. The papillary dermis is then abraded. Once pinpoint bleeding is seen, this signifies the reticular dermis. If continued downward, fat will appear indicating that the reticular dermis has been breached. Full-thickness loss of reticular dermis will result in scarring. The ideal plane is at the level of the rete pegs. After the areas have been dermabraded, a topical hemostatic agent may be applied such as thrombin spray or adrenaline-soaked gauze sponges. After adequate hemostasis has been achieved, a nonadherent dressing such as Vigilon (a polyoxide gel) can be applied. Gauze sponges are placed over this and then overwrapped with Kerlix. Alternatively, bacitracin ointment and telfa dressings may also be applied. These dressings are changed after 1 day and removed after 2 days. The patient then showers three times per day and an antibiotic ointment is applied to minimize crusting. This is done for approximately 2 weeks. Direct sun exposure should be avoided for at least 3 months to minimize the risk of hyperpigmentation. Complete sun protection with sunblock and a wide brimmed hat should be utilized after reepithelialization has occurred if outside contact is contemplated.

Keloids and Hypertrophic Scars

Many patients will have excessively large scars despite adequate treatment at the time of acute injury. Certain ethnic groups, such as people of Mediterranean descent, and racial groups such as African-Americans, are prone to exuberant scar formation. The functional differences between keloids and hypertrophic scars are not well appreciated. The etiology of keloids and hypertrophic scarring is not known and it is difficult to predict which patients will get these. By evaluating burn patients with the laser Doppler flowmeter, Ehrlich and Kelley[21] found that healed sites that developed into hypertrophic scars sustained higher blood flows than those that developed into normal scars. Blood flow in these developing scars had an up, down, up pattern, which indicated a disruption in the remodeling phase of wound repair.

Various therapies have evolved including radiation therapy, surgical excision, pressure application, intralesional steroid injections, and topically applied silicone sheeting or gels.[22–25] All are associated with high recurrence rates and/or well-defined morbidities or drawbacks. In a 10-year follow-up study, Darzi et al[22] looked at radiation with and without reoperation, as well as triamcinolone acetonide (Kenalog) injection. Radiation alone was associated with symptomatic relief but did not reduce the size of the lesion. Excision of the scar, followed by radiation (400 cGy twice per week for a total of 16 Gy) in the early postoperative period, was found to give both symptomatic and cosmetic improvement that was significantly better than radiation alone. Injections with triamcinolone acetonide (total 20 to 120 mg, 4 injections spaced every 1 to 2 weeks) gave comparable results to excision and postoperative radiation, however, it was not as well tolerated as the other regimes for larger lesions owing to the frequent number of needle sticks. They recommend triamcinolone acetonide injection for small scars and excision followed by postoperative radiation for larger lesions.

Silicone sheeting or gels are a relatively new treatment for keloids and hypertrophic scarring. Sawada and Sone[23] obtained good results by covering the lesion with a silicone cream. This study was repeated utilizing only the carrier vehicle without the silicone and similar results were obtained.[24] They concluded that the beneficial effects were not secondary to the use of silicone but that the hydration and occlusion caused by their cream was the reason for the improvement. Sproat et al[25] compared triamcinolone acetonide injections with silicone sheeting each applied to different halves of the same scar. Although both techniques resulted in scar improvement, the improvement seen in the silicone-treated side was superior both subjectively and objectively. The mean time to symptomatic improvement in the silicone sheeting side was found to be approximately one half that of the triamcinolone acetonide-treated side.

Loss of Soft Tissue

Occasionally, the surgeon and patient are confronted with the problem of soft tissue loss in the acute situation. Most small defects can be closed primarily. The primary use of advancement, transposition, rotation flaps, and skin grafts should be scrupulously avoided unless needed for cover of a vital structure or adjacent to a mobile structure which, following contraction, would result in functional sequela. Most wounds can be left to heal by secondary intent. These will subsequently contract and will be amenable to revision at a future time.

Although there is a negligible role for flaps in the acute phase, they are of use in scar revision such as when scars are too wide for other revision procedures already detailed. Fusiform excision of a scar with angles of closure greater than 60° will cause a dog ear and may give rise to an unacceptable scar in itself. The patient may not wish to undergo the multiple procedures entailed in serial excision. When this is the case, a local flap reconstruction is indicated. Local flaps provide excellent matching of skin texture and color because neighboring skin is rotated into the defect.

The flap that is most applicable to scar revision techniques and closure of small wound defects is the rhomboid or rhombic flap[26] (Fig. 8–5). First described by Limberg[27] and later revised by Dufourmental[28] the rhombic flap has become widely used because of its simplicity and versatility. This is a form of transposition flap that is designed according to a form of transposition flap that is designed according to precise geometric principles and skin biomechanics. A rhombus is an obliquely angled parallelogram possessing a short axis and a long axis. When classically designed, the flap has two parallel lines that follow the LME, with two other lines drawn to intersect these. This results in opposing angles of 60° and 120°. Next, lines are drawn on either side of the 120° angle as a continuation of the short axis of the rhomboid. These lines are equal in length to the lines of excision already demarcated. Last, a line equal in length and parallel to the rhomboid shape already delineated is outlined. Therefore, four possible flaps can be created. Local anatomy will indicate which version of the flap to use as rotation of tissue may cause some distortion. Also, when designing these flaps, one should strive to place two of the incisions parallel to the RSTLs. The major force of tension is at the closure of the donor site, therefore, the line connecting the far base of the flap and the 120° angle should be placed in the LME. Once outlined, the flap is incised and the rhombic defect excised. The area is undermined and the flap is transposed. It is closed in layers with intradermal and skin sutures.[26,29,30]

The most common variation of Limberg's flap was designed originally by Dufourmental.[28] This alters the angle of the flap itself. Instead of being a continuation of the short axis, the flap is angled away. This is done when designing the flap by creating an angle through extension of a line along the short axis and intersecting it with a line extending from one of the sides. This angle is bisected and extended the same length as one of the sides of the rhomboid. A line is then drawn from the end of this, which is of equal length, and parallel to the long axis of the rhomboid. This variation is more difficult to design but

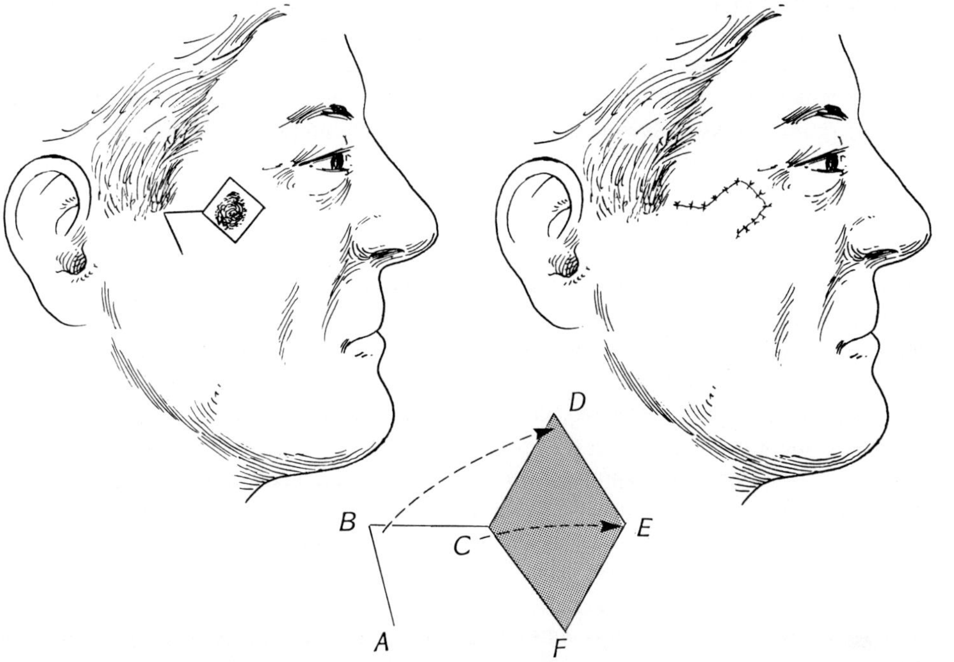

Figure 8–5. Rhombic flap (after Dufourmental).[28] The shaded area (inferior diagram) is to be excised. Dufourmental's variation of Limber's[27] flap offers easier closure and increased blood supply to transposed flap (A–C, F) as base is wider. Complete closure is shown on right.

has the advantages of a widened flap base (to enhance blood supply to the flap), allowance for a smaller donor flap to minimize tissue scarring, and sharing of closure tensions. Both types of rhombic flaps can be combined with an M-plasty to further minimize tissue loss.

Special Areas

Although the previously mentioned techniques work well in most areas of the face, the same areas that posed problems in basic wound management (ie, eyes and nose) are also difficult secondary problems to manage. The eyelids present special problems with tissue loss because protection of the globe and vision is vitally important. Approaches for repair of fractures utilize periorbital or transconjunctional incisions. This may be complicated by ectropion or entropion during healing. Trauma to the naso-orbital area can result in traumatic telecanthus. The nose, positioned as a prominent feature of the face and lying in the central portion of the paranasal sinuses, it frequently fractured in association with sinus injuries. Cosmetic defects may only involve skin, the nasal support alone, or both.

Ectropion

Ectropion is defined as excessive scleral show caused by eversion of the lid margin.[21] Because most posttraumatic ectropion involves the lower lids, this will be the focus of this section. The position of the lower eyelid is the result of a balance of forces: (1) the pulling of the tarsus and canthal ligaments against gravity; (2) support of the eyelid by pretarsal fibers of the orbicularis muscles; and (3) cicatricial forces of the skin, orbital septum, and capsulopalpebral fascia pulling inferiorly.[32] Disruption of these complex vectors may be secondary to lid laceration, postoperative scarring after reduction of an orbital fracture, or from traumatic tissue loss. When ectropion is severe enough it will interfere with the lacrimal drainage system. Epiphora may result when the canaliculus is pulled away from the globe. In the postoperative period, excessive scleral show can be caused by tethering of the lower orbital septum from an imprecise periosteal closure. Mild ectropion can be treated conservatively with periorbital massage up to 6 months postoperatively.[32] If it appears that there is some local inflammation, intralesional steroid injections may be employed. Dosage varies according to author; however, low doses are usually used owing to the risk of blindness following periorbital steroid injection.[33] Failure of the ectropion to resolve with conservative measures, or more severe ectropion, necessitates more aggressive surgical therapy.

Surgical treatment of ectropion is aimed at the specific anatomic cause (ie, lower lid laxity, scarring or adhesions involving the orbital septum, or traumatic tissue loss). Lid laxity is believed to be most commonly the result of lateral tendon laxity,[34] however, this is more of a concern in cosmetic blepharoplasty. Mild lower lid laxity can be corrected with lateral wedge tarsectomy.[32] This is performed through a subciliary incision, elevating a skin flap and preserving the orbicularis muscle. The muscle overlying the portion of tarsus to correct the laxity is sharply removed with iris scissors. The tarsus is closed with 5-0 polyglactin 910 (Vicryl) and the lid margin with 6-0 nylon. The orbicularis muscle is then gently cauterized so that it will contract. The skin is then closed with 6-0 nylon or Prolene.

In the postoperative or posttraumatic setting, lower lid retraction is often due to tethering of the orbital septum or vertical shortening secondary to accidental division or resection of the orbital septum. Hamako and Baylis[35] described a simple procedure for correction of this problem (Fig. 8–6). This is performed through a lateral canthotomy incision, through skin and orbicularis muscle, extending to the posterior aspect of the lateral orbital rim. The inferior limb of the lateral canthal tendon is divided at its insertion into the orbital rim. The skin of the lower eyelid is then undermined. The scar band that causes the retraction is then palpated with scissors and divided adjacent to the orbital rim, extending as far medially as necessary to facilitate adequate mobilization of the lower lid. The lower lid is then placed into its new position, identifying the new lateral canthal angle. The eyelid margin is then excised from the overlap of the eyelid skin, and the conjunctiva is dissected off the posterior aspect of the lateral canthal tendon. The conjunctiva that remains on the upper aspect of the tarsus is deepithelialized. A posteriorly based periosteal flap is then outlined on the lateral orbital rim where placement of the lateral canthal tendon will cause some slight overcorrection of the lower lid. Each arm of a double-armed 4-0 silk suture is then placed through the lateral canthal tendon from anterior to posterior. Each arm of the suture is then passed through the base of the periosteal flap and the sutures are tightened to draw the eyelid into position. Each arm of the suture is then brought upward under the orbicularis muscle to exit the skin at the lateral margin of the eyebrow. The sutures are tied over a bolster. The lateral canthal tendon is further secured to the periosteum with 5-0 polyglycolic acid (Dexon). The skin is then closed loosely.

A more significant problem exists when there is tissue loss.[31] Ectropion due to skin loss will need to be skin grafted. For small defects of the lower lid, full-thickness grafts are

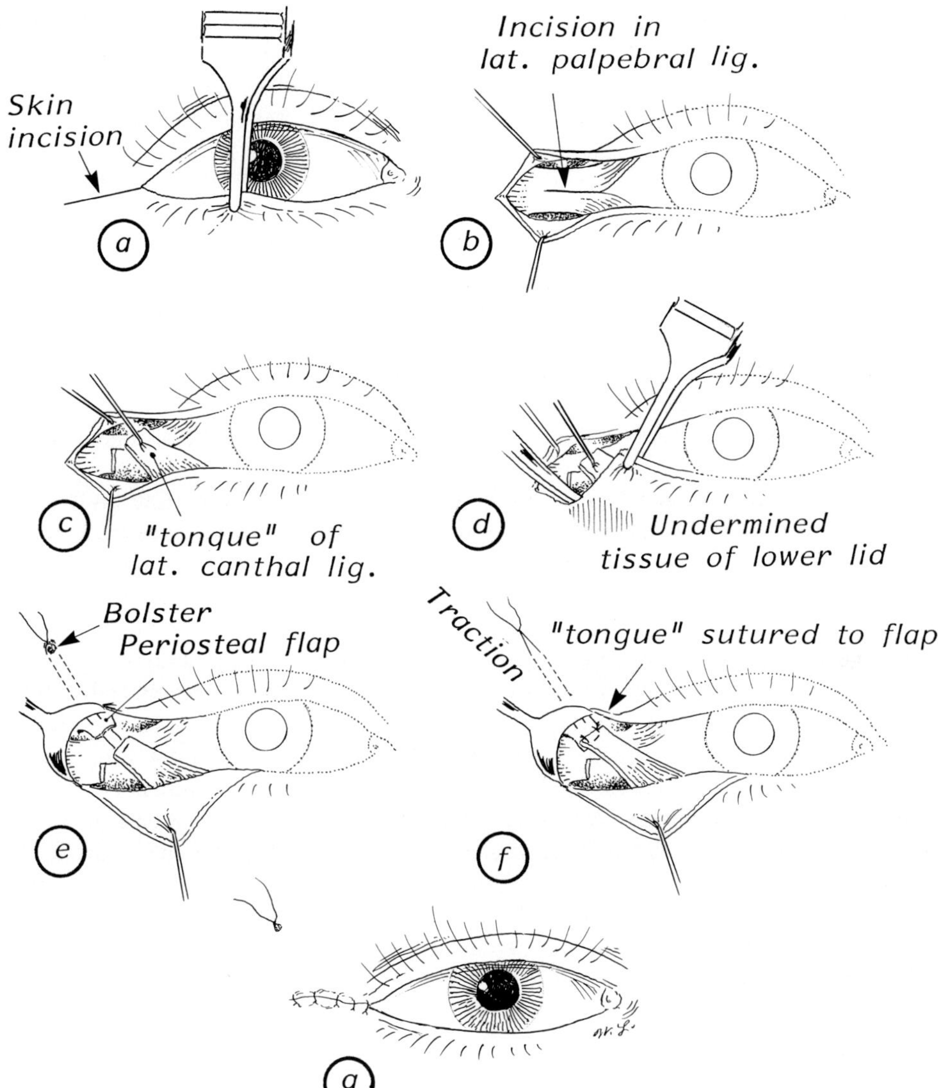

Figure 8–6. Release of ectropion (after Hamako and Baylis[35]). (a). Lateral canthotomy incision. (b). Skin is undermined and lateral canthotomy performed. (c). The lower lid can be mobilized following inferior cantholysis. A tongue of lateral canthal tendon and lateral tarsus is developed. (d). Skin is undermined, excess skin excised, and new lateral canthal angle determined. (e,f). Suture through "tongue" and periosteal flap is brought out through skin and fixed to bolster. (g). Incision is closed, slightly overcorrected.

preferable to provide adequate support. Skin can be used from the upper eyelid, retroauricular skin, or supraclavicular skin. If the defects are large, a split-thickness skin graft may be used. Split-thickness skin grafts are also preferred for upper eyelid ectropion. Surgery is performed after a suitable amount of time has elapsed to allow stabilization of the wound. The scar is outlined and excised, trying to keep the lines in the RSTLs of the lids. The appropriate donor site is identified and a matching full-thickness graft is outlined and incised. The graft is then sutured in with silk sutures that are tied and left long. These ties are then placed over a bolster that is then secured to maintain pressure over the graft for 5 to 7 days. If the defect is so large that a split-thickness graft is needed, this is usually harvested from the neck (but may also be taken from buttock or thigh) with an air- powered dermatome.

Traumatic tissue loss of eyelid tissue greater than 25% usually cannot be closed primarily. A local flap is then needed for repair.[2,3] A variety of flaps are available that are all variations on the advancement flap. The Mustard flap is a technique utilizing a cheek advancement rotation flap for large defects of the lower lid. If necessary, a septal or auricular composite graft can be taken to recreate the support of the missing tarsal plate. The cheek flap is outlined from the lateral canthus laterally, extending in a slight upward arc into the preauricular skin. The flap is then undermined and rotated into the defect. Extension of the incision inferiorly into the preauricular crease can increase the arc of flap rotation if necessary. A permanent stay suture should be placed from the dermis of the flap, overlying the lateral canthus, into the lateral orbital periosteum (to provide upward support and avoid downward tension on the lower lid structures). The composite graft is then sutured into the defect and the remainder of the flap is closed to recreate the lower lid.

The medial canthus is at particular risk for cosmetic deformity in naso-orbital injuries. This typically involves ethmoid sinus fracture(s), which in turn disrupts the attachment of the medial canthal tendon. Scar formation may cause webbing over the medial canthus. Other injuries specifically involving the nose will be discussed under nasal deformities.

Epicanthus is the formation of a web, either congenitally or traumatically, which obscures the medial canthus. This may extend from the nasal bridge to the eyebrow or varying places on the lid. Converse and Smith[36] described a double-opposing Z-plasty technique that effectively lengthens the webbed contracture. The Z-plasties are designed such that the central members are aligned parallel to the web, essentially perpendicular to the long axis of the eye. Mirror image limbs are then designed, which are oriented about the supratarsal and infratarsal creases extending laterally. The final limbs are added superiorly and inferiorly, extending medially, again in mirror image apposition to each other. The flaps are incised, undermined, and the triangles transposed to release the webbed contracture. The wound is then closed as for any Z-plasty technique.

Contour Defects

The soft tissues of the face define the underlying skeleton because it is the soft tissues that we observe and measure directly.[37] Any alteration in the supporting framework of the face, therefore, is transferred to the soft tissues, and it is these that become the defining point for both pre and postoperative evaluations. The keys to successful management of contour deformities resulting from paranasal sinus fracture are a thorough understanding of the anatomy, comprehensive pretreatment data base, carefully thought out preoperative plans, as well as experience in maxillofacial surgery.

Analysis

A detailed history of the timing, type, and mechanism of fracture allows for better understanding of the post-traumatic deformity. A thorough head and neck examination is undertaken. Inspection for contour deformities is made easier by dividing the face into equal thirds, evaluating each area separately, and then taking the sum of these parts and seeing how they relate as a whole.[37,38] Each third of the face is approximately equal in length. In the upper third of the face, the forehead is assessed for asymmetries and depressions. Assessment of the middle third of the facial skeleton is somewhat less straightforward, given the unique three-dimensional relationships between the zygomatic arches, malar eminences, and the nose. Special attention is also paid to the orbital area. The intrapalpebral fissure distance, intercanthal distance, and interpupillary distance should be noted if indicated. Position of the globe is assessed. The nose is examined for external and internal deformities. The patient's occlusion is checked. Profile examination helps to establish deviations in facial subunit projection, angular relationships between topographical structures, and maxillomandibular disharmony. All areas should be compared with each other for symmetry and balance. The surgeon should be well acquainted with the range of normal, as well as what is considered aesthetically appealing, taking into account the patient's race and ethnic origin.

Preoperative photodocumentation is essential. Standard views of the face (frontal, lateral, and oblique) are taken as well as bird's eye and worm's eye views. Often overlooked, but frequently very important, is a photograph of the patient's premorbid appearance. This is not only helpful for contour deformities but in cases where there exist only soft tissue lesions.

Radiographic imaging is also fundamental to thoughtful preoperative planning, as it is helpful to know the full extent of bony injury. Traditional plain films of the facial skeleton are useful in the acute stage; however, diagnosis of late deformities is often difficult. Cephalometrograms supply large amounts of data about facial morphology. Unfortunately this is limited to the profile and are also subject to magnification errors.

Computed tomographic (CT) scans have been a valuable adjunct in the management of facial fractures. Traditional CT scans are taken in two dimensions, axial and coronal. Reconstruction of facial contours, however, requires three-dimensional analysis. Extrapolation of images into the third dimension has traditionally been left to the surgeon. Because recontouring of the visible soft tissues is highly dependent on adequate reshaping of the facial skeletal defect, adequate radiological imaging of the bony anatomy and its soft tissue relationships is crucial. Anticipation of soft tissue changes is poor using regular biplanar analysis.[39] Fortunately, conventional CT scans can now be reformatted into three-dimensional images, with additional software packages available on most new generation scanners.[40]

High resolution CT scans can be obtained using tightly collimated (1 to 2 mm) cuts. Often these scans are already a part of the patient's record. The reconstruction program extracts the bone and soft tissue interface and then replicates it in three dimensions. These reformatted images can then be rotated through 360° or the angle of illumination about the face can be changed to better contrast one side with the other. This allows improved quantification of facial asymmetries.[39]

To further facilitate the analyses of facial asymmetries, a vertical plane may be introduced in the midline with a mirror image of the normal side rotated and superimposed onto the side of the defect. A subtraction analyses program then compares the normal and damaged sides and produces a negative that corresponds to the missing or defective anatomy. Precise volumetric analysis can then be done.[41] Newer programs are able to reconstruct soft tissue contours to evaluate theoretical postoperative appearance. Such measurements allow the surgeon preoperatively to determine placement of osteotomies[42] and to more accurately predict the size and dimensions of required grafts and alloplastic implants.[42–44] By facilitating preoperative planning, intraoperative time is reduced, which lowers morbidity and provides a more precise reconstruction. New technologies are not a substitute, however, for thoughtful preoperative planning and surgical skill.

Reconstruction

There are essentially three modes of correcting posttraumatic facial contour: (1) osteotomies and reduction in true anatomic alignment; (2) recontouring with autogenous grafts or allopastic onlay implants; or (3) a combination of osteotomies and implants. Osteotomies are usually reserved for severe defects involving the orbit or zygomaticomaxillary complex, otherwise simple onlay techniques will usually suffice.[38] This section will concentrate on implant types and techniques.

Alloplasts

The controversies related to implant types, autogenous versus alloplastic, pervade the literature. There are essentially three types of solid alloplastic implants that are in use today for facial contouring: Supramid mesh, Proplast, and Silastic. Supramid is a polyamide mesh that is prepackaged as a woven sheet that is shaped by folding or suturing. Beekhuis[45] claimed good success with dorsal nasal augmentation; however, recent reports claim a high rate of resorption in the long term. Proplast is a porous polytetrafluorene polymer that is somewhat soft and easy to shape with a scalpel. The pores allow for tissue ingrowth and are thought to contribute to implant stability. Proplast is available in two types. Proplast I is black whereas Proplast II is white by the inclusion of aluminum oxide fibers. Silastic is solid medical grade silicone that is nonporous. It is contoured with a scalpel but is more difficult than Proplast because it is more rigid. Both Proplast and Silastic come in ready-to-carve blocks and preformed implants. Tissue response to Proplast has been thought to be fibrous ingrowth due to its porosity, a characteristic that is thought to make it more difficult to remove if indicated.[46] Silastic is nonporous and therefore becomes embellished in a thin fibrous tissue capsule. Both of these findings have been confirmed in animal studies.[47]

Advantages of alloplastic implants include the absence of additional donor site morbidity and a one-stage reconstruction. Also, the implants remain relatively stable and the correction achieved with these tends to be predictable. Disadvantages include the presence of a foreign body, potential for extrusion, and infection. Silastic has a theoretical advantage in that its relative lack of pores may confer an increased resistance to infection. However, infection rates of 2.4 to 4% are seen with Proplast use.[38,48] In general, alloplastic implants should never be used in the presence of a communication between the nose and paranasal sinuses because of the potential for infection.

Autogenous materials are still considered by most as the preferred reconstructive implant because of their lack of immunogenic response and low incidence of migration and extrusion. This needs to be counterbalanced against the disadvantages of unpredictable resorption over time, donor site morbidity, and limited stock of safely available bone and cartilage. Potential donor sites include calvarium, rib, and iliac crest for bone; and rib, septum, and conchal bowl for cartilage. Banked irradiated human cartilage may also be utilized. Advantages of autogenous implants are biocompatibility, and therefore reduced risk of extrusion, infection, and potential failure.

Autogenous bone grafts can be best understood in terms of embryological origin or morphological description. Embryologically, osteogenesis occurs in one of two ways, through membranous or endochondral formation. The majority of the craniofacial skeleton develops from the former. Morphologically, bone is composed of two types, dense cortical bone and the less dense trabeculated cancellous bone. Regardless of origin or type, free bone grafts are incorporated into their host bed by osteoconduction through a process of "creeping substitution." This is the process whereby the grafted bone essentially provides a scaffold for the ingrowth of blood vessels, osteoblasts, and osteoclasts to remodel and lay down new bone. Cancellous grafts are revascularized earlier. In the craniofacial skeleton it appears that membranous bone also revascularizes earlier and maintains volume in greater proportions than endochondral bone. Petroff et al[49] believe that the similarity between cranial bone and the recipient facial bones may account for its increased survival. Other authors believe that the better results obtained with membranous bone, specifically calvarium, have more to do with the increased ratio of cortical bone to cancellous bone.[50]

Hydroxyapatite (HA) is a calcium phosphate compound that contributes a large portion of rigid mineral structure to bones and teeth.[51] It has been used in the ceramic or solid form for the past 20 years. It does not have any osteoinductive properties but does permit osteoconduction to a degree.[51] Salyer and Hall[52] used porous HA as an onlay graft in the maxillofacial area. Using a subjective grading scale, they saw no significant difference between HA onlays and patients who had received a bone graft. Hydroxyapatite was found to be difficult to sculpt, prone to extrusion with thin soft tissue coverage, and experienced problems with delayed fixation of the graft. They concluded that HA was an alternative and not a substitute for bone.

Recently, hydroxyapatite cement (HAC) has been developed.[53] This is a nonceramic form of HA that is able to be applied as a paste so that it crystallizes or hardens in vivo. It is thus able to be shaped intraoperatively, bypassing the problems associated with the solid or ceramic form of HA. The strength of HAC is not as great as that of ceramic HA; however, the authors state it appears to be sufficient for reconstruction of nonstressed bone. Friedman et al[54] used HAC to obliterate the frontal sinus in cats and found partial replacement of the HAC with new bone without volume loss and adequate fixation. Shindo et al[55] found similar results using HAC to augment the facial skeleton (supraorbital ridge) in dogs. Hydroxyapatite cement is still experimental but appears to offer encouraging preliminary data in animals that ultimately may be applicable to humans.

Induced osteogenesis is another area where recent investigations appear to offer promising results. It has been known for some time that devitalized, demineralized bone, although not possessing any osteoprogenitor cells, clearly induces new bone growth in bone and soft tissue.[56] Mullikan and Glowacki[57] showed that demineralized bone grafts and powders consistently induced osteogenesis in rat calvaria. This process does not appear to be species specific. Glowacki et al[58] took this one step further and utilized demineralized banked bone to repair craniofacial defects in humans. They reported rapid ossification of large bony defects. Several proteins are known to be present in demineralized bone. Recently, bone morphogenetic protein 2(BMP2) has been found in demineralized bone and can be produced utilizing recombinant DNA technology. Toriumi et al[59] have used BMP2 to reconstruct 3 cm full-thickness defects in canine mandibles. They found new bone growth that was significant enough to allow removal of the reconstruction plate and the dogs to successfully tolerate a regular diet. Further work is needed but clearly this represents one of the exciting future venues in maxillofacial reconstruction.

Bone may be harvested as a vascularized or nonvascularized graft. The choice of which to use depends on the size of the defect as well as the condition of the recipient bed. Small defects can be reconstructed with good results utilizing nonvascularized bone. Larger defects should be reconstructed with vascularized bone grafts. Vascularized bone grafts have the advantage of bringing in their own blood supply, which is especially important in those cases where the recipient bed is contaminated or the blood supply is compromised. Disadvantages are similar to those of other autogenous grafts, in addition to increased donor site morbidity and limitation of potential donor sites for pedicled grafts. Free vascularized grafts allow more versatility than pedicled grafts but are technically more arduous. To maximize graft survival for any free graft, the recipient site should be prepared to maximize graft–recipient bed interface, eliminate dead space, and provide adequate graft stabilization.[50]

Incisions

Incisions should be planned so that they are as cosmetically acceptable as possible. Often in facial trauma there is a preexisting scar that may be utilized. However, if the possibility of an implant is entertained, then a more distant incision should be undertaken to minimize the potential risks of suture line extrusion and bacterial inoculation. In general, access for recontouring facial defects is similar to that of standard acute traumatic care. The incisions typically utilized are the bicoronal, subciliary, transconjunctival, and gingivobuccal/ gingivolabial.

Forehead

Trauma to the frontal sinus can lead to significant cosmetic deformity. Serious comminution of the fracture, or loss of bone and soft tissues, can contribute to a less than optimal aesthetic result compared with other facial regions. Contour defects in this area may be more perceptible because there is minimal subcutaneous tissue. The type and size of the defect will dictate the type of repair. Recontouring of the forehead can be accomplished by bone reduction, augmentation, or both. Bone reduction can be achieved with the rotating bur tip of a hand-held drill to optimize contour as long as the inner cortex is preserved. For small defects, Proplast implants can be used. For larger defects, methyl methacrylate can be applied directly over the defect and modeled with a spatula.[44] Displacement of the acrylic can be avoided by placement of two small screws that are tapped into the inner cortex of the skull and left partially exposed. The screws are incorporated into the acrylic and provide a solid attachment.[60] Epker and Stella[61] used a method in which a positive impression was made directly on the patient with a kit. This positive template was then sent to the manufacturer (Dow) where a prefabricated implant was constructed from silicone.

Autogenous onlay grafts also work well in the frontal sinus area. Outer table cranial bone is preferred because of ease of harvest and minimal donor site morbidity because it can be harvested through the same bicoronal incision. A relatively large volume of cranial bone is available for reconstruction. For large defects, en bloc reconstruction may help in achieving a smooth more natural appearing contour.[62]

Casanova et al[63] found, by injection studies in cadavers, that random but predictable perforating vessels vascularize what they call the innominate fascia, temporal aponeurosis, and outer table calvarium. Using this information, Psillakis et al[64] transferred vascularized grafts to the upper facial skeleton on a pedicle of only temporal aponeurosis, periosteum, and fascia. This pedicle can theoretically be designed to reach the mandible. At 36 months follow-up, they did not appreciate any volume loss. In cases of loss of soft tissue, the rotation of periosteum into the defect will support a skin graft.[65,66] For purely soft tissue augmentation, pericranial and galeal flaps can be utilized.[67–69]

Malar-Midface

Probably the most consistent complaint relating to the cheek region following trauma is persistent malar flattening.[48] It is in this area that asymmetries are most manifest in oblique projection. Proper evaluation and analysis of the mid-third of the face will identify precisely the type of malar deficiency. Various approaches have evolved for pinpointing where the malar eminence should lay. Wilkinson,[70] Hinderer,[71] Powell et al,[72] Mladick,[46] and Whitaker[38] have all proposed algorithms for finding the perfect malar eminence. The method of Powell et al is probably the most applicable to the posttraumatic situation. They propose separating the malar region into two distinct areas. An anterior segment consists of infraorbital rim and the most anterior projection of the malar bone. The lateral segment consists of the malar eminence, lateral orbital rim, and zygomatic arch. These areas should be evaluated separately because recontouring of either of these segments will result in a distinctly different appearance. The anterior area is the one most often involved in trauma.

The choice of implant is dictated by the extent of injury, the surgeon's preference, as well as the patient's desires. Block et al[48] and Whitaker[38] prefer Proplast implants for malar augmentation. Hinderer[71] and Brennan[73] report good results with the use of Silastic implants whereas Wolfe and Vitenas[74] prefer the use of vascularized bone grafts. Proponents of alloplastic malar implants do not report any evidence of bony resorption beneath the implant. Regardless of the type of implant that is chosen, successful use of alloplastic implants is dependent on placement of the implant in an appropriately developed subperiosteal pocket. Subcutaneous placement does not give the natural contour of subperiosteal placement.[70] If the pocket is too large the implant will be mobile, and if too small the implant may fold or the edges may bend. Handling of the implants should be kept to a minimum as Proplast can be crushed thereby ruining its micropores. If inserted through an intraoral incision, there will be no visible scar. Concerns about contamination can be allayed if the implant is impregnated with antibiotics and the patient is placed on both pre and postoperative antibiotics.

Buccal Fat Pad

Although lipoaugmentation utilizing the buccal fat pad is controversial, it remains a frequently overlooked tool to correct malar contour. The buccal fat pad is a four-lobed structure that is contained in a fascial envelope derived from the masseteric fascia. Although it tends to diminish in size as the facial structures grow around it, it can provide a significant amount of enhancement for soft tissue defects requiring minimal to moderate bulk.[75] The size of the fat pad did not correlate well with overall body adiposity in cadaveric studies.[76] Stuzin et al[77] used a nonvascularized free buccal fat pad graft, with good results, to recontour cheek defects. The fat pad is well vascularized and can be used to line defects without coverage, and has been shown to reepethelialize or support a skin graft.[78]

Complex Defects

Complex defects with loss of major soft tissue and bony components typically require more than only grafts to restore maxillofacial contour. In these types of injuries, local vascular supply is often suboptimal owing to dense scar tissue. There may be contamination with intrasinus or intraoral contents. In these situations, free nonvascularized bone grafts and alloplastic implants are at risk for failure, and a pedicled[79] or free vascularized flap[80] may be the only recourse to adequately restore contour. Using facial moulage as a guide to plan free scapular flaps, Upton et al[81] still found the necessity to secondarily augment certain deficiencies of the malar complex even though the scapular and parascapular flaps can deliver up to 25×35 cm of tissue. To help with the preoperative planning of complex facial defects, the technology of three-dimensional CT reconstructions has been integrated with microvascular reconstruction.[43,62] Again, subtraction analysis of the defect is used to provide a negative corresponding to the missing or deformed part. The encoded message is then sent to a computer controlled, three-axis milling machine that constructs a wax mold. An acrylic template is then fabricated and sterilized for use intraoperatively. Fit is claimed to be accurate to within 2%. Similar technology has been used for fabrication of alloplastic orbital implants.[82] The cost of these implants is prohibitive, therefore, they are not indicated in the majority of patients requiring recontouring. However, in patients with complex defects, this removes much of the guesswork in the operating room, reduces intraoperative time, and can be fit with minimal manipulation.

Nasal Defects

Given the close relationship between the nose and paranasal sinuses, it is understandable that cosmetic deformities of the nose can be a sequela of sinus fracture. This may be in the form of soft tissue loss from penetrating trauma, ranging to loss of support as seen in complex naso-orbital fractures. Reconstructive rhinoplasty is the art and science of restoring aesthetic nasal contour. Even seemingly simple nasal defects may pose complex reconstructive problems. This is because of the central location and prominence of the nose, as well as its three-layered structure composed of skin, rigid support, and lining. It is not enough to restore tissue in the center of the face. The reestablishment of a functional airway and balanced aesthetic form are essential components of a successful repair. The nose needs to maintain the function of inspiring air as well as being as normal looking as possible. Reconstruction of the posttraumatic nose is usually most easily performed through the "open" approach.

Burget and Menick[83] point out that in reality it is not actually possible to recreate a nose. The reconstructive surgeon's role is to fashion bits and pieces of other expendable tissue into facsimiles of cover, lining, and support that give the appearance of a normal nose. In general, autogenous grafts are the most dependable materials for reconstruction of the nose. Many alloplasts have been tried in the past; however, they present potential problems with infection and extrusion that make it a less than ideal implant. Skin grafts, cartilage grafts, bone grafts, and composite grafts are the mainstays of the reconstructive surgeon's armanentarium. The most internal layer, the lining, is important in that it provides coverage of the raw undersurface, minimizing wound contraction and helping to maintain airway patency. Reconstruction of this layer may be accomplished with flaps of vestibular skin or septal mucosa.

Other skin flaps tend to be took bulky. Cartilage grafts provide thin but stable support. Septal cartilage is usually the preferred source owing to its ease of harvest. It is easily shaped and does not distort easily. It is well suited for struts, battons, and filling material for depressions. Auricular (conchal) cartilage can also be utilized. A significant amount can be harvested, approximately 6 cm^2 per side. Auricular cartilage is flexible and possesses a curved surface, making it most useful for tip onlay grafts and alar support. Rib grafts provide an alternate source of cartilage, however, they are not used with much regularity if there is adequate septal or auricular cartilage available. Rib cartilage warps easily over time, is rigid, and is associated with significant donor site morbidity. Skin coverage is probably best provided by local flaps owing to the superior color and texture match. For large defects of soft tissue, the paramedian forehead flap[84] has been shown to be effective in providing adequate skin coverage as well as giving a good aesthetic result. Full-thickness skin grafts may also be utilized. The use of split-thickness skin grafts on the nose is limited owing to poor color match, inadequate bulk, and tendency to contract.

The nose has been divided into subunits.[85] These include the dorsum, nasal tip, the alae, nasal side walls, and the soft triangles. Scars that are raised or depressed tend to be more conspicuous on the nose as a result of light reflections and shadows created off uneven surfaces. The subunit principle takes advantage of these differences in topography when replacing tissue or positioning scars, so that these reflect light in such a way as to fool the observer into perceiving a normal nasal contour.

Saddle-Nose Deformity

Loss of bony or cartilaginous support causes depression of the nasal dorsum. Improvement in dorsal height to achieve a change in profile is the goal. This is most easily accomplished with implants. Alloplastic implants have been available for a long time but continue to suffer from high rates of infection and extrusion. Autogenous grafts continue to be the implant of choice. Controversy still exists as to the most appropriate type of autograft to use. For small defects, septal cartilage is probably a good donor source because of reasons detailed previously. If inadequate septal cartilage is available, it may be supplemented with conchal cartilage. Some defects will be too large for septal or conchal cartilage alone. Autografts such as rib or costal cartilage can be used. Rib grafts have a tendency to warp over time and have a higher donor site morbidity. Irradiated cadaveric costal cartilage has been frequently utilized;[86] however, Welling et al in a long-term follow-up of cadaveric implants show a high rate of resorption after 10 years. The implantation can be accomplished through an external rhinoplasty approach or through an intercartilaginous incision. The grafts are harvested, and depending on the extent of augmentation required, can be coapted in a tiered fashion and suture fixated.

Alternatively, the grafts may be folded on each other, sutured, and then wrapped in temporalis fascia. This technique helps to smooth out irregularities, especially in patients with thin skin and minimal subcutaneous tissue.[88] A subperiosteal pocket is created for graft placement and stabilization. Particular attention is paid to splinting the nasal dorsum to prevent migration of the grafts. They will eventually be surrounded by a fibrous capsule. Alternately, temporalis fascia alone may be used for augmentation. It has a great deal of tensile strength, is not associated with an inflammatory reaction, and is easily harvested with minimal donor site morbidity and scar. An approximate volume of 2 cm^3 per side can be obtained. These grafts will readily conform to the area requiring augmentation. As a result of their flexibility, mattress sutures are necessary to hold the grafts in place. Fascia grafts can also provide tissue for forehead contour.[88,89]

In noses where there is insufficient projection because of a retruded maxilla, the lower nasal base can be brought forward by the placement of an implant at this inferior location. Hinderer[71] has developed an implant that consists of a central segment that is positioned against the lower nasal spine beneath the columella-lip angle. Smaller segments lay under the nostrils to elevate them and the perialar groove. The implant can be placed through a transfixion or Rethi-type incision into a subperiosteal pocket without any further fixation.

Severe defects of the bony dorsum may require bone grafts for adequate dorsal support. The donor source may be rib, iliac crest, split, or full-thickness calvarial bone. Rib has a tendency to curl. Iliac crest grafts have enjoyed the most popularity until recently. Newer rigid fixation techniques, utilizing lag screws and miniplates, have given excellent results with split-calvarial bone grafts.[90]

In summary, there are many cosmetic problems that can result from paranasal sinus trauma; however, there are many more methods for their correction. A well thought out logistic approach, technical facility, and an updated awareness of surgical refinements and technology will help make this a less difficult problem to deal with. In the end, success is predicated on how well we understand and are able to achieve what the patient desires.

REFERENCES

1. Gunter JL. Revision of scars of the head and neck. *Otolaryngol Clin North Am.* 1974; 7:119–131.
2. Converse JM, Smith B. The eyelids and their adnexa. In: Converse JM, ed. *Reconstructive Plastic Surgery.* Philadelphia, Pa: WB Saunders Co., 1977;2:858–874.
3. Custer PL. Conceptual approach to eyelid reconstruction. *Otolaryngol Clin North Am.* 1990;23:991–1002.
4. Schultz RC. *Facial Injuries.* Chicago, Ill: Year Book Medical; 1988:181–185.
5. Borges AE. Scar analysis and objectives of revision procedures. *Clin Plast Surg.* 1977;4:223–237.
6. Thomas JR, Ehlert TK. Scar revision and camouflage. *Otolaryngol Clin North Am.* 1990;23:963–973.
7. Thomas JR, Holt GR. *Facial scars, incision, Revision and Camouflage.* St Louis, Mo: CV Mosby; 1989:103–122.
8. Baker SR, Swanson NA. Clinical applications of tissue expansion in head and neck surgery. *Laryngoscope.* 1990;100:313–319.
9. Baker SR, Swanson NA. Rapid Intraoperative tissue expansion in reconstruction of the head and neck. *Arch Otolaryngol Head Neck Surg.* 1990;116:1431–1434.
10. Horner WF. Clinical report on the surgical department of the Philadelphia Hospital. *Am J Med Sci.* 1837;21:99–112.
11. Davis WE, Shchrick RE, Templer J. An Introduction to Z Plasty. *Ear Nose Throat J.* 1981;60:29–34.
12. Webster RC, Davidson TM, Smith RC. Broken line scar revision. *Clin Plast Surg.* 1977;4:263–274.

13. Newman J, Dolsky RL, Nguyen A. Facial profileplasty by liposuction extraction. *Otolaryngol Head Neck Surg*. 1985;93:718–731.
14. Spira M, Rosen T. Injectable soft tissue substitutes. *Clin Plast Surg*. 1993;20:181–188.
15. Shumrick KA, Kridel RWH. Comparison of injectable silicone versus collagen for soft tissue augmentation. *J Dermatol Surg Oncol*. 1988;14:66–72.
16. Bailin MD, Bailin PL. Correction of surgical scars, acne scars, and rhytids with Zyderm and Zyplast implants. *J Dermatol Surg Oncol*. 1988;14:31–33.
17. Bailin PI, Bailin MD. Collagen implantation: clinical applications and lesion selection. *J Dermatol Surg Oncol*. 1988;14:21–26.
18. Klein AW. Indications and implantation techniques for the various formulations of injectable collagen. *J Dermatol Surg Oncol*. 1988;14:27–30.
19. Millikan L. Long term safety and efficacy with Fibrel in the treatment of cutaneous scars. *J Dermatol Surg Oncol*. 1989;15:837–842.
20. Koranda FK. Dermabrasion. In: Thomas JR, Holt GR, eds. *Facial Scars, Incision, Revision and Camouflage*. St. Louis, Mo: CV Mosby: 1989:123–136.
21. Ehrlich HP, Kelley SF. Hypertrophic scar: an interruption in the remodeling of repair- a laser Doppler blood flow study. *Plast Reconstr Surg*. 1992;90:993–998.
22. Darzi MA, Chowdri A, Kaul SK, Khan M: Evaluation of various methods of treating keloids and hypertrophic scars: a 10 year follow up study. *Br J Plast Surg*. 1992;45:374–379.
23. Sawada Y, Sone K. Treatment of scars and keloids using a cream containing silicone oil. *Br J Plast Surg*. 1990;40:683.
24. Sawada Y, Sone K. Hydration and occlusion treatment for hypertrophic scars and keloids. *Br J Plast Surg*. 1992;45:599–603.
25. Sproat JE, Dalcin A, Weitauer N, Roberts R. Hypertrophic sternal scars: silicone gel sheet versus Kenalog injection treatment. *Plast Reconstr Surg*. 1992;90:988–992.
26. Fee WE, Gunter JP, Carder HM. Rhomboid flap principles and common variations. *Laryngoscope*. 1975;86: 1706–1711.
27. Limberg AA. Design of local flaps. In: Gibson T, ed. *Modern Trends in Plastic Surgery*. London: Butterworths; 1966:38–61.
28. Dufourmental C. An L shaped flap for loss in shape defects. *Trans Third International Congress on Plastic Surgery*. Amsterdam: Excerpta Medical Foundation, 1963.
29. Borges AF. The rhombic flap. *Plast Reconstr Surg*. 1981;67:458–466.
30. Becker FF. Rhomboid flap in facial reconstruction. *Arch Otolaryngol*. 1979;105:569–573.
31. Rees TD. *Aesthetic Plastic Surgery*. Philadelphia, Pa: WB Saunders Co; 1980.
32. Carraway JH, Mellow CG. The prevention and treatment of lower lid ectropion following blepharoplasty. *Plast Reconstr Surg*. 1990;85:971–981.
33. Thomas EL, Laborde RP. Retinal and choroidal vascular occlusion following intralesional corticosteroid injection of a chalazion. *Ophthalmology*. 1986;93:405–410.
34. Ousterhout DK, Weil RB. The role of the lateral canthal tendon in lower eyelid laxity. *Plast Reconstr Surg*. 1982;69:620–622.
35. Hamako C, Baylis HI. Lower eyelid retraction after blepharoplasty. *Am J Ophthalmol*. 1980;89:517–521.
36. Converse JM, Smith B. The eyelids and their adnexa. In: Converse JM, ed. *Reconstructive Plastic Surgery*. Philadelphia, Pa: WB Saunders Co; 1977;2:940–942.
37. Bartlett SP, Wornom I, Whitaker LA. Evaluation of facial aesthetics and surgical planning. *Clin Plast Surg*. 1991;18:1–9.
38. Whitaker LA. Aesthetic augmentation of the malar-midface structures. *Plast Reconstr Surg* 1987;80:337–346.
39. Marsh JL, Vannoer MW. The "Third" dimension in craniofacial surgery. *Plast Reconstr Surg*. 1983;71:759–767.
40. Vannier MW, Marsh JL, Warren JO. Three dimensional CT reconstruction images for craniofacial surgical planning and evaluation. *Radiology*. 1984;150:179–184.
41. Hemmy DC, David DJ, Herman GT. Three dimensional reconstruction of craniofacial deformity using computed tomography. *Neurosurgery*. 1983;13:534–541.
42. Cutting C, Bookstein FL, Grayson B, Fellingham L, McCarthy JG. Three dimensional computer assisted design of craniofacial surgical procedures:optimization and interaction with cephalometric and CT based models. *Plast Reconstr Surg*. 1986;77:877–885.
43. Rose EH, Norris MS, Rosen JM. Application of high technology three dimensional imaging and computer generated models in complex facial reconstructions with vascularized bone grafts. *Plast Reconstr Surg*. 1993;91:252–264.
44. Hardesty RA, Coffey JA. Secondary craniomaxillofacial deformities, current principles of management. *Clin Plast Surg*. 1992;19:275–300.
45. Beekhuis GJ. Polyamide mesh used in facial plastic surgery. *Arch Otolaryngol*. 1980;106:642–644.

46. Mladick RA. Alloplastic cheek augmentation. *Clin Plast Surg*. 1991;18:2929–38.
47. Maas CS, Merwin GE, Wilson J, Frey MD, Maves MD. Comparison of biomaterials for facial bone augmentation. *Arch Otolaryngol Head Neck Surg*. 1990;116:551–556.
48. Black MS, Zide MF, Kent JN. Proplast augmentation for post-traumatic zygomatic deficiency. *Oral Surg Oral Med Oral Pathol*. 1984;57:123–131.
49. Petroff MA, Burgess LPA, Lau P, Anonsen CK, Goode RL. Cranial bone grafts for post-traumatic facial defects. *Laryngoscope*. 1987;97:1249–1253.
50. Arden RL, Burgio DL. Bone grafting of the craniofacial skeleton: clinical and biological considerations. *Am J Otolaryngol*. 1992;13:328–341.
51. Klinge B, Alberius P, Isaksson S, Jonsson J. Osseous response to implanted natural bone mineral and synthetic hydroxylapatite ceramic in the repair of experimental skull bone defects. *J Oral Maxillofac Surg*. 1992;50:241–249.
52. Salyer KE, Hall CE. Porous hydroxypapatite as an onlay bone-graft substitute for maxillofacial surgery. *Plast Reconstr Surg*. 1989;84:236–244.
53. Constantino PD, Friedman CD, Jones K, Chow LC, Pelzer HJ, Sisson GA. Hydroxyapatite cement I. Basic chemistry and histologic properties. *Arch Otolaryngol Head Neck Surg* 1991;117:379–384.
54. Friedman CD, Constantino PD, Jones K, Chow LC, Pelzer HJ, Sisson GA. Hydroxyapatite cement II. Obliteration and reconstruction of the cat frontal sinus. *Arch Otolaryngol Head Neck Surg*. 1991;117:385–389.
55. Shindo ML, Constantino PD, Friedman CD, Chow LC. Facial skeletal augmentation using hydroxyapatite cement. *Arch Otolaryngol Head Neck Surg*. 1993;119:185–190.
56. Urist MR. Surface decalcified allogeneic bone (SDAB) implants. A preliminary report of 10 cases and 25 comparable operations with undecalcified lyophilized bone implants. *Clin Orthop Rel Res*. 1968;56:37–50.
57. Mullikan JB, Glowacki J. Induced osteogenesis for repair and construction in the craniofacial region. *Plast Reconstr Surg*. 1980;65:553–559.
58. Glowacki J, Murray JE, Kaban LB, Folkman J, Mulliken JB. Application of the biological principle of induced osteogenesis for craniofacial defects. *Lancet* 1981;1:959–962.
59. Toriumi DM, Kotler HS, Luxenberg DB, Holtrop ME, Wang EA. Mandibular reconstruction with a recombinant bone-inducing factor. *Arch Otolaryngol Head Neck Surg*. 1991;117:1101–1112.
60. Monasterio FO. Aesthetic Surgery of the facial Skeleton: the forehead. *Clin Plast Surg*. 1991;18:19–27.
61. Epker BN, Stella JP. Reconstruction of frontal and frontal-nasal deformities with prefabricated custom implants. *J Oral Maxillofac Surg*. 1989;47:1272–1276.
62. Elisavich, Bite U. En bloc forehead reconstruction with split-thickness cranial bone. *Surg Neurol*. 1991;35: 384–388.
63. Casanova R, Cavalcante D, Grotting JC, Vasconez LO, Psillakis JM. Anatomic basis for vascularized outer-table calavarial bone flaps. *Plast Reconstr Surg*. 1986;78:300–308.
64. Psillakis JM, Grotting JC, Casanova R, Cavalcante D, Vasconez LO. Vascularized outer-table bone flaps. *Plast Reconstr Surg*. 1986;78:309–317.
65. Flint PW, Cummings CW. The pericranial turndown flap for coverage of soft tissue defects. *Laryngoscope*. 1991;101:92–94.
66. Terranova W. The use of periosteal flaps in scalp and forehead reconstruction. *Ann Plast Surg*. 1990;25: 450–456.
67. Carstens MH, Greco RJ, Hurwitz DJ, Tolhurst DE. Clinical applications of the subgaleal fascia. *Plast Reconstr Surg*. 1991;87:615–626.
68. Jackson IT, Adham MN, Marsh WR. Use of the galeal-frontalis myofascial flap in craniofacial surgery. *Plast Reconstr Surg*. 1986;77:905–910.
69. Argenta LC, Friedman RJ, Dingman RO, Duus EC. The versatility of pericranial flaps. *Plast Reconstr Surg*. 1985;76:695–702.
70. Wilkinson TS. Complications in aesthetic malar augmentation. *Plast Reconstr Surg*. 1983;71:643–647.
71. Hinderer UT. Nasal base, maxillary and infraorbital implants-alloplastic. *Clin Plast Surg*. 1991;18:87–105.
72. Powell NB, Riley RW, Laub DR. A new approach to evaluation and surgery of the malar complex. *Ann Plast Surg*. 1988;20:31–39.
73. Brennan HG. Augmentation malarplasty. *Arch Otolaryngol*. 1982;108:441–444.
74. Wolfe SA, Vitenas P. Malar augmentation using autogenous materials. *Clin Plast Surg*. 1991;18:39–54.
75. Neder A. Use of buccal fat pad for grafts. *Oral Surg*. 1983;55:349–350.
76. Herring SM. Reconstruction of facial contour deformity with the buccal fat pad flap. *Ann Plast Surg*. 1992;29:450–453.
77. Stuzin JM, Wagstrom MD, Kawamoto HK, Maker TJ, Wolfe SA. The anatomy and clinical applications of the buccal fat pad. *Plast Reconstr Surg*. 1990;85:29–37.
78. Tideman H, Bosanquet A, Scott J. Use of the buccal fat pad as a pedicled graft. *J Oral Maxillofac Surg*. 1986;44:435–440.
79. Govila A. Restoration of facial contour with deepethelized pectoralis major musculocutaneous flap. *Ann Plast Surg*. 1991;27:80–86.

80. Smith AA, Manktelow RT. The Use of free tissue transfer to restore facial contour. *Clin Plast Surg*. 1990;17:655–661.
81. Upton J, Albin RE, Mulliken JB, Murray JE. The use of the scapular and parascapular flaps for cheek reconstruction. *Plast Reconstr Surg*. 1992;90:959–971.
82. Toth BA, Ellis DS, Stewart WB. Computer-designed prosthesis for orbitiocranial reconstruction. *Plast Reconstr Surg*. 1988;81:315–322.
83. Burget GC, Menick FJ. Nasal reconstruction: seeking a fourth dimension. *Plast Reconstr Surg*. 1986;78: 145–157.
84. Menick FJ. Aesthetic refinements in use of forehead for nasal reconstruction: the paramedian forehead flap. *Clin Plast Surg*. 1990;17:607–622.
85. Burget GC, Menick FJ. The subunit principle in nasal reconstruction. *Plast Reconstr Surg*. 1985;76:239–247.
86. Murakami CS, Cook TA, Guida RA. Nasal reconstruction with articulated irradiated rib cartilage. *Arch Otolaryngol Head Neck Surg*. 1991;117:327–330.
87. Welling DB, Maves MD, Schuller DE. Irradiated homologous cartilage grafts; long term results. *Arch Otolaryngol Head Neck Surg*. 1988;114:291–295.
88. Guerrerosantos J. Nose and paranasal augmentation: autogenous, fascia and cartilage. *Clin Plast Surg*. 1991;18:65–86.
89. Miller TA. Temporalis fascia grafts for facial and nasal contour augmentation. *Plast Reconstr Surg*. 1988;81:524–533.
90. Posnick JC, Seagle MB, Armstrong D. Nasal reconstruction with full-thickness cranial bone grafts and rigid internal fixation through a coronal incision. *Plast Reconstr Surg*. 1990;86:894–904.

9

Cerebrospinal Fluid Fistula

DON L. BURGIO, M.S., M.D.
STEVEN C. MARKS, M.D.

Cerebrospinal fluid (CSF) leakage occurs whenever dural and arachnoidal tears in combination with a bony defect or fracture of the skull base allow escape of CSF from the subarachnoid space. When CSF leaks persist, a fistula is present. Spontaneous CSF rhinorrhea was first described by Willis[1] in 1676, but posttraumatic CSF rhinorrhea was not reported until Bidloo[2] in 1700. In 1923, Grant[3] was the first to attempt to surgically close a CSF fistula. The patient was a 19-year-old man with a frontal sinus fracture, and the attempt at closure was aborted owing to profuse bleeding, likely from the superior sagittal sinus. The first successful operative closure of a CSF fistula was reported by Dandy[4] in 1926. The patient had a dural tear associated with a frontal sinus fracture, and the defect was repaired through a direct approach with a muscle and fascia lata graft. In 1948, Dohlman[5] reported closure of CSF fistula via the intranasal transethmoid approach using septal and turbinate mucosal flaps.

Posttraumatic CSF leak is estimated to occur in 2 to 3% of all patients with head injuries, in 5% of all patients with skull base fractures, and in 25 to 50% of all patients with anterior skull base fractures.[6–9] Trauma associated with motor vehicle accidents and interpersonal violence is the most common cause of CSF fistula.[10–12] Penetrating trauma to the skull base often creates defects that lead to CSF fistula, but most of these injuries are fatal, minimizing the importance of this mechanism in creating CSF leaks.

PATHOPHYSIOLOGY

All posttraumatic CSF fistulas share several common features that include pia-arachnoid perforation, dural perforation, and a bony defect. Although this type of injury can occur anywhere along the dural covering of the central nervous system, it is most often located along the skull base. The most common site for posttraumatic CSF fistula is the floor of the frontal fossa particularly in the region surrounding the cribriform plate.[7,13] The bone in this region is very thin and fragile, and the dura is tightly adherent, predisposing this area to CSF fistula formation. Rootlets of the olfactory nerve with small investing arachnoid pouches pass through foramina in the cribriform plate, which may be a factor in the formation of both traumatic and nontraumatic CSF rhinorrhea.

The cribriform plate and crista galli are relatively thick and strong bones as compared with the thin bone of the surrounding ethmoid labyrinth. It is likely that many cribriform plate fractures associated with CSF leaks are actually due to fractures at its junction with the ethmoid labyrinth, or due to pia-arachnoid fistulization along the preformed pathways formed by the olfactory rootlets.[11] Traumatic CSF fistula can also occur with direct involvement of the ethmoid, frontal, or sphenoid sinuses, all of which have adherent overlying dura. Depending on the pattern of pneumatization, the fovea ethmoidalis can comprise a significant portion of the anterior skull base and is a common site of CSF fistula. The size and configuration of the frontal sinus are highly variable. For CSF fistula to occur here, a fracture of the posterior wall must be present. Sphenoid sinus fracture with CSF fistula is uncommon and usually associated with other severe craniofacial fractures. Lateral extensions of the sphenoid sinus into the middle cranial fossa can make detection of a fistula in that location difficult.[14]

The incidence of CSF fistula following head injury is likely greater than is reported. The arachnoid mesh is a vascular tissue with great reparative capability, and can seal most small tears within the first 24 to 48 hours.[15] CSF leakage may go unnoticed during this period because of other serious concomitant injuries. Additionally, reduction of the associated fracture will frequently stop the CSF leak without further intervention.[8]

The majority of posttraumatic CSF fistulas present within several days to weeks of the injury. Approximately 70% of patients with CSF fistula will present within 1 week of injury, and up to 90% will be evident within 1 month of injury.[9,16,17]

Although the majority of CSF fistula present within 1 month of the inciting injury, some will present later, and a small number will be intermittent. Reports of patients presenting from 1 to 35 years after injury are not uncommon.[9,16–19] Meningitis is frequently the heralding sign in a patient with a delayed CSF fistula.

Early delayed leaks (within 1 month) are likely due to resolution of edema and inflammation at the fracture site that had been obstructing the flow of CSF.[13] Late delayed leaks can result from dural tears which, when healed, are weak and susceptible to delayed perforation with sudden increases in CSF pressure.[7] A second possible mechanism of delayed leak is the herniation of nonlacerated dura into a fracture site. Over time the effects of intracranial pressure pulsations cause separation of the dural fibers and CSF leakage.[6] Another mechanism of delayed leak may be liquefaction of herniated brain tissue and/or absorption of blood clot, either of which may have been sealing a dural defect.

Intermittent leaks are also not uncommon. In one review, the incidence of intermittent leak was 7% at a mean follow-up of 6.5 years.[20] Intermittent leaks may be due to ball valving at the fracture site by dura, brain, or other adjacent tissue.

COMPLICATIONS

The two most frequent clinical findings associated with CSF fistula are meningitis and pneumocephalus. Meningitis is the most common severe complication of CSF fistula, and its reported incidence varies from 3 to 50%.[7,9,16,17,20] The bacteria associated with meningitis is these patients are shown in Table 9–1. These organisms are largely the same as found in any sinogenic meningitis.[11,16,17,21] The mortality rate for adults is less than 10%,[13,20–22] but at least one report indicates that children with CSF fistula associated meningitis may have a poorer prognosis, and therefore should be treated more aggressively.[23] Several studies have indicated that the incidence of meningitis in delayed-onset leaks is much greater than in cases of immediate or early-onset leaks, and recommend early intervention in cases of delayed fistula.[11,20]

The routine use of prophylactic antibiotics in the management of posttraumatic CSF fistula is controversial.[7,13,20,24] Although meningitis may be avoided with prophylactic antibiotics, there is a risk of producing infection with drug-resistant organisms. Two prospective randomized studies of antimicrobial prophylaxis in patients with acute traumatic CSF fistulas failed to show any statistically significant difference between treatment and nontreatment groups.[25,26] Cases have been reported in which meningitis developed despite prophylactic treatment with antibiotics to which the isolated organisms were sensitive. Antibiotic treatment is definitely indicated in cases with penetrating brain injury, retention of a foreign body, or cortical laceration.[7]

Pneumocephalus occurs in approximately 30% of patients with posttraumatic CSF fistula.[11,17,20] The presence of intracranial air is usually the consequence of a relatively large dural tear, and associated CSF leaks may be less likely to resolve spontaneously. It is not clear if pneumocephalus increases the risk of developing meningitis, as reports both supporting and refuting this contention appear in the literature.[11,20] Tension pneumocephalus is an unusual and potentially fatal complication. This occurs when the defect at the injury site produces a ball-valve effect, not allowing leakage of air or CSF out of the subarachnoid space. With increased pressure in the sinus, as during coughing or sneezing, air is forced intracranially causing the effects of a mass lesion. This usually manifests as a sudden decline in mental status or syncope and requires emergency evacuation of the air and closure of the dural defect.

DIAGNOSIS

A CSF fistula should be suspected in all patients presenting with head trauma, and in all adults with a history of head trauma who subsequently develop meningitis. Aside from those fistulas associated with an external defect, posttraumatic CSF fistulas from anterior skull base trauma usually present as intermittent clear rhinorrhea, and are more likely to

Table 9–1. Causative Organisms in Meningitis Associated with Traumatic CSF Fistula

ORGANISM	INCIDENCE (%)
Streptococcus pneumoniae	50–85
Other streptococci	10–15
Haemophilus influenzae	10–15
Neisseria meningitidis	5–10
Staphylococcus aureus	5–10
Enteric gram-negative bacilli	3–7
Staphylococcus epidermidis	<5
Others	<5

actively leak when the patient is standing or leaning forward. In the reclining or supine positions CSF leakage may decrease or go unnoticed if it drains posteriorly into the nasopharynx.

The reservoir sign is the voluntary elicitation of rhinorrhea with changes in head position. The patient is placed supine for a period of time and then brought upright with the neck flexed. A sudden flow of clear fluid is indicative of a CSF fistula. This clinical test can be augmented by the Valsalva's maneuver, which increases intracranial pressure by straining against a closed glottis and may be useful for collecting fluid for laboratory analysis.

The double-ring or target sign[13] is another finding indicative of, but not specific for, CSF fistula. The CSF rhinorrhea specimen (assumed to be contaminated with at least a small amount of blood) is placed on filter paper or the patient's pillowcase. The CSF migrates farther than blood from the center of the application and thus produces a double-ring or bull's-eye appearance.

The glucose level of rhinorrhea fluid may be used for confirmation that a CSF leak is present. Normal CSF will have a glucose level greater than 30 mg/dL whereas nasal secretions should contain less than 10 mg/dL.[27] Glucose oxidase reagent strips have been used for this determination. However this test is associated with a high false-positive rate and should not be used as the sole technique.[28–31] Comparison of quantitative glucose level of rhinorrhea fluid with simultaneously collected blood or lumbar CSF glucose level has been performed. If the rhinorrhea is CSF, the glucose level should be very close to the lumbar specimen and 40 to 60% of the blood level. In one report of 16 cases, the sensitivity of quantitative glucose analysis was found to be 88%.[11]

A more recent method of CSF determination is based on identification of beta-2 transferrin (tau-protein), a protein that is almost unique to CSF. With the exception of rare genetic variants and liver cirrhosis, beta-2 transferrin is not found in serum, nasal secretion, tears, or saliva, and has only been detected in CSF and the vitreous fluid of the eye.[32,33] The determination is made using immunoelectrophoresis, which requires between 1 and 50 μL of specimen.[33–36] It is important to examine a sample of the patient's serum and CSF as well as the rhinorrhea specimen to eliminate false-positives. The presence of high serum protein content or hemoglobin in the specimen can effect the determination, but newer methods may be less sensitive to specimen contamination.[33]

The intrathecal injection of vital dyes to verify and localize CSF leaks is another useful technique. Methylene blue, indigo carmine, Evans blue, phenolthalein, and fluorescein have all been used.[37] Many of these dyes were associated with frequent and severe neurological complications, and today fluorescein is the only one still used intrathecally.[38,39] Typically 0.2 to 2.0 mL of 5% injectable fluorescein (usually mixed with CSF) is slowly injected through a lumbar puncture. Cottonoid pledgets are placed in the nose after decongestion and anesthesia, usually in the following locations: (1) roof of nasal cavity (cribriform area); (2) sphenoethmoid recess; (3) middle meatus; and (4) posterior floor (eustachian tube orifice; Fig. 9–1). The patient is placed in a supine recumbent position for 30 minutes to several hours, depending on the size of the leak, to allow for diffusion of fluorescein throughout the CSF. The pledgets are then removed and examined (with ultraviolet light if needed) for the presence of fluorescein staining. Reliability of fistula localization using this technique is dependent on accurate placement of the pledgets, and size of the leak, and the amount of nasal secretions. For very slow leaks, identification of fluorescein on the pledgets using gel electrophoresis has been described.[34]

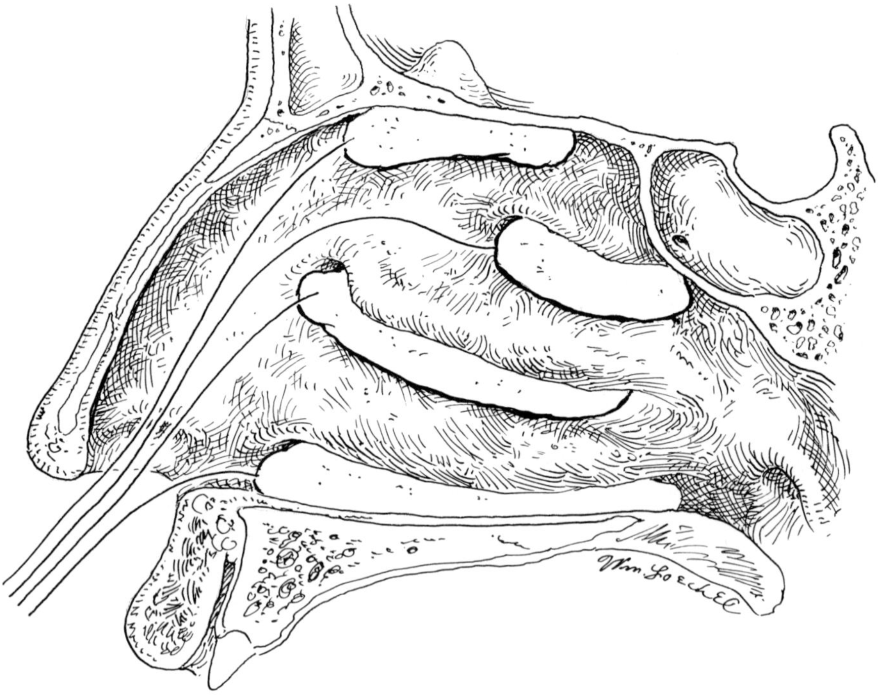

Figure 9–1. Placement of pledgets for radionucleide detection of CSF leak.

More recently, intrathecal fluorescein followed by intraoperative endoscopic nasal examination has been described as a sensitive method for leak detection and localization.[34,40] The standard light source of the endoscopic telescope is usually adequate for fluorescein identification. Thirty minutes to 1 hour after the intrathecal injection a complete endoscopic examination is performed. Detection of fluorescein stained discharge from a sinus ostium or the nasal roof can reliably predict the site of CSF leakage.

The radiological demonstration and localization of CSF fistulas is dependent on the intrathecal administration of contrast or tracer, followed by an imaging study. Today, the study of choice for initial demonstration and localization of a CSF leak is cisternography with a water soluble contrast agent (metrizamide) in combination with high resolution computer tomography (CT) scanning. All patients should have a high-resolution axial and coronal CT scan of the brain, skull base, and paranasal sinuses as a part of the initial evaluation. The contrast is then injected, and the CT scan repeated. Using this technique the success rate of CSF leak identification appears to be high, 85% or greater in many series.[41–46] Metrizamide CT cisternography is well tolerated by patients, with headache, nausea, and vomiting being the most common side effects. The shortcoming of CT cisternography is that visualization of contrast within the fistulous tract may be difficult owing to the static nature of the image. The exact site of the leak must sometimes be inferred from the location of the extrathecal contrast media. Digital subtraction fluoroscopic cisternography, a dynamic evaluation of the contrast media, may be a useful addition to CT cisternography.[47,48]

Radioisotope cisternography can be of value in evaluating patients with possible slow or intermittent leaks in whom metrizamide CT studies have been negative. Cottonoid pledgets are placed in the nose (see Fig. 9–1), and a radiopharmaceutical tracer agent is introduced into the subarachnoid space. The patient can be placed in the position thought most likely to induce the leak, and can also perform Valsalva's maneuver to increase the probability of demonstrating the leak. After approximately 24 hours the pledgets are removed, labeled, and their radioactivity counted to determine if tracer is present. The morbidity is very low, the sensitivity for detection appears to be as high as 80%, but localization is less accurate than with other techniques.[49–52] The use of simultaneous isotope and CT cisternography can be performed and may be useful in selected cases.[53]

If CT and isotope cisternography are both negative but there is good evidence for the presence of a CSF leak, overpressure cisternography can be used. Through a lumbar puncture radioisotope or contrast is administered, and normal saline is slowly infused until a leak is demonstrated or the intracranial pressure reaches 600 mm H_2O. This technique will demonstrate some leaks not apparent on other studies and appears to be safe when performed carefully.[54,55]

Current magnetic resonance (MR) techniques are inadequate for demonstrating CSF leaks. Studies in dogs indicate MR gadolinium cisternography may be useful in demonstrating CSF leaks,[56] but gadolinium-DTPA is not currently approved for use as an intrathecal tracer in humans.

MANAGEMENT

Management of traumatic CSF fistulas can be either operative or nonoperative. The majority of CSF leaks will be self-limited and stop spontaneously within 2 to 7 days of the traumatic event.[13] Of those that do not, reduction of the associated fracture (if possible) will often stop or decrease the leak.[8]

Nonoperative Management

In most circumstances, a period of 7 to 10 days of nonoperative therapy will be utilized before proceeding to operative repair. The basis of nonoperative management of CSF leaks is lowering the CSF pressure at the fistula site, which should decrease flow through the defect and allow the fistula to spontaneously heal. Management includes bed rest with elevation of the head, and the avoidance of straining (stool softeners may be given), nose blowing, sneezing, and coughing. Fluid restriction and medications to decrease CSF production (acetazolamide or dexamethasone) can be used, but their role has not been clearly defined.[7] In addition, CSF drainage from the subarachnoid space is an effective method of decreasing CSF pressure. The simplest means to do so is repeated lumbar punctures. The intent of each puncture is to lower the CSF pressure to approximately atmospheric pressure. Alternatively, continuous drainage of CSF using an indwelling lumbar catheter for 5 to 10 days has been reported in patients with post-traumatic leaks with good success.[57,58] Continuous spinal drainage, though, can have serious complications including meningitis, pneumocephalus, and herniation, and should be performed under close monitoring with a knowledgeable nursing staff.[59] Long-term percutaneous lumboperitoneal shunting for recalcitrant CSF leaks and surgical failures has been reported in nine patients of whom 8 had resolution of their leaks.[60] Cerebrospinal fluid drainage can be useful following operative repair to decrease recurrent postoperative leaks, especially in cases with large dural defects.

Operative Management

Failure of nonoperative management is an indication for surgical repair. The duration of nonoperative measures before electing direct repair depends on several factors including size of the defect, stability of the patient, and associated injuries. In most cases 10 to 14 days are required. Many surgeons favor early operative repair on the basis that operative morbidity and mortality are a lesser risk than that of meningitis, but this relationship has not been clearly established. Any patient with neurosurgical indications for operation will have repair of the fistula at the same time. Other definite indications for operation include profuse leaks, pneumocephalus, delayed and intermittent leaks, and recurrent meningitis.[13] In cases of intermittent leaks and leaks that cannot be demonstrated on imaging or dye studies, operative exploration may be the only way of identifying the fistula site.

Operative management of CSF fistula can be approached through an intracranial or extracranial route. The intracranial approach allows direct visualization of the dural tear and the adjacent cortical tissue. Also, following dural repair any graft placed over the defect will be tamponaded in place by the overlying brain tissue.[7] This approach requires a craniotomy and brain retraction, and has the risks of the associated morbidity and complications including anosmia. Extracranial techniques have less associated morbidity, although exposure of the anterior skull base is limited, and the leak must be patched from the outside. In selected cases a combined intracranial and extracranial approach can be used allowing superior exposure and better management of sinus injury. The choice of appropriate approach will be determined by the location of the leak, extent of the fracture, and the associated injuries.

Intracranial Approach

The intracranial approach is recommended when associated injuries mandate neurosurgical intervention and for leaks with very large defects. A third indication is in situations when multiple extracranial approaches have failed to successfully close the leak despite aggressive CSF drainage and supportive measures. The intracranial approach to the floor of the frontal fossa employs a frontal craniotomy through a coronal scalp incision. Bifrontal craniotomy has anosmia as a frequent complication, so a unilateral frontal craniotomy should be used when possible. The floor is approached intradurally, which allows greater exposure, avoids the need for tedious dural elevation, and facilitates repair of the dural defect with less risk of injuring adjacent cortex.[13] The extradural approach is well suited for leaks from the posterior wall of the frontal sinus. After identification of the dural defect, the associated bony defect should be evaluated. A large bony defect may require repair with bone or cartilage grafts. Dural defects have been repaired with many materials including temporalis fascia, fascia lata, lyophilized dura, and pericranial flaps (Fig. 9–2).

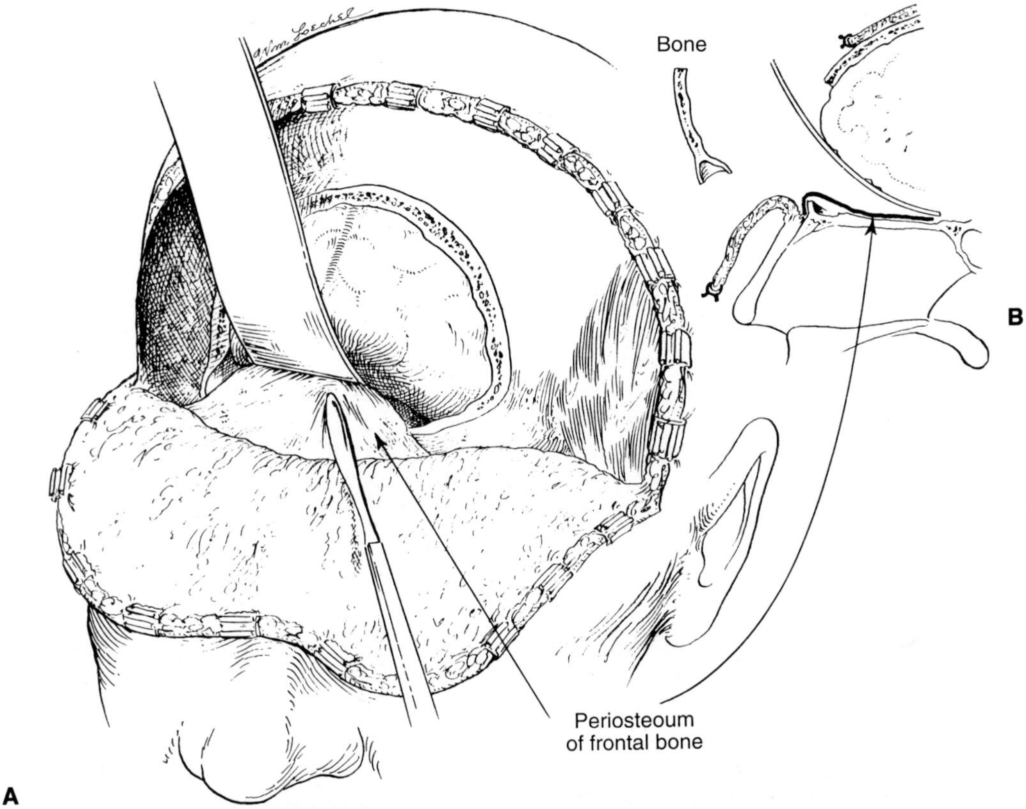

Figure 9–2. Intracranial approach for repair of CSF leak. (A). Surgical view of pericranial flap covering defect. (B). Saggital view of pericranial flap in place.

Extracranial Approach

Extracranial approaches have less associated morbidity and minimal risk of anosmia. These techniques are usually employed as initial operative intervention before the more invasive and morbid intracranial procedures are considered. A number of different approaches have been successfully applied including external approach for frontal sinus and ethmoidal defects, direct intranasal approach for cribriform plate or ethmoid leaks, and transseptal transsphenoidal approach for sphenoidal defects.[6–13,15,17,61–65] Most recently, intranasal endoscopic techniques have been utilized for a number of different locations with good success.[40,66–69] As an adjunct, fibrin glue is becoming more widely used in closure of CSF leaks, and has been used both intracranially and extracranially to augment closure of defects.[70,71]

Endoscopic Approach

Intranasal endoscopic repair is the preferred method for extracranial closure of small anterior cranial fossa posttraumatic CSF fistulas in our hands. Rigid endonasal telescopes provide superior illumination and visualization of the skull base. An additional advantage over the operating microscope is that endoscopes provide visualization of areas that are not in the direct line of vision. Also, endoscopic techniques allow precise placement of grafts and packing material over the defect.

If possible, local anesthesia with intravenous sedation is used for the procedure. This "twilight" anesthesia will eliminate the possibility of coughing and bucking during extubation, which could increase intracranial pressure and bleeding, and cause the graft to dislodge. Topical 4% cocaine solution or cocaine flakes are applied to the nasal mucosa and middle meatus using cotton pledgets or applicators. After decongestion (5 to 10 minutes), the middle turbinate and the uncinate process are injected with 1% xylocaine with 1:100,000 epinephrine. Five percent fluorescein for intrathecal injection should be available for cases where localization of the fistula is difficult.

A CSF fistula of the ethmoid roof is approached using an anterior to posterior dissection. After appropriate anesthesia, the middle turbinate is medialized to increase the view of the middle meatus, and complete nasal endoscopy is performed. The uncinate process is incised and resected. This exposes the infundibulum and the anterior wall of the ethmoid bulla. The ethmoid bulla is then entered and resected. The medial orbital wall should be identified and skeletonized. At this point, the posterior limit of the dissection is the basal (ground) lamella, which is the attachment of the middle turbinate to the skull base. This relatively dense ridge of bone separates the anterior and posterior ethmoid cells and extends from the middle turbinate to the lamina papyracea. If the defect is posterior, a complete posterior ethmoidectomy should be performed. The ground lamella is entered medially and inferiorly, and dissection continues along the edge of the middle turbinate until the anterior wall of the sphenoid sinus is identified. A complete posterior ethmoidectomy can now be safely performed using the previously identified landmarks with complete skeletonization of the skull base. The sphenoid sinus can be exposed, if needed, after completion of the posterior ethmoidectomy. The natural sphenoid ostium should be identified and then enlarged in a medial and inferior direction. If the natural ostium cannot be located, the sphenoid sinus can be entered 1 cm above the posterior choana at the posterior end of the middle turbinate.

Defects along the anterior ethmoidal roof may require complete dissection of the frontal recess. Improved exposure is achieved by removal of the anterior attachment of the middle turbinate and opening of the agger nasi cells. This allows complete exposure of the anterior skull base with identification of the anterior ethmoid artery and the ostium of the frontal sinus.

With skeletonization of the anterior skull base complete, the CSF fistula can be identified and managed. After the site of CSF leak is identified, mucosa surrounding the defect is removed approximately 5 mm in all directions (Fig. 9–3b).This is done because residual mucosa will prevent adhesion of the mucosal graft.[40] (Fig. 9–3c) A bone graft from the septum or turbinate can be fashioned to plug the defect before placement of the mucosal graft. Mucosal grafts can be harvested from the nasoseptum, turbinate, or buccal mucosa. A pedicled septal or turbinate flap can be used if a large graft is required.[72] The mucous membrane remaining around the defect is elevated, and the graft is placed over the defect with the edges tucked under the mucosal edge (Fig. 9–3d). Fibrin glue can be used to secure the position of the graft, and the graft is then held in place with Gelfoam impregnated with antibiotic ointment (Fig. 9–3e). The nose is then packed with antibiotic-impregnated gauze strips that are left in place for 3 to 7 days.

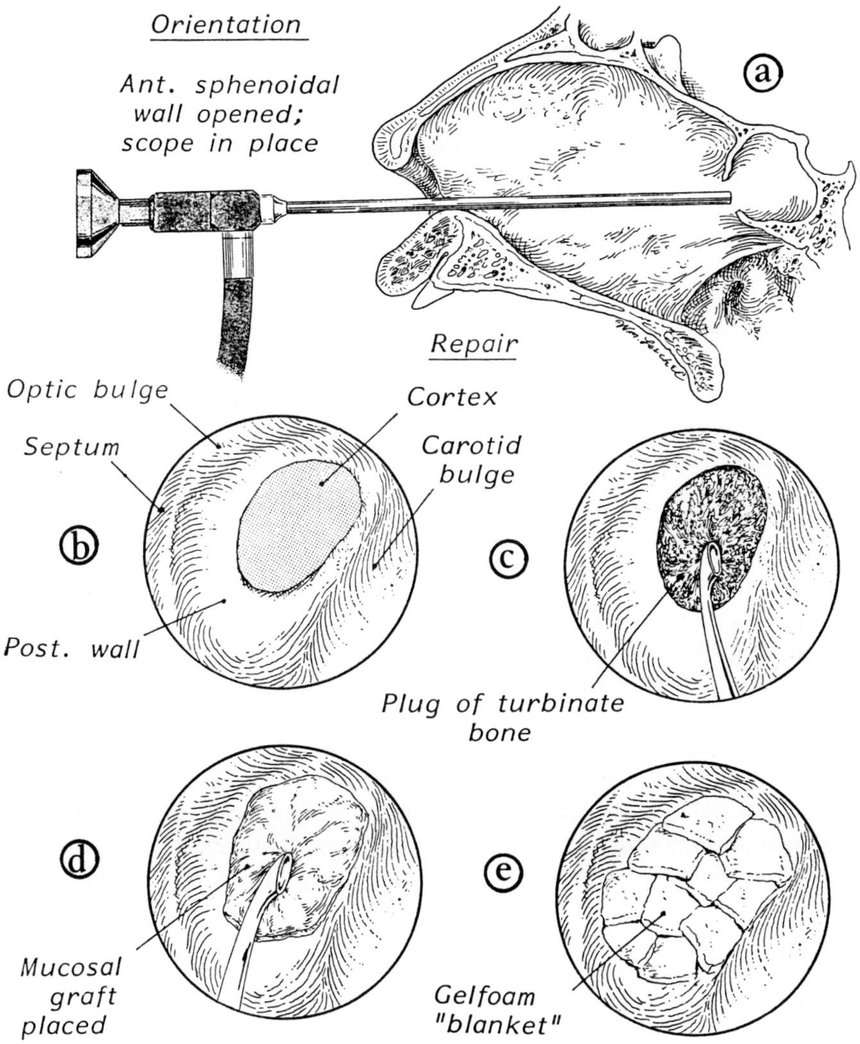

Figure 9–3. Endoscopic repair of CSF leak. (a). Endoscopic exposure of sphenoid sinus. (b). Endoscopic view of bony defect. (c). Placement of bone graft. (d). Placement of mucosal graft. (e). Covering graft with disolvable packing.

Postoperatively, patients are placed on broad spectrum antibiotics until the nasal packing is removed. Bed rest is instituted, and the head of bed is elevated to avoid increases in intracranial pressure. Additionally, stool softeners can be used and patients are instructed not to blow their nose. Alternatively, lumbar drainage can be instituted to assure low CSF pressure at the repair site.

Transsphenoidal Approach

Cerebrospinal fluid leaks from the sphenoid sinus can also be managed through a transseptal-transsphenoidal approach. We would prefer this technique when significant trauma to the septum requires operative repair or when preexisting septal deviation limits exposure to the sphenoid through the transnasal route. However, sphenoid fractures are usually the result of severe trauma and may be associated with multiple fractures and dural tears necessitating an intracranial or combined approach. A sublabial or transnasal approach to the nasoseptum can be used. A mucoperichondrial flap is developed and carried to the sphenoid rostrum. The cartilaginous septum is separated from its posterior and inferior bony attachments, and is swung out of the field in a trap-door fashion. The perpendicular plate of the ethmoid and the vomer is removed until adequate visualization of the anterior sphenoid is obtained and a self-retaining retractor is placed. An operating microscope is used to examine the sphenoid and to identify the ostium. The anterior wall and the intersinus septum are removed, exposing the posterior wall. The leak is identified and the sinus mucosa is removed surrounding the defect. A fascia or mucoperichondrial graft is placed over the dural tear and the sinus is packed with fat or muscle. The anterior sphenoid wall can be reconstructed, if desired, with bone or cartilage followed by the application of nasal packing.

External Approaches

Traumatic leaks of the cribriform plate and ethmoid roof that are very large, or where an endoscopic approach is unsuccessful, can be approached through an external ethmoidectomy or frontoethmoidal approach using the operating microscope for visualization.[73] A medial canthal incision is used, and for the frontoethmoidal approach, the floor of the frontal sinus is entered using a cutting bur, and the opening is enlarged to expose the floor to the nasofrontal duct. A complete ethmoidectomy is then performed using curettes and rongeurs. After completion of the ethmoidectomy, the dural defect is exposed and the leak can be repaired (Fig. 9–4b). A mucoperiosteal flap can be developed from the middle turbinate[61] or posterior septum[62,72] (Fig. 9–4c). The flap is rotated against the defect, reinforced with Gelfoam if desired (Fig. 9–4d), and secured with nasal packing for 5 to 10 days.[6]

Frontal Sinus

The posterior table of the frontal sinus is best approached using an osteoplastic flap technique, through fractures present from the inciting injury, or combination of both. This approach provides wide exposure of the posterior and inferior walls of the frontal sinus. The coronal incision affords excellent exposure and allows development of pericranial flaps that may be needed to repair dural defects. Limited fractures of the posterior table can be managed with obliteration of the sinus (as described in Chapter 3). The site of the CSF leak can be exposed by removal of bone fragments or thinning the bone with a diamond bur. The leak can then be directly repaired with suture or fascial grafts.[4,8,73]

Extremely comminuted posterior table fractures should be managed with a combined approach with neurosurgery. When reconstruction and stabilization of the posterior table are not feasible, the sinus is cranialized. The posterior table and all sinus mucosa are removed and the nasofrontal ducts are plugged with muscle or fascia. Dural defects are directly repaired and the brain is allowed to expand to fill the space occupied by the sinus.

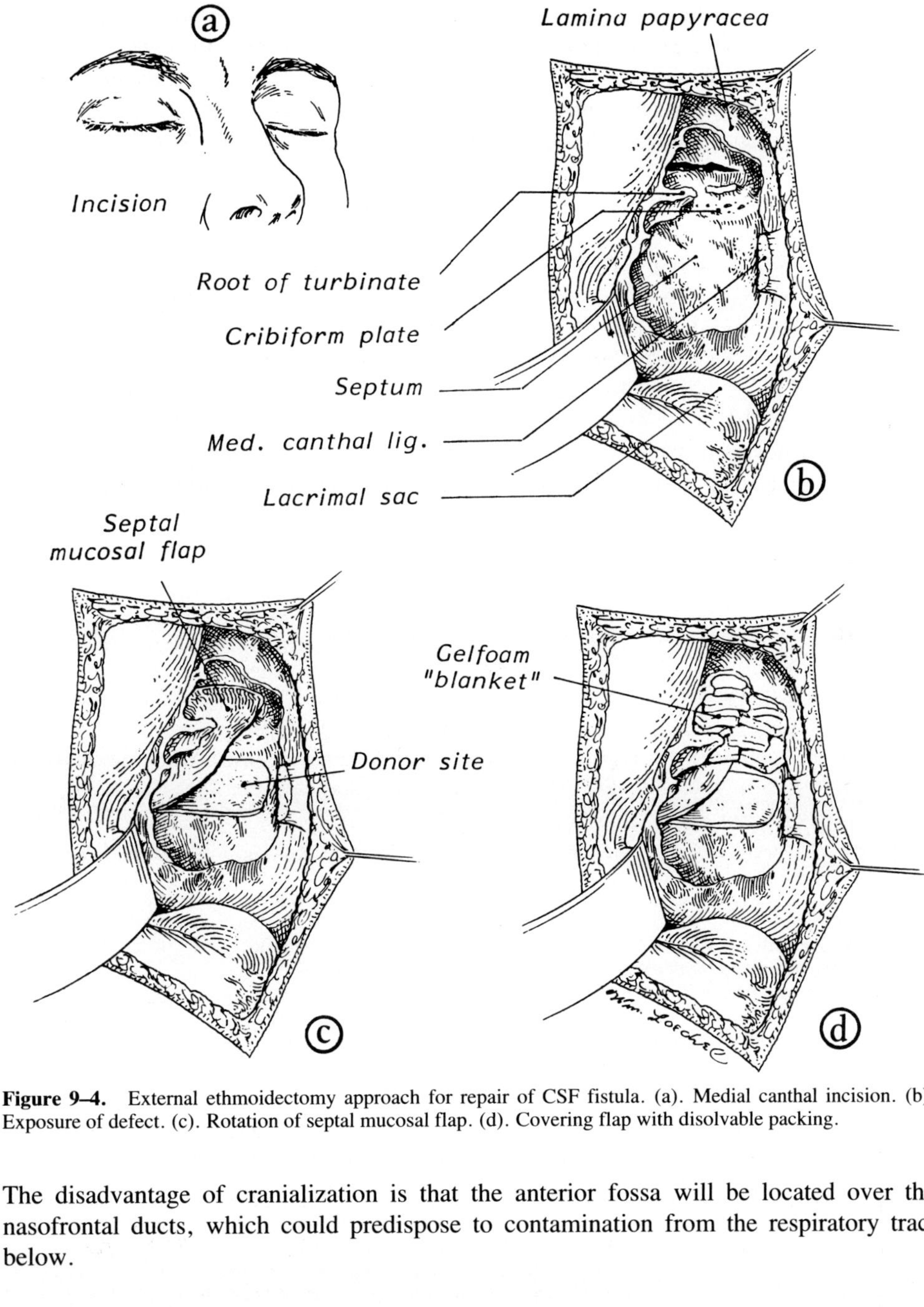

Figure 9–4. External ethmoidectomy approach for repair of CSF fistula. (a). Medial canthal incision. (b). Exposure of defect. (c). Rotation of septal mucosal flap. (d). Covering flap with disolvable packing.

The disadvantage of cranialization is that the anterior fossa will be located over the nasofrontal ducts, which could predispose to contamination from the respiratory tract below.

Nonlocalized Fistula

Occasionally, the site of a CSF fistula (an obvious leak or recurrent meningitis with a history of head trauma) cannot be established despite the use of multiple diagnostic tests.

Operative exploration of the anterior fossa through a bifrontal craniotomy has been the procedure used in these cases. If the fistula cannot be demonstrated, the cribriform plates are covered with grafts and the sphenoid sinus is obliterated.[7] The role of the extracranial approach for the nonlocalized fistula is not clearly defined.

PROGNOSIS

The analysis of outcome for CSF fistula is difficult owing to the varied nature of the injuries and management protocols and the different operative techniques. For those patients who are candidates for conservative management, success rates vary widely from 34 to 96%.[11,17,71] Success in operative closure of post-traumatic CSF fistulas has been reported from 60 to over 90%, with the occurrence of postoperative meningitis ranging from 1 to 10%.[6,11,17,71–73]

The prognosis for patients with closed (spontaneously or operatively) CSF fistula is excellent, having a small risk of delayed recurrence or meningitis. Many of these patients are lost to follow-up. However, any patient who has had closure of a CSF fistula should be followed for many years to check for delayed recurrence or complications of the closure such as mucocele and encephalocele.

REFERENCES

1. Willis T. Opera omina; cerebri antomia, nervorumque descriptio et usus. *Geneva*. 1676.
2. Morley TP, Hetherington RF. Traumatic cerebrospinal fluid rhinorrhea and otorrhea, pneumocephalus and meningitis. *Surg Gynecol Obstet*. 1957;104:88–98.
3. Grant FC. Intracranial aerocele following fracture of the skull. Report of a case and review of the literature. *Surg Gynecol Obstet*. 1923;36:251–255.
4. Dandy WE. Pneumocephalus (intracranial pneumatocele or aerocele). *Arch Surg*. 1926;12:949–982.
5. Dohlman G. Spontaneous cerebral spinal rhinorrhea. *Acta Otolaryngol (Suppl)*. 1948;67:20–23.
6. Calcaterra TC. Extracranial surgical repair of cerebrospinal rhinorrhea. *Anal Otol Rhinol Laryngol*. 1980;89: 108–116.
7. Spetzler RF, Zabramski JM. Cerebrospinal fluid fistulae: their management and repair. In: Youmans JR, ed. *Neurological Surgery*. Philadelphia, Pa: WB Saunders Co; 1990;74:2269–2289.
8. Mathog RH, Rosenberg Z. Complications in the treatment of facial fractures. *Otolaryngol Clin North Am*. 1976;9:533–552.
9. Lewin W. Cerebrospinal fluid rhinorrhea in closed head injuries. *Br J Surg*. 1954;42:1–18.
10. Briant TDR, Bird R. Extracranial repair of cerebrospinal fluid fistulae. *J Otolaryngol*. 1982;11:191–197.
11. Park JI, Strelzow VV, Friedman WH. Current management of cerebrospinal fluid rhinorrhea. *Laryngoscope*. 1983;93:1294–1300.
12. Charles DA, Snell D. Cerebrospinal fluid rhinorrhea. *Laryngoscope*. 1979;89:822–826.
13. Marentette LJ, Valentino J. Traumatic anterior fossa cerebrospinal fluid fistulae and craniofacial considerations. *Otolaryngol Clin North Am*. 1991;24:151–163.
14. Morley TP, Wortzman G. The importance of the lateral extensions of the sphenoidal sinus in post-traumatic cerebrospinal rhinorrhea and meningitis. *J Neurosurg*. 1965;22:326–332.
15. Chandler JR. Traumatic cerebrospinal fluid leakage. *Otolarngol Clin North Am*. 1983;16:623–632.
16. Lewin W. Cerebrospinal fluid rhinorrhea in nonmissle head injuries. *Clin Neurosurg*. 1966;12:237–252.
17. Westmore GA, Whittam DE. Cerebrospinal fluid rhinorrhea and its management. *Br J Surg*. 1982;69:489–492.
18. Russell T, Cummins BH. Cerebrospinal fluid rhinorrhea 34 years after trauma: a case report and review of the literature. *Neurosurgery*. 1984;15:705, 706.
19. Pandya PM, Keogh AJ. Traumatic cerebrospinal fluid rhinorrhea: a timely reminder. *Br J Accident Surg*. 1991;22:492–493.
20. Eljamel MS, Foy PM. Acute traumatic CSF fistulae: the risk of intracranial infection. *Br J Neurosurg*. 1991;4:381–385.

21. Hand WL, Sanford JP. Posttraumatic bacterial meningitis. *Ann Intern Med*. 1970;72:869–874.
22. Appelbaum E. Meningitis following trauma to the head and face. *JAMA*. 1960;173:1818–1822.
23. Caldicott WJH, North JB, Simpson DA. Traumatic cerebrospinal fluid fistulas in children. *J Neurosurg*. 1973;38:1–9.
24. Ignelzi RJ, Vanderark GD. Analysis of the treatment of basilar skull fractures with and without antibiotics. *J Neurosurg*. 1975;43:721–726.
25. Macgee EE, Cauthen JC, Brackett CE. Meningitis following acute traumatic cerebrospinal fluid fistula. *J Neurosurg*. 1970;33:312–316.
26. Klatersky J, Sadeghi M, Brihaye J. Antimicrobial prophylaxis in patients with rhinorrhea or otorrhea: a double blind study. *Surg Neurol*. 1976;6:111–114.
27. Kosoy J, Trieff NM, Winkleman P, Bailey BJ. Glucose in nasal secretions. *Arch Otolaryngol*. 1972;95:225–229.
28. Steedman DJ, Gordon M. CSF rhinorrhea: significance of the glucose oxidase strip test. *Injury*. 1987;18: 327–328.
29. Hull HF, Morrow G. Glucorrhea revisited. *JAMA*. 1975;234:1052–1053.
30. Katz RT, Kaplan PE. Glucose oxidase sticks and cerebrospinal fluid rhinorrhea. *Arch Phys Med Rehabil*. 1985;66:391–393.
31. Gadeholt H. The reaction of glucose-oxidase test paper in normal nasal secretion. *Acta Otolaryngol*. 1964;58:271–272.
32. Meurman OH, Irjala K, Suonpaa J, Laurent B. A new method for the identification of cerebrospinal fluid leakage. *Acta Otolaryngol*. 1979;87:366–369.
33. Fransen P, Sindic CJM, Thauvoy C, Laterre C, Stroobrandt G. Highly sensitive detection of beta-2 transferrin in rhinorrhea and otorrhea as a marker for cerebrospinal fluid leakage. *Acta Neurochir*. 1991;109: 98–101.
34. Oberascher G. A modern concept of cerebrospinal fluid diagnosis in oto- and rhinorrhea. *Rhinology*. 1988;26:89–103.
35. Yokoyama K, Masegawa M, Hasegawa M, Shiba K. Diagnosis of CSF rhinorrhea: detection of tau-transferrin in nasal discharge. *Otolaryngol Head Neck Surg*. 1988;98:328–332.
36. Reisinger PWM, Hochstraber K. The diagnosis of CSF fistulae on the basis of beta-2 transferrin by polyacrylamide gel electrophoresis and immunoblotting. *J Clin Chem Clin Biochem*. 1989;27:169–172.
37. Duckert LG, Mathog RH. Diagnosis in persistent cerebrospinal fluid fistulas. *Laryngoscope*. 1960;70:921–930.
38. Mahalay MS, Odom GL. Complication following intrathecal injection of fluorescein: case report. *J Neurosurg*. 1968;25:298, 299.
39. Wallace JD, Weintraub MI, Mattson RH, Rosnagle R. Status epilepticus as a complication of intrathecal fluorescein: a case report. *J Neurosurg*. 1972;36:659–670.
40. Mattox DE, Kennedy DW. Endoscopic management of cerebrospinal fluid leaks and cephaloceles. *Laryngoscope*. 1990;100:857–862.
41. Ozgen IH, Tekkek A, Erzen C. CT cisternography in evaluation of cerebrospinal fluid rhinorrhea. *Neuroradiology*. 1990;32:481–484.
42. Chow JM, Goodman D, Mafee M. Evaluation of CSF rhinorrhea by computerized tomography with metrizamide. *Otolaryngol Head Neck Surg*. 1989;100:99–105.
43. Ahmadi JA, Weiss M, Segall H. Evaluation of cerebrospinal fluid rhinorrhea by metrizamide computed tomographic cisternography. *Neurosurgery*. 1985;16:54–60.
44. Nabawi P, Mafee M, Phillips J, Capek V. The success rate of metrizamide CT in the evaluation of cerebrospinal fluid rhinorrhea. *Comput Radiol*. 1982;6:343–354.
45. Manelfe C, Cellerier P, Sobel D, Prevost C, Bonafe A. Cerebrospinal fluid rhinorrhea: evaluation with metrizamide cisternography. *AJR*. 1982;138:471–476.
46. Brandt F, Nahser HC, Hartjes H, Kunitsch G. The value of metrizamide CT cisternography in the diagnosis of CSF fistulae. *Acta Neurochir* (Wien). 1983;69:37–42.
47. Byrne JV, Ingram CE, Macvicar D, Sullivan FM, Uttley D. Digital subtraction cisternography: a new approach to fistula localization in cerebrospinal fluid rhinorrhea. *Neurol Neurosurg Psychiatry*. 1990;53: 1072–1075.
48. Takahashi T, Kunishio K, Sunami N. Localization of dural fistulas using metrizamide digital subtraction fluoroscopic cisternography. *J Neurosurg*. 1988;68:721–725.
49. Yamamoto Y, Mutsuga N, Aoki T. Identification of CSF fistulas by radionuclide counting. *AJNR*. 1990;11: 823–826.
50. Flynn BM, Butler S, Quinn R. Radionuclide cisternography in the diagnosis and management of cerebrospinal fluid leaks. *Med J Aust*. 1987;146:82–84.
51. Mamo L, Cophignon J, Rey A, Thurel C. A new radionuclide method for the diagnosis of posttraumatic fistulas. *J Neurosurg*. 1982;57:92–98.
52. Lantz EJ, Forbes GS, Brown ML, Laws ER. Radiology of cerebrospinal fluid rhinorrhea. *AJR*. 1980;135: 1023–1030.

53. Piepgras U, Huber G. Simultaneous isotope and CT cisternography in the diagnosis and evaluation of cerebral fluid rhinorrhea. *Acta Radiol Suppl (Stockh)*. 1986;369:290–291.
54. Magnaes B, Solheim D. Controlled overpressure cisternography to localize cerebrospinal fluid rhinorrhea. *Diag Nucl Med*. 1977;18:109–111.
55. Curnes JT, Vincent LM, Kowalsky RJ, Mccartney WH, Staab EV. CSF rhinorrhea: detection and localization using overpressure cisternography with Tc-99m-DTPA. *Radiology*. 1985;154:795–799.
56. Wakhloo AK, Velthoven VV, Schumacher M, Krauss JK. Evaluation of MR imaging, digital subtraction cisternography, and CT cisternography in diagnosing CSF fistula. *Acta Neurochir (Wien)*. 1991;111:119–127.
57. Shapiro SA, Scully T. Closed continuous drainage of cerebrospinal fluid via a lumbar subarachnoid catheter for treatment or prevention of cranial/spinal cerebrospinal fluid fistula. *Neurosurgery*. 1992;30:241–245.
58. Swanson SE, Chandler WF, Kocan MJ, Bogdasarian RS. Flow-regulated continuous spinal drainage in the management of cerebrospinal fluid fistulas. *Laryngoscope*. 1985;95:104–106.
59. Graf CJ, Gross CE, Beck DE. Complications of spinal drainage in the management of cerebrospinal fluid fistula. *J Neurosurg*. 1981;54:392–395.
60. Bret P, Hor F, Huppert J, Lapras C, Fischer G. Treatment of cerebrospinal fluid rhinorrhea by percutaneous lumboperitoneal shunting: review of 15 cases. *Neurosurgery*. 1985;16:44–47.
61. Yessenow RS, Mccabe BF. The osteo-mucoperiosteal flap in repair of cerebrospinal fluid rhinorrhea: a 20 year experience. *Otolaryngol Head Neck Surg*. 1989;101:555–558.
62. Montgomery WW. Cerebrospinal fluid rhinorrhea. *Otolaryngol Clin North Am*. 1973;6:757–771.
63. Obrien MD, Reade PC. The management of dural tear resulting from mid-facial fracture. *Head Neck Surg*. 1984;6:810–818.
64. Eljamel MSM, Foy PM. Post-traumatic CSF fistula, the case for surgical repair. *Br J Neurosurg*. 1990;4: 479–483.
65. Persky MS, Rothstein S, Breda S. Extracranial repair of cerebrospinal fluid fistula otorhinorrhea. *Laryngoscope*. 1991;101:134–136.
66. Papay FA, Maggiano H, Dominquez S. Rigid endoscopic repair of paranasal sinus cerebrospinal fluid fistulas. *Laryngoscope*. 1989;99:1195–1201.
67. Stankiewicz JA. Complications of endoscopic intranasal ethmoidectomy. *Laryngoscope*. 1987;97:1270–1273.
68. Stankiewicz JA. Complications in endoscopic intranasal ethmoidectomy: an update. *Laryngoscope*. 1989;99: 686–690.
69. Papay F, Benninger M. Transnasal transseptal endoscopic repair of sphenoidal cerebral spinal fluid fistula. *Otolaryngol Head Neck Surg*. 1989;101:595–597.
70. Nishihira S, Mccaffrey TV. The use of fibrin glue for the repair of experimental CSF rhinorrhea. *Laryngoscope*. 1988;98:625–627.
71. Pomeranz S, Constantini S, Umansky F. The use of fibrin sealant in cerebrospinal fluid leakage. *Neurochirurgia*. 1991;34:166–169.
72. Weisman RA. Septal chondromucosal flap with preservation of septal integrity. *Laryngoscope*. 1989;99: 267–271.
73. Mathog RH. *Atlas of Craniofacial Trauma*. Philadelphia, Pa: WB Saunders Co; 1992;72,73:363–372.

10

Nasal Obstruction

RICHARD L. ARDEN, M.D.
GARY B. COLEMAN, M.D.

Nasal obstruction following external trauma can be acute or delayed. Nasal airway obstruction resulting from sufficient external nasal trauma to produce internal derangement is related to mucosal hyperactivity and bony cartilaginous abnormalities. The most common cause of airway obstruction in the immediate posttraumatic period is nasal mucosal edema. Functional difficulties, however, may extend beyond the acute reactive phase. Illum's[1] study of 86 patients with nasal fractures revealed in incidence of objective nasal obstruction in 22%, 3 years status posttreatment. Chronic nasal obstruction typically involves nasoseptal abnormalities that may include deformities of:

1. Septum
   a. Osseous
      1) Perpendicular plate of ethmoid
      2) Vomer
   b. Cartilaginous
      1) Quadrangular cartilage
      2) Columella
2. Bony pyramid
   a. Maxillary spine/crest
   b. Frontal process of maxilla
   c. Paired nasal bones

PHYSIOLOGICAL CONSIDERATIONS

As the cross-sectional area of the nasal airway widens or narrows, airflow will decrease or increase, respectively (Bernoulli's principle). The change in flow will be directly proportional to the radius to the fourth power (Poiseuille's law). Thus, minor alterations in the cross-sectional area of the nasal airway following injury can result in major effects on airflow.

During low flow states nasal airflow is laminar; lateral airflow is nearly motionless compared with the rapid central current. With increased flow rates, however, flow becomes turbulent. In turbulent flow the air column progresses as a whole, with eddy currents and changing velocity. Greater pressure gradients are required in turbulent flow than in laminar flow to maintain identical flow rates.

CLINICAL EVALUATION

Assessment of nasal breathing begins with an appropriate history. The next step includes both external and internal examination. Rhinoscopy should involve careful assessment of the septum for deflections, duplications, thickenings, and buckling. Turbinate orientation, caliber, and degree of mucosal reactivity should be noted as well. Rhinoscopy should be performed before and after maximal decongestion with 2% phenylephrine or a similar vasoconstrictive agent. It then becomes possible to determine the relative importance of mucosal versus structural nasal obstruction.

Disturbances in nasal breathing are affected by many factors and conditions. Often, patients are not able to subjectively assess their own nasal breathing function.[2] Vaino-Mattila[3] observed 26% of normal individuals had septal deflections, yet only 10% had airway obstruction attributed to their deviations.

Rhinomanometry has been developed to objectively assess nasal obstruction. Nasal airway resistance, as discussed previously, is calculated via pressure and airflow measurements. McCaffrey[4] has shown a correlation between nasal resistance and subjective anatomic assessment. Bachmann[5] stressed the two tests should be performed together to provide useful information about nasal airflow.

MUCOSAL CHANGES

In the immediate posttraumatic phase, mucosal hyperactivity is the most common cause of nasal obstruction. Posttraumatic edema of the nasal mucosa and inflammatory secretions should be treated with both oral and topical decongestants. This form of partial nasal obstruction is transient, usually resolving spontaneously within several weeks.[6]

Inspissated blood or crusting may be present immediately posttrauma. Nasal mucosa should be treated actively and prophylactically with normal saline douches (Ocean Spray/ Nasal). Topical intranasal steroid sprays are not recommended in the acute posttraumatic period because of the possibility of retarding wound healing and promoting local infection.[7]

Following nasal trauma, both retained nasal packing and foreign body impaction must be considered as a possible cause for nasal obstruction and treated accordingly. Patients with preexisting nasal inflammatory disease may have an exacerbation of their underlying condition following trauma. Sherman[8] showed preexisting allergy lowered the chance of obtaining a "good airway" following nasal surgery. He reported 86% of 99 nonallergic patients undergoing nasal surgery ultimately achieved a "clear airway." This compares favorably to the 58 cases with preexisting allergy, of which only 68% were clear following nasal surgery.

Beekhuis[9] found approximately 10% of patients postrhinoplasty had persistent nasal obstruction due to "vasomotor" turbinate hypertrophy. Roos[10] believed this "obstructive rhinitis" to be the result of dysfunction in vagal and orthosympathetic turbinate innervation. This obstruction began immediately postoperatively and persisted indefinitely. Topical intranasal steroids and anticholinergics remain the treatment of choice for medical management.

An alternate technique of administering intranasal steroid therapy is by intraturbinal injections. Beekhuis[8] and Baker and Strauss[11] report 90% and 80% relief of symptoms, respectively, following intraturbinal injections. Allen[12] does not consider turbinate injections beneficial on a long-term basis if steroidal nasal sprays do not offer initial relief.

Eleven cases of blindness have been reported following turbinate injection and are thought to be secondary to retinal embolization or vasospasm. The mechanism appears to be inadvertent intra-arterial injections into the ethmoidal arteries with retrograde flow to the ophthalmic artery.[13] To preclude this complication it is recommended to utilize steroid preparations with size particles of less than 10 μm,[14] aspirate before injection, use small needles, and inject without undue pressure following mucosal decongestion.[15]

SEPTAL HEMATOMA

Complete nasal airway obstruction resulting from septal hematoma formation can occur following nasal trauma. If the nasal mucosa remains intact, bleeding can develop in the submucoperichondrial plane of the septum. With septal fractures, blood can dissect to the opposite side and form bilateral hematomas. If the hematoma is not drained, the sequelae of cartilage necrosis, abscess formation, and distortion of the nasal architecture can occur. Septal cartilage is dependent on the mucoperichondrium for its nutrition. Pressure on the cartilage, coupled with a reduced blood supply from the elevated perichondrium, makes the tissue more susceptible to ischemic necrosis and infection. Cartilage loss can occur in 3 to 4 days, leading ultimately to saddle deformity and columellar retraction.

Incidence

Although septal hematomas can occur in all age groups, it is a more frequent complication of nasal injury in children. It is suspected that the softer cartilage of children predisposes to a more significant injury without fracture.[16] East and O'Donaghue[17] reported a 2% incidence of bilateral hematoma in 50 consecutive children with nasal injury. Holt[18] reported only one case of major septal hematoma in 112 consecutive adults with nasal fracture.

Diagnosis

Diagnosis requires careful endonasal examination after topical decongestion with 4% cocaine hydrochloride. General anesthesia is usually required for children younger than 12 years old for diagnosis as well as treatment.[18] Persistent pain, in the form of anterior midline headache,[19] and nasal obstruction secondary to septal swelling are cardinal symptoms. Usually the nasoseptum in children is straight and measures 2 to 4 mm thick.[20] Palpation with a cotton-tipped applicator will determine compressibility. Aspiration with a 27-gauge needle will be diagnostic.

Management

Management should include immediate drainage. One or several small tangential incisions should be made paralleling the nasoseptal blood supply (septal branch of superior labial, anterior ethmoidal, and sphenopalatine arteries). Drainage is through the mucoperichondrium to allow evacuation of blood and prevention of further accumulation. In early cases of hematoma formation, aspiration alone can be performed under direct vision with an 18-gauge needle.

To preclude further hematoma formation, the surgeon should leave the incision on the septum open or suture a 1/4-in Penrose drain into the incision site. Suction drainage can be applied but gentle, firm pressure from plastic splints or intranasal packing is simple and effective. Antibiotic coverage is essential to prevent infection. Kern[21] recommends reexamination within 24 hours if treated on an outpatient basis.

An unrecognized septal hematoma, even in the absence of infection, can lead to cartilage necrosis after only 24 to 48 hours.[22] Rapid aseptic liquefaction is thought secondary to the inflow of tissue collagenases.[22] Healing following cartilage loss is by fibrous tissue formation, not chondroneogenesis. Saddle-nose deformity (dorsal strut affected), columellar retraction (caudal strut affected), septal perforation, and nasal base widening can be resultant sequelae.

If significant cartilage loss exists at the time of treatment, open techniques are usually indicated. Holt[18] has recommended immediate autogenous auricular cartilage grafts to disrupt the fibrous tissue contractile forces. If sufficient, however, the patient's own septal cartilage may be reimplanted. Both rib cartilage[23] and the perpendicular plate of the ethmoid have also been suggested as appropriate implants.[20]

SEPTAL ABSCESS

Fortunately, infections of the nose rarely occur following trauma. Excellent regional blood supply accounts for this low infection rate. Septal hematomas are particularly susceptible to abscess formation. Patients incapacitated by chronic disease or malnutrition are also predisposed to infection following trauma.

Early diagnosis of nasal infection and timely treatment remain critical. Persistent pain, elevated temperature, edema, and erythema are important signs and symptoms. Adequate drainage is important and nasal packing should be used sparingly. Intravenous broad spectrum antibiotics are administered to cover nasal flora as well as *Staphylococcus aureus*, pending culture and sensitivity results. Local heat application is also recommended. Life-threatening complications include meningitis, cerebral abscess, septic cavernous sinus thrombosis, subdural empyema, endocarditis, central nervous system histoplasmosis, and localized cerebritis.[24–29]

Toxic shock syndrome (TSS) has also been reported following submucous resection and rhinoplasty.[30] This results from *S aureus* produced exotoxin (TSS toxin 1). Jacobson and Kasworm[31] attribute the pathogenesis of TSS to four unlikely events including: (1) colonization or infection with *S aureus*; (2) TSS toxin 1 production; (3) alteration in the skin or mucosa at the site of colonization; and (4) absence of the antibody or susceptibility to the toxin affects.

Cartilage necrosis may ensue within 24 to 48 hours even in the absence of abscess formation.[22] Nasoseptal reconstruction is required to prevent the sequelae of functional and cosmetic complications. Kemble[32] reported that in children up to age 6 years, the nasoseptum was necessary to preclude maxillary hypoplasia.

Huizing[33] proposed immediate septal reconstruction with autogenous perpendicular plate bone grafts at the time of incision and drainage. Pirsig[34] concluded that saddle- nose deformity is largely prevented by immediate reconstruction with homologous cartilage in the acute phase of septal abscess. There remains the theoretical concern, however, that cartilage resorption will occur with direct communication of the free graft with the contaminated pocket.

ADHESIONS

Following nasal trauma, continued nasal obstruction can be related to intranasal synechiae formation. Because most nasal fractures are associated with lacerations of the mucosa, scar-band formation is not uncommon. Mucosal abrasions from nasal packing can also be responsible.[9]

Intranasal adhesions usually present between the lateral nasal wall (usually the inferior turbinate) and the septum. Alternatively, or concomitantly, the contractile forces of scar maturation may cause septal deflections.

Management

Treatment can include simple division of small adhesions following local anesthesia with 4% cocaine hydrochloride. Synechiae formation can also be reduced in the acute phase post-trauma with meticulous nasal hygiene and vasoconstrictor agents. The judicious use of nasal saline douches clears fibrin strands that form the basis of adhesions.[35]

As previously discussed, more mature synechiae will require interposition of a Silastic stent between opposing surfaces. For extensive adhesions, the plastic plate should remain sutured to the septum until epithelization is complete (2 weeks).[9]

TURBINATE HYPERTROPHY

Persistent, posttraumatic nasal obstruction can result from hypertrophic inferior turbinate mucosa. Septal deflections following nasal insult may result in compensatory turbinate hypertrophy. Turbinate hypertrophy may also be related to vasomotor dysfunction or unrecognized allergic rhinitis. Following rhinoplasty, prolonged nasal obstruction may be related to a vasomotor turbinate hypertrophy. Haight and Cole[36] reported that two thirds of nasal resistance occurred in the bony cavum and was produced largely from mucosal congestion of the anterior end of the inferior turbinate.

Management

Surgical management of nasal obstruction secondary to hypertrophied inferior turbinates has included a plethora of treatment modalities. Radical trimming of the inferior turbinate remains a controversial technique owing to the possible loss of physiological functioning.[37] However, Wight et al[38] compared anterior resection and radical trimming of the inferior turbinate in 118 patients with chronic rhinitis. Although radical trimming significantly decreased both subjective and objective nasal obstruction, anterior trimming alone decreased objective nasal resistance only. Courtiss et al[39] have recommended partial inferior turbinate resection. They reported only two failures in 88 patients following turbinectomy. No untoward sequelae or intranasal pathology resulted.

More recently, the method of submucous resection of the inferior turbinate has been undertaken to provide a more physiological outcome. Thickened bone can be removed while sparing functioning mucosa, affording more consistent, long-lasting, and predictably favorable results.

Finally, Thompson[40] reported the effectiveness and safety of surgical reduction of the inferior turbinate in 22 children with severe nasal obstruction.

NASOSEPTAL DEFORMITY

Anatomic Considerations

The nasoseptum is the single most important structure for determining both the functional and cosmetic aspects of the nose. In patients following nasal trauma (external or iatrogenic), residual deformity with or without nasal obstruction may persist. This may include those patients treated in the acute phase with open or closed reduction of nasoseptal fractures.

Mayell[41] reported good functional and cosmetic results in only one third of the cases selected for closed reduction. In Harrison's[42] retrospective review of 40 cases, only 13 were found to have obtained perfect results. Harrison attributes the progressing deformity to a lack of centralization of the displaced septal fracture. Murray and Moran[43] reported a failure rate of 30 to 40%. Murray et al[44] in a subsequent article attributed the poor results to an unrecognized and unmanaged C-shaped septal fracture. They also attributed late failures (deviations) to the interlocking of these fractured septal segments, which would drag the mobile nasal bones toward their initially displaced positions. Murray and Moran[45] acknowledged that the septal component of the nasal fracture must be reduced in an open fashion when there is significant deviation of the bony dorsum. However, according to Fry,[46,47] who evaluated cadaveric cartilage and retrospective clinical data, injury to the septal surface can activate interlocked stresses that can cause the cartilage to twist (Fig. 10–1).

Timing

If residual nasal obstruction or deformity persists following closed reduction of nasoseptal fractures, site-specific open reduction should be performed as soon as possible. Patients who desire a reduction rhinoplasty when a posttraumatic deformity is to be corrected will require a controlled septorhinoplasty. The ideal period for such corrective surgery is usually 3 to 6 months postinjury.[48–51] Mathog[52] considers earlier repair if there is (1) obstruction; (2) a simple deformity requiring minimal correction; and (3) severe deformity affecting the patient's well-being.

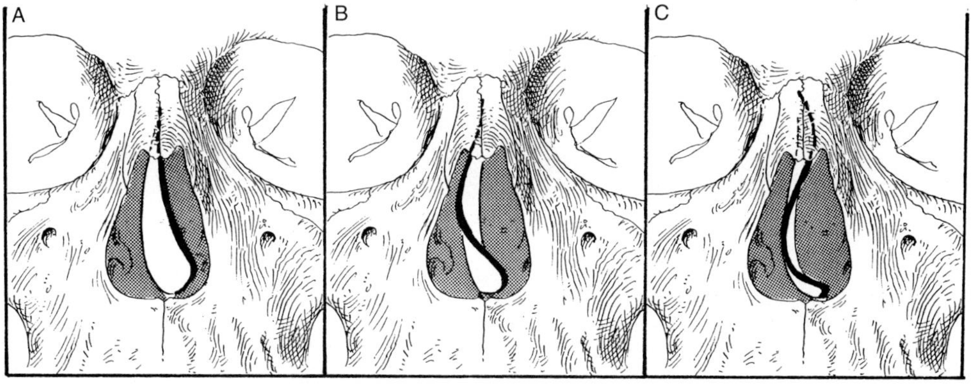

Figure 10–1. Various septal configurations created subsequent to asymmetrical internal stresses on quadrangular cartilage.

In children, timing of revisional surgery remains controversial. If the deformity is minimal, surgery can be delayed until the child is 15 to 16 years of age when facial growth is nearly complete. However, if significant deformity or dysfunction exists, early intervention is indicated.[53]

Management

Open techniques to correct previously existing nasal deformity or malunion are via intercartilaginous or intracartilaginous incisions that are extended into a transfixion incision. The same transfixion incision also allows exposure for septoplasty. Marginal incisions are reserved for cases in which small implants are to be inserted over the cartilages (and/or dorsum) and for employing tip projection techniques.[52] An alternative technique using open rhinoplasty is afforded via transcolumellar and marginal incisions. This technique is best used when the deformity is complex or there is confusion as to the etiology of the deformity.[52]

Septoplasty, employing separate pockets, is carried out through either an intermembranous incision (between the columella and septum) or a Killian incision placed 1.5 to 2.0 cm cephalad to the caudal border of the septum. These incisions should be positioned caudal to the area of deflection (Fig. 10–2).

The dorsal nasal skin is elevated from the upper lateral cartilages (ULC) in the supraperichondrial plane, with further cephalad dissection proceeding in the subperiosteal plane to expose the nasal bones directly. Care should be exercised in the extent of lateral undermining, such that the soft tissue is elevated only slightly beyond the fracture lines. In this way, some degree of external stabilization is afforded by the soft tissue/periosteal attachments.

Septoplasty is usually performed at this stage in the combined septorhinoplasty. A mucoperichondrial flap should be raised on one side of the septum. Once the deviation is encountered, a crossover incision is made through the septal cartilage. Dissection is continued subperichondrially and subperiosteally cephalad on the contralateral side. Devi-

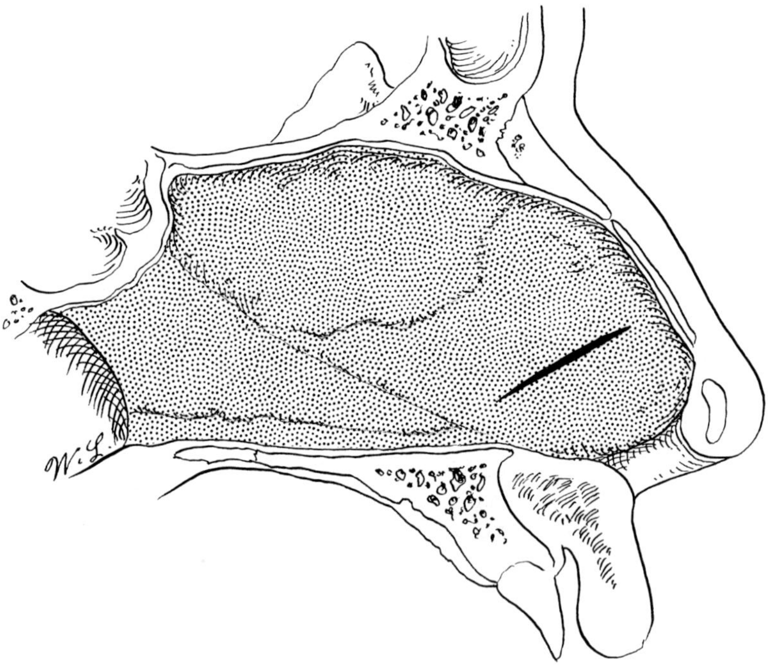

Figure 10–2. Classic Killian incision employed for access to septal space.

ated portions of cartilage and/or bone can be removed with Takahashi rongeurs. Harrison[42] noted good results with resection of both horizontal and vertical components along the c-shaped septal fracture line. Occasionally, an inferior slip of cartilage must be removed from the maxillary crest to allow cartilage rotation back to the midline. Scoring, or even wedge resection, can release interlocked stresses on the concave side of the cartilaginous septum.[46,47] Reshaping is accomplished by creating partial cuts in the concavity of the cartilage with a Beaver knife (Fig. 10–3). In addition, a small batten of surplus cartilage or vomerine bone on the unscored side can act as a reinforcing batten[54] (Fig. 10–4). Morselization, as described by Rubin,[55] is another method to straighten bowed cartilage but is discouraged in the most caudal aspect of the septum owing to the potential for loss of tip support.

Finally, several full-thickness cartilage incisions, parallel to the maxillary crest, can be created. These free segments can then be maintained in a midline position using suture techniques described by Wright.[56] A similar suture technique is useful for maintaining the septum in position along the maxillary crest and anterior nasal spine (Fig. 10–5).

The rhinoplasty portion of the procedure is now carried out, as indicated, for associated deformities. Modeling of the nasal tip and dorsal hump reduction are performed before addressing the nasal pyramid. Management of bony defects significant enough to produce nasal obstruction requires mobilization and repositioning of the nasal bones. Fine, narrow osteotomies are carried out after extending the plane of undermining beyond the fracture zone(s).

Schultz,[51] however, reported periodically accomplishing closed reduction of nasal fractures 1 or more years following surgery. He proposed an inverse correlation between

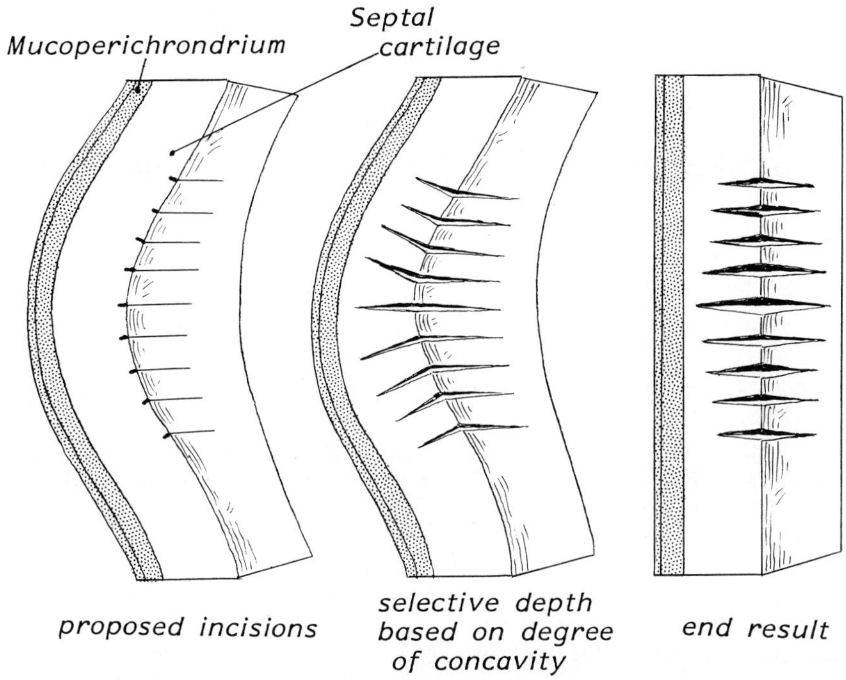

Figure 10–3. Release of internal stresses by parallel incisions on concave surface of septal deflection.

displacement of the bony fragments and strength of the fibrous union, thereby allowing for closed manipulation in many cases.

Paramedian osteotomies are performed first, initially on the depressed side,[57] utilizing a graduated 6 to 7 mm osteotome. The osteotome is inserted at the caudal border of the nasal bone, along the septum, and driven in the paramedian plane to the glabellar angle. Thomas et al[58] described a fading, medial oblique osteotomy to prevent the formation of

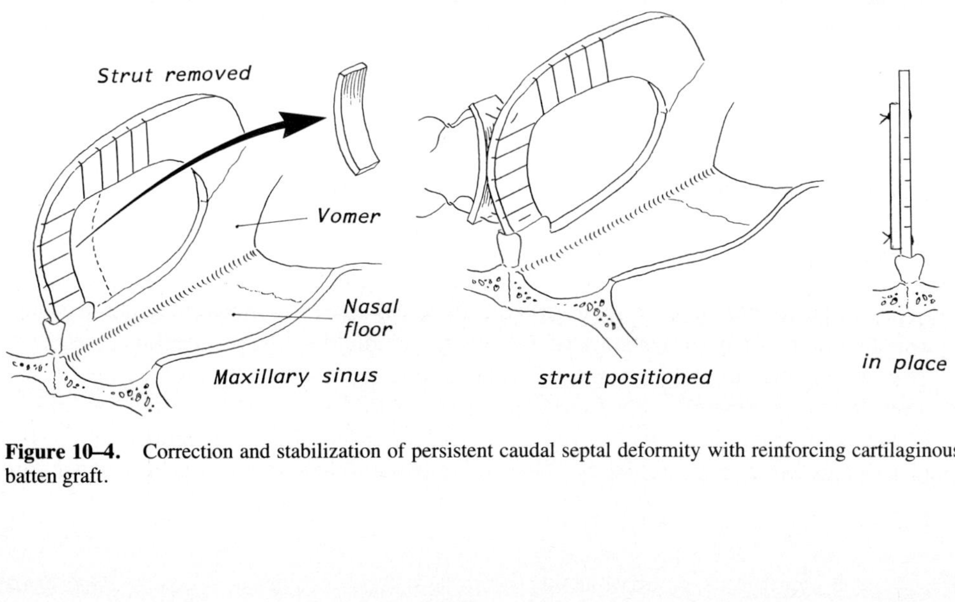

Figure 10–4. Correction and stabilization of persistent caudal septal deformity with reinforcing cartilaginous batten graft.

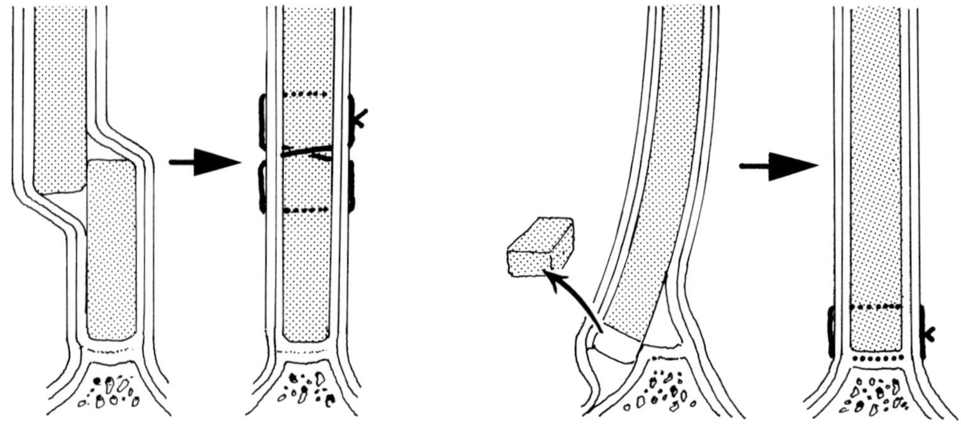

Figure 10–5. Maintenance of septal repositioning with suture fixation. (Left). Figure-of-eight suture employed to prevent overriding of free cartilage edges. (Right). Horizontal mattress suture through septal cartilage and maxillary crest periosteum to stabilize inferior septal attachment.

the rocker deformity. The osteotome is directed toward the nasion, outlining an oblique fade. Sharp instrumentation and precise execution are required as there exists a propensity for uncontrolled fracture at the time of osteotomy, usually occurring in the lines of previous fracture.

Lateral osteotomies can be performed with offset saws (discouraged), or more preferably, with 3 to 4 mm osteotomes. A stab incision is made just caudal to the inferior turbinate over the margin of the pyriform aperture. Ideally, the osteotomy should only transect periosteum and bone on the inner side of the nose, leaving the lateral investing periosteum intact. The osteotome is driven approximately 6 mm to the inferior margin of the nasomaxillary process. The osteotome is then repositioned and advanced superomedially to the level of the intercanthal line where the medial osteotomy is joined. This low-curved, lateral osteotomy leaves a triangular piece of bone at the pyriform aperature, thereby avoiding steplike prominences, and precludes narrowing in the region of the nasal vault that can contribute to nasal obstruction[59] (Fig. 10–6). The report by Rozner[60] detailed this complication resultant from restriction of the lateral bony nasal inlet. He reported an 80% relief following excision of the anterior free margin of the bony nasal pyramid.

SEPTAL PERFORATIONS

Etiology

Nasoseptal perforation (NSP) involves full-thickness losses of quandrangular cartilage (most commonly) and/or portions of the vomeroethmoidal bones, together with their respective mucoperichondrial/mucoperiosteal coverings. Despite its low metabolic rate and nutritive requirements, septal cartilage once denuded of its blood supply will invariably undergo chondrolysis, which eventuates in perforation. The exact incidence of NSP is unknown and difficult to estimate because most perforations are small, usually asymptom-

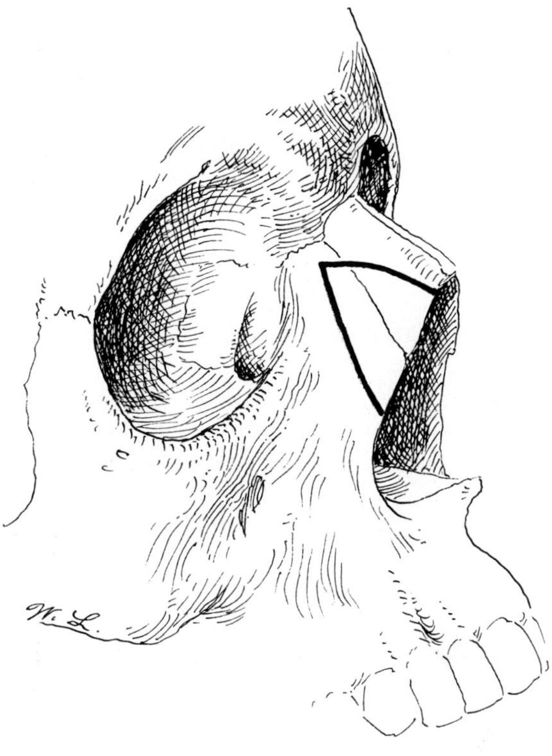

Figure 10–6. Proposed lines of osteotomy for resetting of bony nasal pyramid employing fading medial oblique and curved low lateral osteotomies.

atic, and either go undetected or unreported. In the series of Ismail[61] and Frey and Weinang,[62] this incidence was reported at slightly over 1%.

Although multiple causes of NSP exist,[63–65] direct nasal trauma accounts for the largest category, of which prior nasoseptal surgery is the most common cause. In Facer and Kern's[66] study of 73 patients with septal perforation, surgical trauma accounted for 48% and external trauma 19% of the cases. Similar studies by Brain,[67] Fairbanks and Fairbanks,[68] and Pallanch et al[69] demonstrate collective ranges of incidence of 30 to 80% and 10 to 20% for surgical trauma and external trauma, respectively. Meyer and Berghaus[70] subdivided traumatically induced perforations into three broad categories: (1) facial macro and septal microtraumas; (2) iatrogenic septal defects, and (3) occupationally induced causes.

Macrotraumas to the septum typically involve nasoseptal or septal fractures with resultant hematoma formation within the septal space. Inoculation of this nutrient medium by pathogenic bacteria may result in septal abscess formation and subsequent cartilage necrosis. This process may ensue as early as 24 to 48 hours later if not recognized and managed appropriately.[71] Penetrating stab and gunshot wounds to the nose are a rarely occurring cause of septal macrotrauma.

Septal microtraumas, which include nose picking, and chronic exposures to dry air, heat, and dust have, as their common denominator, mucosal irritation, inflammation, and eventual superficial ulceration. As a result of compromised local mucosal blood supply, ischemic changes to the intervening cartilage develop leading to septal perforation. Iatrogenic perforations typically occur following improperly executed septoplasty. This is particularly true when a Killian submucous resection is employed in conjunction with a swivel knife, where the potential for bilateral mucosal tears is increased. Even with careful technique, the mucosal thinning and surface desiccation overlying sharp septal spurs or deflections predispose to iatrogenic injury during flap elevation. Previous surgical exploration with scarred tissue planes, or improper elevation in a supraperichondrial plane, further compounds the risk. Occupational exposures to inhalent irritants leading to NSP have been well described[64,72] and follow pathophysiological sequences similar to septal microtraumas.

Medical Management

It is generally recognized that the majority of patients with NSPs remain asymptomatic. When symptoms do occur, the size and location of the perforation are often determinate of degree. In his series of 67 patients, Brain[67] demonstrated symptomatic correlation with increases in size of the NSP to be 10%, 33%, and 81% for small, medium, and large defects, respectively. Based on Cottle's topographical classification of the nasoseptum, Brain also showed a tendency for increased likelihood of symptoms the further anterior the perforation was. Bridger[73] offered the explanation that anterior perforations are subject to inspired air that has limited time to be warmed and humidified compared with more posteriorly situated perforations. Kuriloff,[71] in summarizing three clinical reports of 334 patients with NSP, found the following symptomatic incidence: crusting (68%), epistaxis (61%), obstruction (45%), pain (22%), whistling (14%), postnasal discharge (7%), rhinorrhea (6%), hyposmia (4%), and voice change (1%). With the exception of whistling, which is associated with smaller anterior perforations and higher associated flow rates (as predicted by Poiseuille's law), the remaining symptoms are typically seen with larger perforations. As a result of crosschambered shunting through the septal perforation, a portion of the laminar flow is converted into turbulent flow with energy lost to eddy currents (Fig. 10–7). Increased turbulence against the edges of the perforation and its opposing mucosa along the lateral nasal vault creates excessive drying, mucosal irritation, and ciliary dysfunction. Reflex mucosal gland hyperactivity, stagnant secretions, and impaired mucociliary clearance contribute to putrid fetor, malodorous discharge, and chronic rhinitis. Subjective nasal obstruction, even in the face of limited septal perforations, has been frequently observed. Multiple causes have been cited to explain this phenomenon:

1. Effective transnasal airflow diminishes at any given intranasal pressure drop due to diverted upstream airflow (ie, through perforation).
2. The presence of crusts, clots, or mucosal inflammatory edema will compromise nasal vault dimensions.
3. Increased intranasal resistances created by the aforementioned conditions may result in premature nasal valve collapse.

In cases of large NSPs involving the dorsal and caudal cartilaginous struts, development of a saddle-nose deformity and columellar retraction may ensue. A ptotic nasal tip, created through loss of caudal support, can limit airflow at the level of the external nares whereas a retrograde overly rotated tip, created through loss of dorsal support, can limit airflow in the mid- cartilaginous vault at the level of the nasal valve (Fig. 10–8).

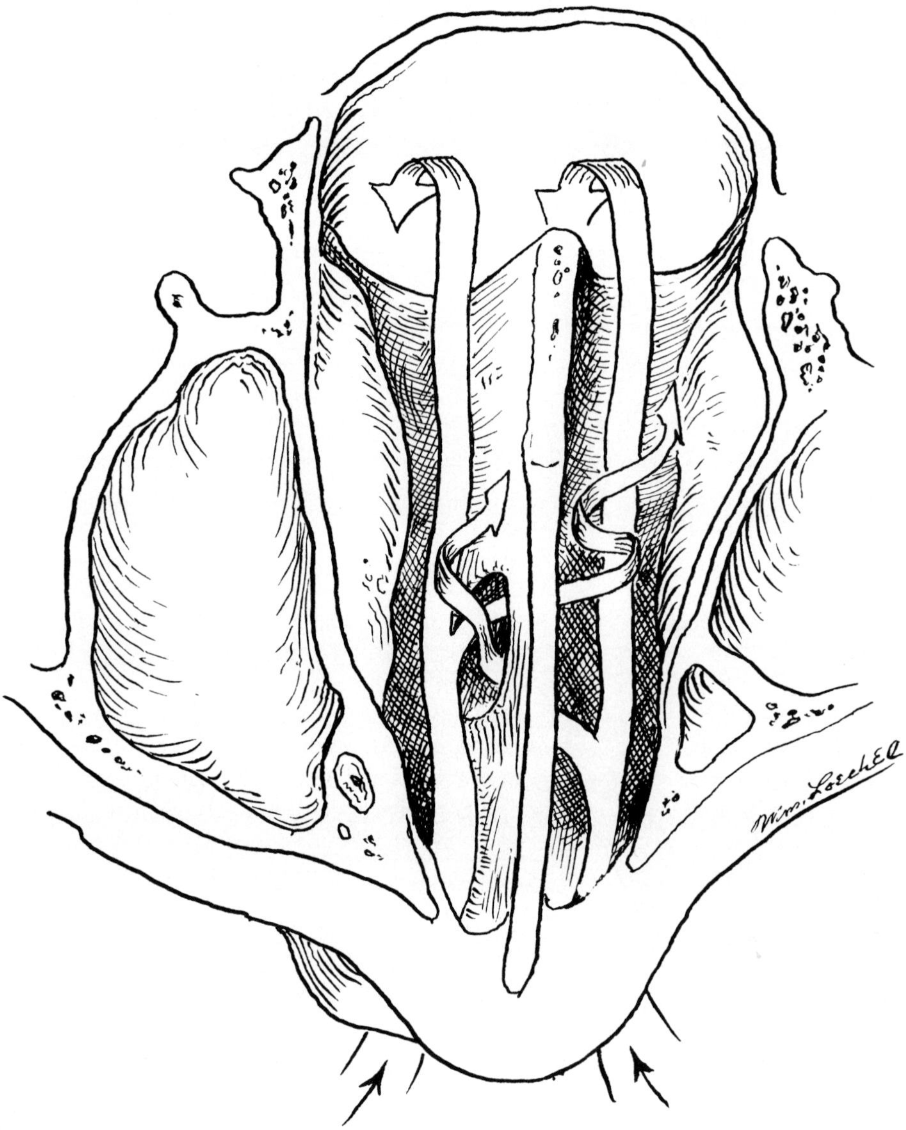

Figure 10–7. Turbulent airflow and eddy currents created through crosschambered airflow shunting.

Irrespective of cause, any symptomatic NSP should be managed initially with a trial of nasal moisturizing sprays and/or irrigations. Commercially available saline sprays (ie, Ayr, Nasal, Ocean Nasal) can be used as needed but tend to evaporate quickly. The addition of propylene glycol to a 0.9% saline solution (25% vol/vol), or Karo syrup (100 mL/L), will provide enhanced duration of moisturizing effect. Extended protection can be afforded by the addition of emollients (ie, petrolatum jelly, bacitracin ointment, Ponaris oil). Adjunctively, Goodman and Strelzow[74] advocated "putting the nose to rest" by plugging the nasal vestibules with ointment-impregnated cotton for 3 hours a day, thereby

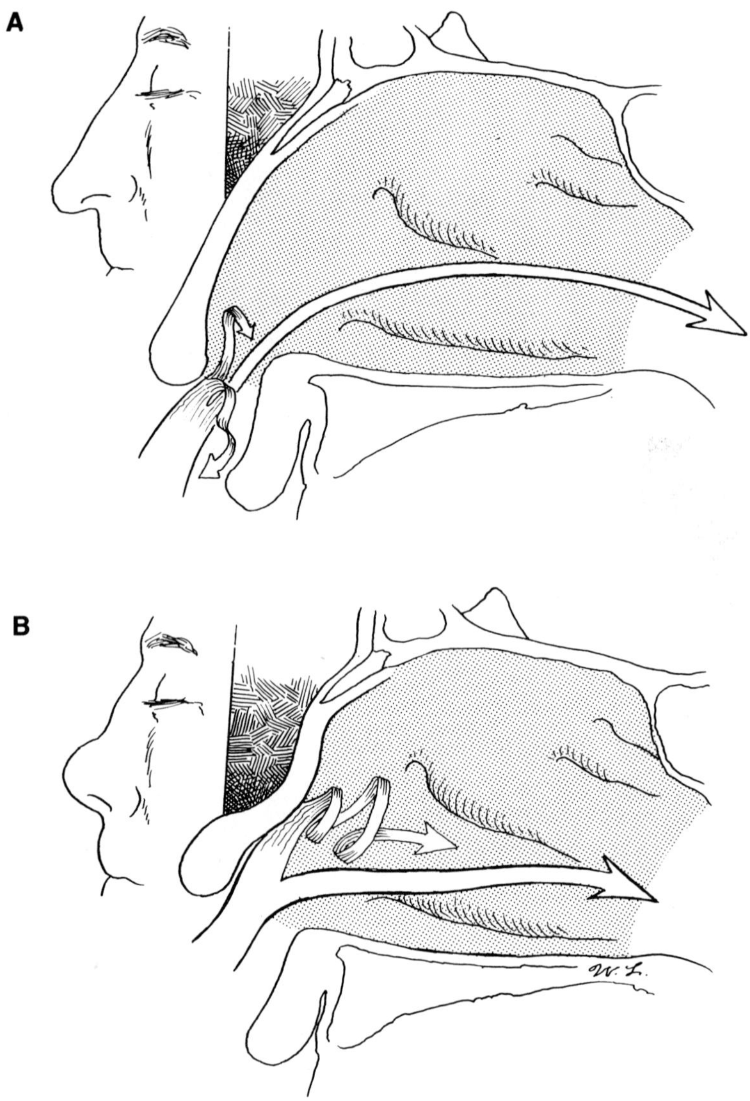

Figure 10–8. Effects of nasal tip positioning on inspiratory airflow. (A). Ptotic tip creating partial obstruction at the level of nasal vestibule. (B). Saddle deformity creating obstruction at middorsal cartilaginous vault.

softening existent crusts. In cases of active discharge (particularly malodorous), or in cases of secondary sinus involvement, a 2-week course of appropriate antimicrobial therapy is indicated. Once the local infection has been eradicated, institution of short-term topical nasal steroids will help quiesce the background of friable, chronically inflamed, edematous mucosa often seen.

Obturators

Patients who present poor operative risks (ongoing or long-term illicit nasal substance abusers, patients with active granulomatous disease, coexistent collagen vascular disorder, recent history of local carcinoma), resist surgical intervention or have failed prior surgical attempts, or are not symptomatically optimized with nasal hygiene maneuvers remain candidates for septal prosthetic placement (Fig. 10–9). Depending on the size and location of the NSP, placement of the prosthesis may be counterproductive, however (Fig. 10–10). Mechancial closure of perforations located high in the cartilaginous vault may obstruct or compromise nasal valve function. Septal deformities may result in poor coaptation of the prosthetic phlange against the perforation margin and exacerbate nasal obstruction. Finally, large or irregularly shaped NSPs may lend themselves to difficult or improper fitting, thereby resulting in migration, extrusion, or poor tolerance. The use of template impressions[66,67] and/or computed tomography scanning[69] may be of assistance in prosthetic fabrication.

The long-term tolerance of septal obturators has been met with variable results. In the study of 73 patients by Facer and Kern,[66] with follow-up evaluations between 6 months and 4 years, a 38% success rate was reported within the first 12 months and 96% thereafter if retained. The earlier failures were attributed by the authors, in part, to the less durable construct initially used. Of the 171 patients reported on by Pallanch et al[69] (1 month to 8 year follow-up), an overall 73% successful closure rate was noted. Of the 34 patients whose buttons were removed, roughly one third were due to persistent discomfort and one fourth due to poor fit. In those prostheses that were tolerated, the benefits most commonly reported were a reduction in epistaxis frequency, decreased crusting, and improved nasal breathing.

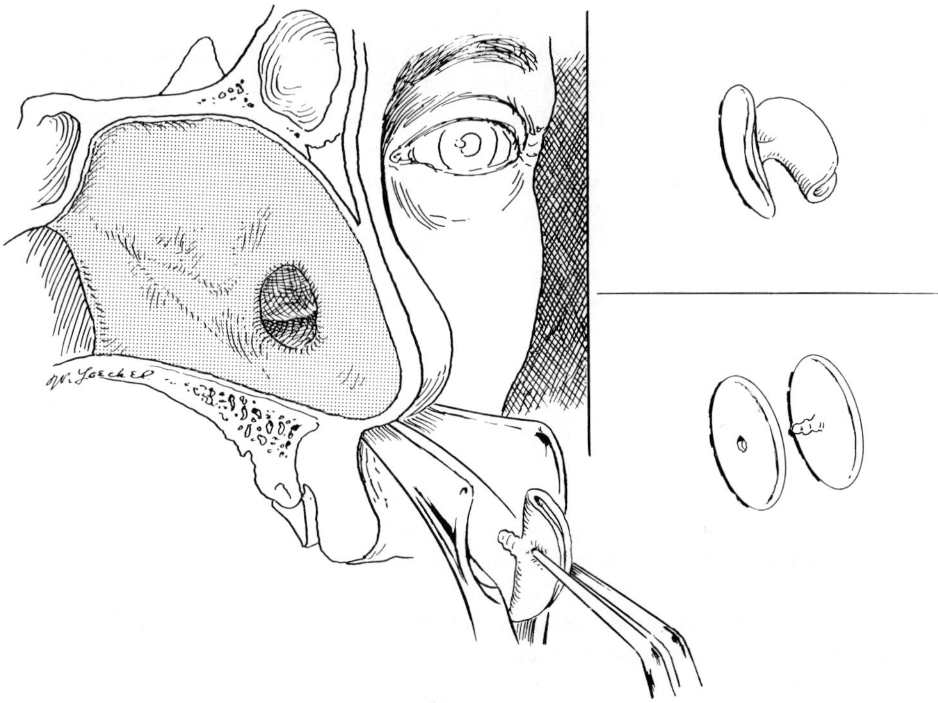

Figure 10–9. Mechanical obturation of septal perforation with Silastic button. (Top right). One-piece button. (Bottom right). Two-piece button.

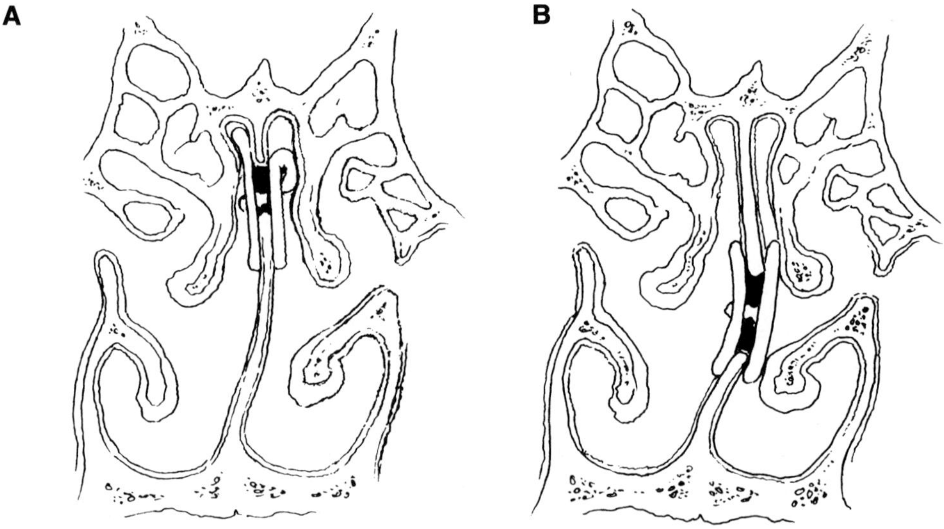

Figure 10–10. Anatomic difficulties encounterable with septal button placement. (A). Potential for prosthesis placement in upper nasal vault to interfere with valve function. (B). Septal deflections contributing to turbinate impaction following prosthetic placement.

Surgical Management

The indications for surgical repair of NSPs include symptomatic patients who fail conservative medical therapy and/or do not tolerate or wish to be considered for prosthetic obturation. Proper preparation of the septal and nasal tissues is essential preoperatively because marginal closure of the perforation with local flaps and free grafts is dependent on unimpeded wound healing. Measures that reduce dryness and crusting, local inflammation and/or infection, and repeated local mucosal trauma will facilitate the repair process.

Multiple surgical approaches have been advocated in the literature using a plethora of flap designs. Underlying each of these treatment modalities, however, are several essential tenets: (1) the base of the mucosal flap(s) should be patterned axially to dominant septal vessels (ethmoidal, sphenopalatine, septal branch of superior labial); (2) surgical exposure should be optimized; and (3) adequate mobilization of the mucosal tissues most be ensured to permit a tension-free coaptation.

Septal perforations may be accessed through four basic routes, each possessing its own inherent advantages and disadvantages. The decision to choose a given approach is usually guided by prior experience, technical facility, and size and location of the perforation. The standard endonasal approach usually combines a hemitransfixion incision with a variety of intranasal mucosal incisions to develop flap coverage (Fig. 10–11). The simplicity of the approach, limited incisions, and reduced operative time provide compelling reasons for its application in small (<2 cm) anteriorly located NSPs. Larger more posteriorly positioned NSPs present technical problems related to depth of field, shadowing, and difficulties related to instrumentation (particularly suturing of flaps and elevation of intact mucoperichondrium posterior to perforation). The use of adjunctive alarotomy to facilitate closure of inferior[67] and anterior[65] NSPs has been described to assist in exposure.

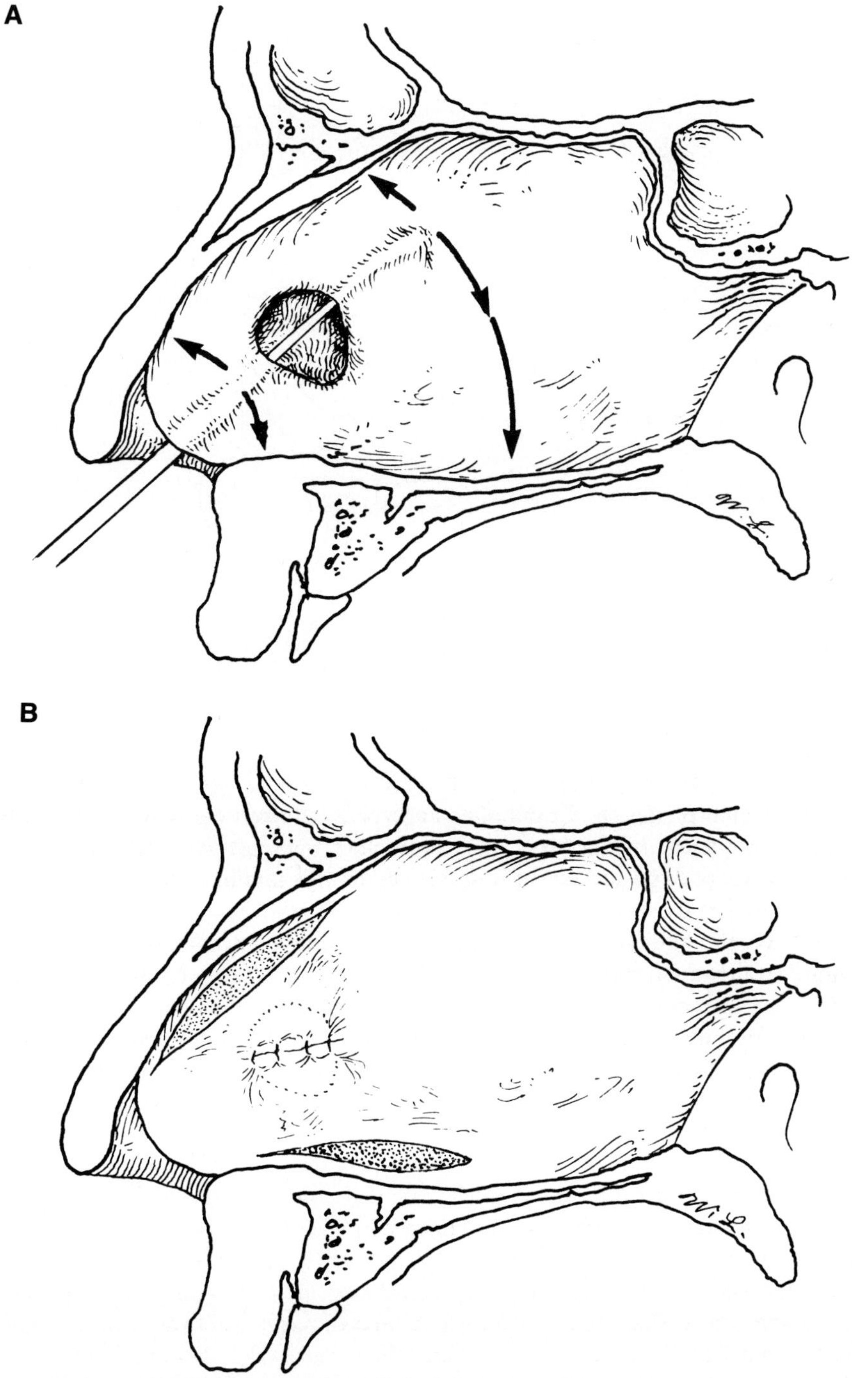

Figure 10–11. Commonly employed advancement and rotation flaps for septal perforation closure. (A). Circumferential mucosal undermining about septal perforation via hemitransfixion incision. (B). Superior and inferior relaxing incisions for direct mucosal advancement. (Figure continued on next page.)

C

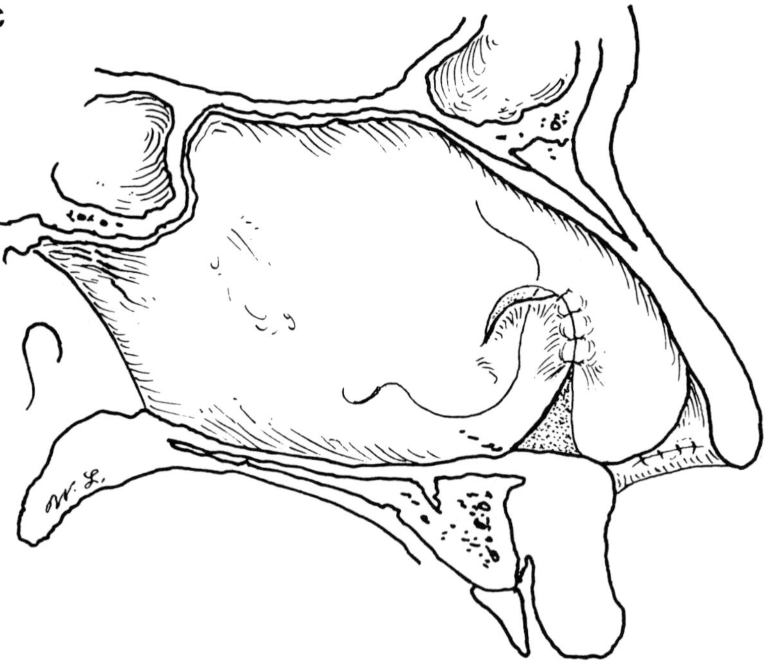

Figure 10–11. *Continued.* (C). Posteriorly based mucosal rotation flap.

The application of the open rhinoplasty approach adopted by Strelzow and Goodman,[75] and subsequently by Kridel et al,[76] overcomes many of the problems related to superior and posterior exposure for larger perforations. By dividing the ULC extramucosally, and separating the lower lateral cartilages (LLC) from their septal attachment, a more direct access to both sides of the septum from above is afforded (Fig. 10–12). The ability to reflect the septal flaps laterally, thereby providing a broader area for instrumentation, provides opportunity for suturing on the septal, nasal, or both sides of the mucoperichondrial/mucoperiosteal flaps. The ability to perform limited rhinoplastic procedures concurrently and the enhanced teaching of residents in academic settings have also been cited as advantages of this approach. Disadvantages include prolonged nasal tip edema and hypoesthesia, columellar scarring, and the potential for alar retraction, asymmetry, and nasal valve dysfunctions (with improper exposure/closure technique). Kuriloff[71] described a technique for lifting the medial crura and columella as a unit in an effort to obviate the tip swelling and numbness associated with the classic approach.

The sublabial-transnasal approach was advocated by Karlan et al[77] as a means of reliably closing large NSPs. They used a gingivolabial incision with submucoperiosteal elevations of the vomer, floor of nose, and lateral inferior nasal wall to develop a periosteal flap based on the septal branch of the superior labial artery (Fig. 10–13). This approach provides direct access to the pyriform aperture and facilitates the development of widely based flaps from the nasal floor. By releasing tension on the base of the flap anteriorly, greater mobility of the flap is afforded. Disadvantages include increased upper lip swelling and constraints similar to the endonasal approach for posterosuperior dissection and

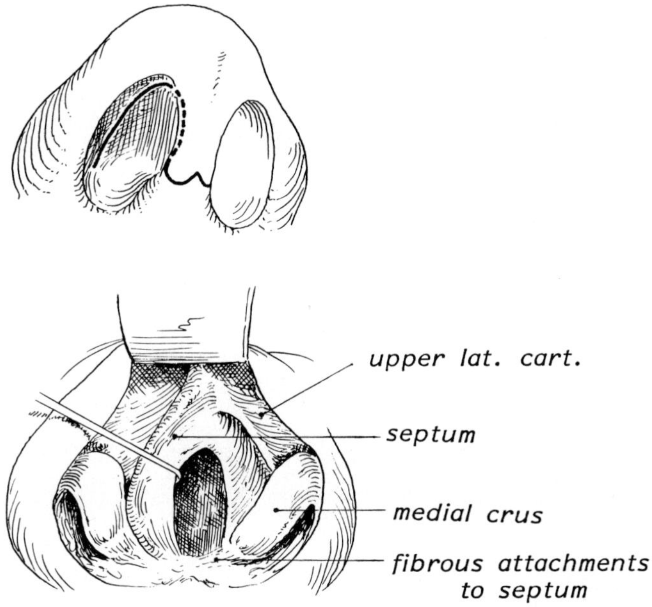

Figure 10–12. Open rhinoplasty approach for closure of septal perforation. Rethi-type external incision combined with marginal incisions (top) illustrated with submucoperichondral separation of ULC and LLC from dorsal and caudal cartilaginous septum, respectively.

suturing. The ability to instrument from above (through either nare) and below concurrently, however, provides decided advantages over the limited exposure associated with the endonasal approach.

Romo et al[78] adopted a midfacial degloving technique for the repair of large NSPs. By providing circumferential exposure of the nasal cavity at the level of the pyriform aperture, a panoramic view of anterior and midseptal perforations is possible (following medial detachment and retraction of the ULC). Development of local flaps from the nasoseptum and floor is facilitated by direct exposure and posterior suturing is made easier by the resultant short transnasal distances. Disadvantages cited by the authors include: (1) need for general anesthesia: (2) longer operative time; (3) greater intraoperative blood loss; (4) potential injury to the infraorbital nerves; and (5) requirement for a postauricular (or other) skin graft to the nasal floor to minimize the risk of vestibular stenosis.

The principles of mobilizing local mucosal and cutaneous tissue, although maintaining an intact blood supply, have been admonished in the literature through the use of advancement, rotation, and transposition flaps. In a comprehensive review of 90 NSPs, Younger and Blokmanis[79] concluded that bilateral rotation or advancement flaps were statistically more successful techniques than unilateral or transpositional flaps, likely secondary to their more favorable width to length ratios. Previously, Fairbanks[64] had observed accelerated healing times with bilateral flap closures.

Direct septal mucosal advancement flaps are generally applicable for small (1 to 1.5 cm) septal defects. Because the amount of mucosa available for closure is inversely proportional to the diameter of the perforation, a midseptal location (with respect to the vertical axis) would more equally distribute the donor tissue requirements for closure.

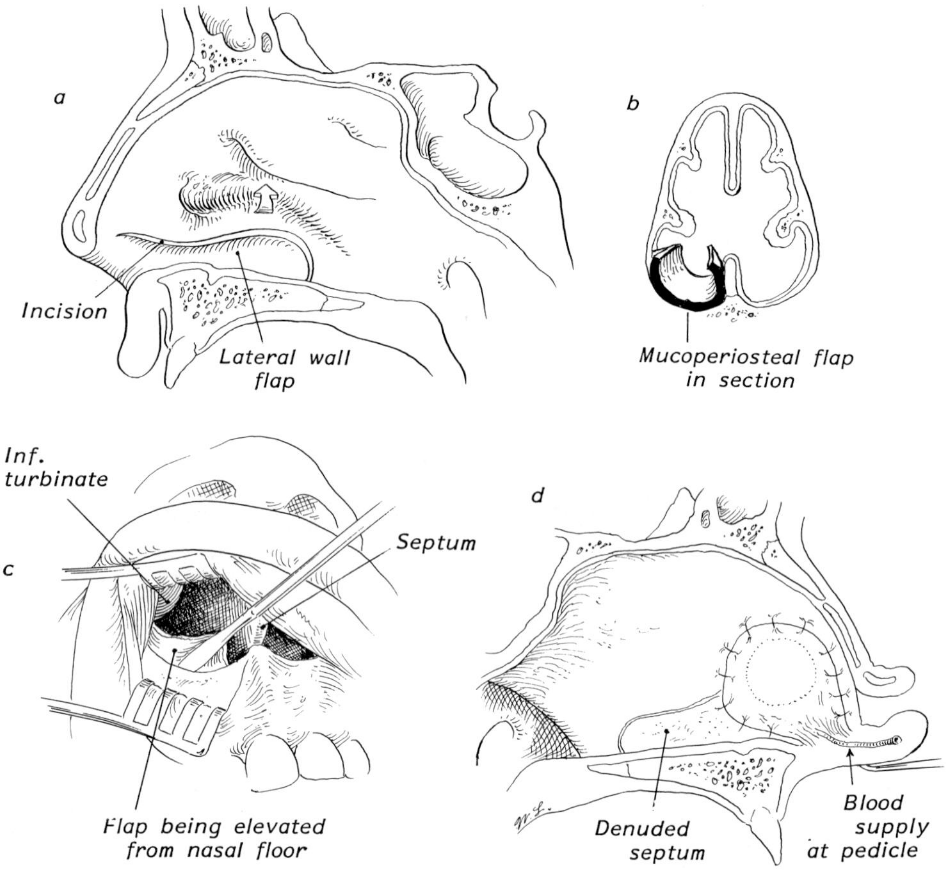

Figure 10–13. Sublabial-transnasal approach for flap closure of anterior septal perforation. (a). Internal lateral view of right nasal cavity demonstrating lateral wall incision and infractured inferior turbinate (arrow) for exposure. (b). Coronal view of nasal floor component of submucoperiosteally developed flap. (c). Sublabial exposure for direct access to pyriform aperture (labial attachment to flap has been omitted for illustration purposes). (d). Sagittal view of right septum following transposition and closure with septal branch of superior labial artery providing axial blood supply.

Perforations located higher in the nasal vault would require more extensive mobilization of mucosal tissue from below with greater surface area requirements for closure. With a longitudinally oriented bipedicle design, mobility is counterbalanced between the obligate anterior and posterior tethering at the base of the flaps and the extent to which relaxing incisions can release these tissue tensions without compromising the incoming blood supply (Fig. 10–14). Inherent in this technique, therefore, is broad mucoperichondrial undermining and the use of appropriately placed relaxing incisions. Horizontally oriented perforations are optimally suited to incisions placed superiorly (junction of ULC and septum) and inferiorly (adjacent to maxillary crest) whereas vertically oriented perforations lend themselves to anterior and posterior relaxing incisions.[75] The use of "mucosal steal," as advocated by Kridel et al,[80] may provide additional tissue from the contralateral side of the perforation but is often unreliable because of the attenuated hypovascular nature

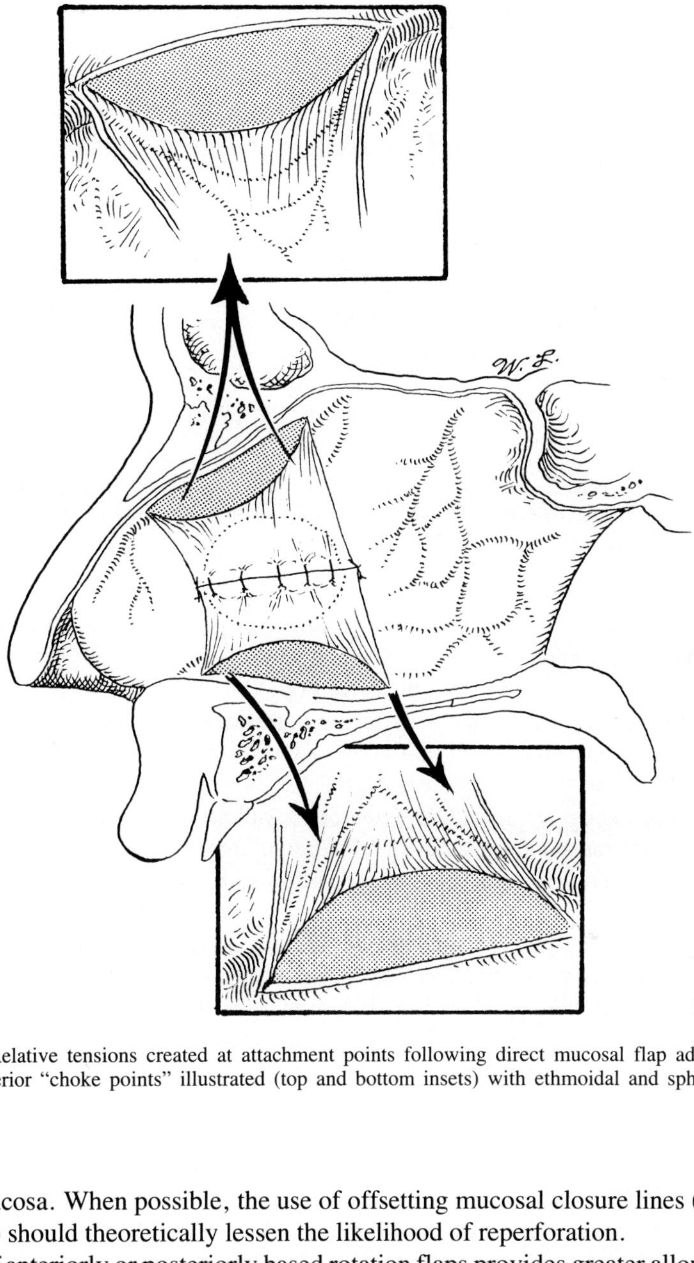

Figure 10–14. Relative tensions created at attachment points following direct mucosal flap advancement. Anterior and posterior "choke points" illustrated (top and bottom insets) with ethmoidal and sphenopalatine vessels (stippled).

of marginal mucosa. When possible, the use of offsetting mucosal closure lines (on either side of septum) should theoretically lessen the likelihood of reperforation.

The use of anteriorly or posteriorly based rotation flaps provides greater allowance for mucosal coverage by virtue of harvesting inherently stronger mucoperiosteal tissue from the floor of nose, inferior meatus, and medial aspect of the inferior turbinate, if needed. Belmont[65] advocated a posteriorly based mucoperiosteal flap developed on the side of the hemitransfixion incision. After resecting the anterior two thirds of the inferior turbinate, a 35-mm wide flap was raised. For anterior (within 1 cm of membranous septum) or very long perforations, Karlan et al[77] preferred an anteriorly based flap from the septal branch of the superior labial artery. This design provides a potential advantage should a dehis-

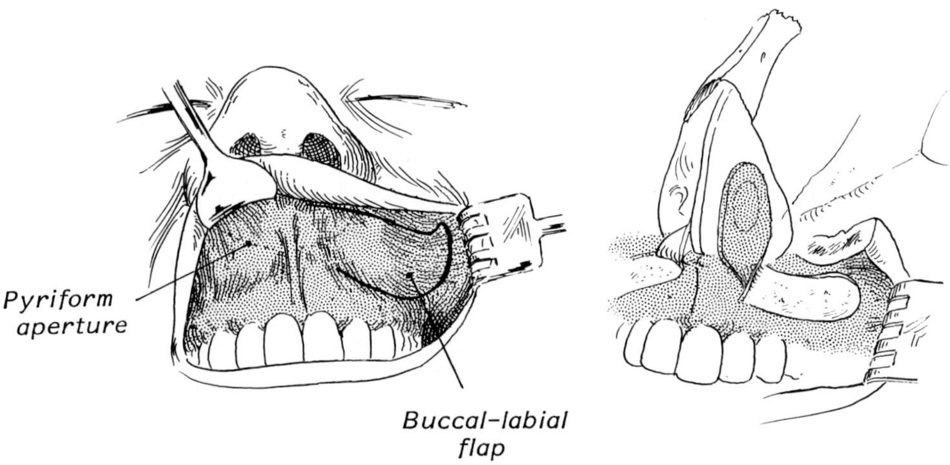

Figure 10–15. Buccolabial transposition flap. (Left). Gingivolabial and gingivobuccal incisions outlined before transposition. Note more medial extension of upper limb to facilitate transposition and provide wider flap base. (Right). Flaps transposed over pyriform aperture and into septal defect.

cence develop along the mucosal closure line because small posterior perforations generally remain asymptomatic.

Transposition flaps require, by definition, the crossing of an intermediary tissue bridge. When used to close a septal perforation, this may result in burying mucoperiochondrium (posterior inverting septal flap[81]), the necessity of a two-stage procedure for pedicle division (nasolabial flap[81]), or the potential for autostrangulation of a tunneled mucosal flap (buccolabial flap[82,83]). Although the buccolabial flap (Fig. 10–15) is the most commonly utilized transposition flap for closure of larger (2 to 4 cm) NSPs, it has the disadvantages of greater bulk, more limited flap width, tendency for contraction over time (in contrast to mucoperiosteal flaps), and a more tenuous submucosal blood supply (in contrast to axial-patterned mucoperichondrial/mucoperiosteal flap designs).

The introduction of the connective tissue intraseptal autograft by Fairbanks and Chen[83] significantly enhanced the predictability and ultimate success of NSP repairs. In 1980, Fairbanks[64] reported a 95% closure rate employing bipedicled mucosal advancement flaps with a fascial or pericranial autograft at 1 to 7 years follow-up. These results were consistent with those of Younger and Blokmanis[79] who noted in their 90 case review an 80% closure rate for small and medium-sized perforations when tissue grafts were utilized (in contrast to 35% success rate without). Kridel et al[76] have pointed out that periosteum, unlike fascia, does not tend to curl and therefore has better handling characteristics with regard to placement and suturing.

The enhanced surgical repair results with interposition grafts are explainable on several counts: (1) Because the free tissue autograft possesses low metabolic requirements, it can be sustained in areas of marginal perfusion (closure lines, perforation edges); (2) the connective tissue graft lends internal stability to the repair and provides a framework for reepithelialization; and (3) its use precludes the need to ensure complete mucosal coverage on both sides of the septum as long as one side of the tissue graft is completely covered. According to Wright,[84] a 2-cm perforation may require up to 2 months for complete reepithelialization.

NASAL VALVE DYSFUNCTION

Anatomic derangements resulting from external nasal trauma, sufficient to displace the bony pyramid, are often associated with some degree of nasal obstruction beyond the acute reactive phase. More marked internal displacements of the nasal bones are generally required, however, to significantly alter nasal resistances. This is in contrast to the nasal valve area, which often becomes dysfunctional with relatively minor deviations of the nasal valve angle. It is generally appreciated that most abnormalities of the nasal valve region result from narrowing of the valve angle secondary to septal deflections, followed in frequency by ULC disturbances and posttraumatic scarring.[85]

Compromised valvular function following nasoseptal trauma often results from direct fracture injury to the upper one-third of the nasal vault with secondary internal displacement of the ULC and/or direct avulsion injuries to the ULC itself (less common). Dislocation of the ULC is more commonly unilateral and may cause a "flutter valve effect" during inspiration as a result of internal prolapse toward the nasoseptum.[86] If unrecognized and/or uncorrected, fibrous adhesions and internal webbing may develop at the level of the limen nasi leading to regulatory disturbances of inspiratory airflow and subsequent problems related to nasal obstruction.

Blunt or penetrating injuries that weaken or disrupt the caudal attachment of the ULC or the lateral attachment of the alar cartilage can result in an inward rotation of the respective cartilages limiting valve mobility. In their review of 304 cases of Moh's surgery involving the nasal unit, Robinson and Burget[87] categorized various defects according to anatomic site, diameter, and depth of resection. Utilizing 5-year follow-up data, they demonstrated a strong association of nasal obstructive symptomatology and defects of the lateral sidewall or alae that were greater than 1 cm diameter and within 1 mm of the alar crease. It can be concluded that recognition and reconstitution of these key anatomic regions are paramount to maintaining baseline physiological nasal function.

Anatomic Considerations

Mink[88] is credited with the first description of the nasal valve, which he applied to the junctional area between the ULC and LLC, representing the site of greatest internal nasal resistance. Employing static model systems and spirometric techniques, Van Dishoeck[89] supported Mink's notion of the nasal valve location at the level of the limen nasi. In an elaborate series of experiments using maximum inspiratory pressure flow methodology, Bridger[90] and Bridger and Proctor[91] defined a "flow-limiting" segment (FLS) corresponding to a triangular aperture 0.5 to 1.0 cm proximal to the junction of the ULC and septum. They compared the behavior of this collapsible segment to a Starling resistor and emphasized the interdependence of nasal valve rigidity/elasticity and changes in critical transmural pressures. Kern[85] determined the normal range of the nasal valve angle to be 10 to 15°. He distinguished this entity from the nasal valve area, which circumscribes the region of the caudal end of the ULC, with its dense fibrous attachment to the septum medially, to its junction laterally with the pyriform aperture. Owing to the presence of fibrofatty tissue, and a variable sesamoid complex in the external lateral nasal wall adjacent to the pyriform aperture, this area represents an inherently weak point in valvular support.

The ULCs receive their greatest support rostrally, where they may underlie the nasal bones for as much as 11 mm,[86] as well as medially, where firm fibrous connective tissue attachments maintain a septal relationship between respective perichondrial ensheathments. Because the caudal end of the ULC also underlies the cephalic border of the LLC, a rigid, outwardly curving orientation of the latter will contribute to additional support of the nasal valve area. Additionally, the phasic activity of the nasal dilator muscles (anterior and posterior dilator naris, levator labii superioris alaque nasi, alar portion of nasalis, depressor septi) counterbalances the tendency for inward collapse of the cartilaginous vault during deep inspirations. The importance of these muscles is underscored by the observations of Van Dishoeck[92] who noted a fourfold increase in nasal resistance associated with forced inspirations in cases of unilateral facial palsy. Despite these supportive mechanisms, the middle one third of the nose maintains a relative mobility (although less so than the lower one third), which consequently affords some degree of protection against blunt external trauma.

Classification

The literature is replete with descriptive references to conditions contributing to functional abnormalities of the nasal valve, yet few reports detail a classification system sufficiently comprehensive that can be easily remembered and cogently applied to clinical diagnosis. Kasperbauer and Kern[93] provided a complex pathologic and clinical classification schema that highlights the variety of anatomic conditions and sites that impact on nasal valve function. More recently, Fanous[94] has simplified the clinical classification of anterior nasal collapse (ie, lateral wall collapse of anterior nasal passages).

Anatomically, anterior collapse can be subdivided into nostril rim, vestibular, and valve collapse. With nostril rim collapse, the external nasal aperture narrows, typically at small negative intranasal pressures, owing to loss of lateral alar rim support. This condition is usually associated with surgical modifications of the lateral crus (excessive volume reduction of cephalic portion or overaggressive rim strip division), and is most likely to occur in patients with narrow elongated nostrils, projected nasal tips, thin skin, underdeveloped alar cartilages, and LLCs with inward curvatures. Vestibular collapse pertains to narrowing of the lateral cartilaginous wall (mainly lateral crus) rendering a slitlike appearance to the nostrils. This circumstance most commonly follows iatrogenic disruption of lateral crural support (ie, lateral extension of intercartilaginous incision, resection of major portion of lateral crus) but may be a component of medial maxillary fractures with inward displacement of a mobile segment. Valvular collapse refers to narrowing of the internal nares due to collapse of the superior cartilaginous vault giving the central portion of the nose a pinched appearance. The conditions leading to abnormalities in this area have been well described[95–98] and usually result from excessive shortening of the caudal ends of the ULCs, excessive narrowing of the nasal vault following infracture, web/stricture/synechial formation at the valve angle, or internal displacements subsequent to nasomaxillary fractures or primary avulsion injuries.

Fanous[94] further subdivided anterior nasal wall collapse pathologically into flaccid and rigid types (referring to a mobile or immobile lateral nasal wall, respectively). Medial wall intrusion, or pseudocollapse, refers to narrowing of the anterior nasal canal secondary to changes in structure and/or position of the anterior septum or columella.

Physiological Considerations

In his classic article, Bridger[90] provided considerable insight into the function of the nasal valve, which serves as a regulator of nasal airflow and resistance. Comparing the internal nose to a rigid tube (osseous nasal cavity), and the external nose to a short collapsible FLS (cartilaginous vault), he purported the nasal valve behaves like a Starling resistor influenced by Bernoulli forces. In this model, nasal airflow across the FLS would be proportionate to the product of the transmural pressure difference (change in pressure = atmospheric pressure minus intranasal pressure) and upstream (toward external nares) resistance(s). Within a defined range of change in pressure, nasal airflow will vary directly with increases in the transluminal pressure gradient. As the pressure gradient becomes larger (owing to increased inspiratory flow rates or increased upstream resistances) the forces acting on the nasal valve area tend to favor collapse. It is at this critical transmural pressure (CTP) that the nasal valve behaves like a Starling resistor and further increases in inspiratory effort do not result in further increases in nasal airflow. This model correctly predicts, therefore, that obstruction distal to or at the level of the nasal valve (ie, hypertrophic turbinates, nasoseptal deviations, synechiae, webs, etc) or weakened support of the valve itself will predispose to smaller CTPs and a reduction in maximal obtainable nasal airflows.

Using anterior mask rhinomanometry in 38 subjects in whom transmural pressure differences and intranasal resistances (total, upstream, and downstream) were obtained, Bonilla et al[99] demonstrated the relationship between nasal obstructive symptomatology and collapsibility of the nasal valve as a function of alterations mainly in upstream and not downstream resistances. The mechanism by which this occurs is explainable by a loss of resiliency of the cartilaginous and fibrous connective tissue in the nasal valve area. Because the first 2 to 3 cm of the nasal cavity represents the area where the pressure drop across the nose is nearly complete,[100] it stands to reason that small alterations in the size or integrity of the nasal valve will have a marked influence on its collapsibility.

Physiological differences in regulation of inspiratory nasal airflow vary with morphometric features and genetic predisposition. In the platyrrhine nose, the FLS lies between the nasoseptum and the anterior portion of the inferior turbinate, with the largest diameter of the ostium internum oriented horizontally. This corresponds to the 4 mm average greater pyriform interaperture distance found between Negro and Caucasian skulls in Williams' study.[101] By contrast, in the leptorrhine nose, the nasal valve represents the narrowest part with the long axis of the os internum oriented vertically.

Clinical Evaluation

Surgical intervention directed at normalizing nasal valvular function must be site specific and determined by careful history and objective clinical determinations. A history of external trauma or surgical intervention that temporally correlates with subjective nasal obstructive symptomatology should be elicited. Knowledge of the direction, magnitude and mechanism of injury, or nasoseptal structures modified/removed (ie, as in rhinoplasty) will often lend insight into the clinical diagnosis. Comorbid factors such as inhalent allergy, endocrine dysfunction, chronic sinusitis, medication effect, alterations of the nasal cycle, and psychogenic causes must be distilled from the history.

Examination should begin with external inspection, focusing particularly on the overall nasal shape (tip projection, rotation, alar base dimensions and orientation, width of osseocartilaginous vault), symmetry, and consistency of the investing integument (ie, skin thickness). Observations of the rate and depth of nasal breathing, and dynamic movements associated with deep inspiration, should be noted. Compromised integrity of the ULC and LLC may result in alar collapse with the clinical appearance of slitlike nostrils on basal view. If the collapse is limited to the ULC only, a pinched appearance to the central cartilaginous vault will often be appreciated in frontal projection. Finally, a history of nasal trauma, with the finding of an indentation between the ULC and nasal bone, may suggest an avulsive injury of the latter.[86]

Internal inspection should include careful evaluation of the septum for internal derangements (deflections, duplications, thickenings, bucklings) particularly in the nasal valve area and its upstream segment. The relationship of the septum with the caudal end of the ULC should be noted (normal 10 to 15°) in such a way as not to distort their normal configuration during the exam. Turbinate caliber, orientation, and degree of mucosal reactivity before and after topical decongestant treatment must be assessed to determine what contribution the "turbinal valve" may play in intranasal resistance. In general, high intranasal resistances, which exist prior to decongestion but which normalize following vasoconstriction application, suggest mucosal hyperactivity whereas the failure to improve often points to a fixed anatomic derangement.[102]

Several provocative maneuvers exist that may aid in establishing the locus/loci of obstruction. Elevation of the nasal tip will often improve subjective nasal breathing in patients with ptotic, boxy, heavy, or counterrotated nasal lobules by redirecting inspiratory air currents in a more streamline fashion over the inferior turbinate and through the middle meatus. The Cottle test has been described as a means of assessing midnasal cartilaginous vault instability.[103] By displacing and supporting the nasofacial skin outward with a finger, a positive Cottle sign is elicited if nasal airflow is improved and suggests primary dysfunction of the nasal valve. A negative Cottle sign is obtained if no improvement in airflow is achieved and implies an abnormality beyond the nasal valve proper (assuming nasal obstruction exists). Kern[85] further qualified test conditions of false-positive response, which may be seen with alar collapse, as well as false-negative responses that can exist with intranasal adhesions or stricture formation in the nasal valve area. Fanous[94] provided a means of clinically distinguishing alar from true valve collapse by use of a probe test. In this description, a positive probe test suggests a flaccid form of collapse and is obtained when a probe (intranasally placed) can easily mobilize a portion of the lateral nasal wall outward and effect a marked improvement in nasal breathing. A positive probe test, limited in position to the alar segment only, would therefore suggest alar collapse. Distinguishing the conditions that may lead to a false-negative Cottle sign can usually be made by careful inspection.

The relative changes in magnitude of nasal airflow can often be assessed following a given provocative maneuver by "poor-man's rhinomanometry" utilizing the cotton whisp method (Fig. 10–16). In this technique, a thin cotton whisp strip is held from the side, with the distal end 1 cm caudal and tangent to the alar base, opposite the nasal cavity to be tested. By observing the to and for movements of the cotton end, information concerning change following unilateral provocation (opposite side occluded) can be inferred. Simultaneous use of cotton whisps between nasal sides may offer comparative information. A more sophisticated and objective method to identify, localize, and quantitate nasal resis-

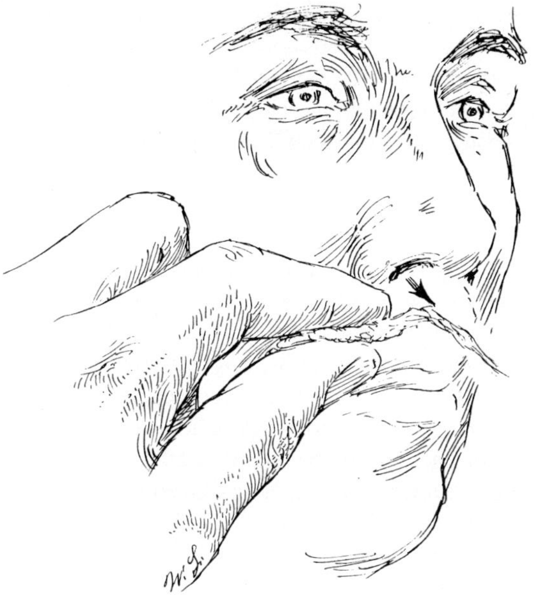

Figure 10–16. "Poor-man's" rhinomanometry using cotton whisp method to assess relative nasal airflow.

tance employs anterior rhinomanometry and has been popularized by Kern.[85,102] Through direct interpretations of the nasal pressure-flow curves (resistance indirectly derived), reversible (mucosal) and irreversible (structural) forms of obstruction can be distinguished, as well as the patterns consistent with alar or valvular collapse (plateau effect on inspiratory flow curve).

Surgical Management

Once arriving at a correct etiologic diagnosis for valvular dysfunction, surgical intervention may be aimed at correction of primary or secondary septal deviations, repositioning of the bony pyramid with its conjoined ULC, segmental reduction and stabilization of the ULC only, and/or lysis and stenting of intranasal synechiae, webs, or strictures. Because reactive subcutaneous/mucosal edema and turbinate hypertrophy often confuse the early clinical diagnosis of posttraumatic valvular derangement, operative manipulations are typically deferred for 5 to 7 days so that a more accurate assessment can be made. Following acute fracture displacement or avulsive injuries to the upper and midnasal vault, reduction and realignment should be accomplished within 2 weeks to avoid any significant callus or fibrous tissue response that may limit mobilization of the involved structures. In these cases, a standard closed nasal reduction approach with intranasal packing for 4 to 5 days is usually sufficient to reposition the malaligned lateral nasal wall segments.

When delayed recognition or presentation of valvular insufficiency exists subsequent to previous trauma, several conditions may be operative. The ULC may be deflected, thickened, or twisted near its medial attachment with the septum compromising its ability to function as a physiological valve. In these cases, Kern[85] has described a technique of conservative triangular wedge resection (apex oriented cephalically) of the caudomedial end of the ULC to enable the valve angel to open up (Fig. 10–17). Adequate intrinsic support and positioning of its more proximal attachments represent selective criteria for its use. In this procedure, an intercartilaginous incision is employed to directly access the ULC after sharp division of its aponeurotic attachments to the LLC. Following submucoperichondrial elevation over its dorsal surface, and extramucosal separation about its undersurface, the caudal aspect of the ULC may be effectively delivered into the nasal vestibule. Direct inspection and anatomic modification of its structure may then be effectively carried out.

Following traumatic avulsion, the ULC is typically displaced inward and maintained in a distorted angulated position by fibrous tissue attachments. Late treatment of this injury, as described by Parkes and Kanodia,[86] involves wide and complete undermining of the avulsed segment through an intercartilaginous incision. Following sharp release of all scar tissue attachments, reduction of the mobilized cartilage is accomplished bluntly, followed by internal and external splinting for 7 days. In those cases where cephalic bony attachment is present, the osseocartilaginous unit should be mobilized by fine narrow osteotomes after extending the plane of undermining beyond the fractured zone. Reduction is usually accomplished with a combination of a Boies elevator and Walsham forceps.

When the existent midnasal cartilaginous framework is inadequate to provide supportive function, either secondary to partial resorption and/or extensive scarring, then septal or conchal cartilage autografts may be strategically placed to lend mechanical stability. Several techniques exist for modifying structural support in this area. Bridger[104] described use of a split rib graft (1 to 1.5 mm thick) inserted percutaneously via the alar-facial crease to treat three cases of alar collapse. In this technique, the costal graft extended from the lateral bony vault to the cephalic margin of the LLCs. Obvious disadvantages of this approach include donor site morbidity associated with graft harvest, potential fullness created about the nasal sidewalls, an external scar placed in a nonshadow zone, and unnatural stiffness created in the lower cartilaginous vault.

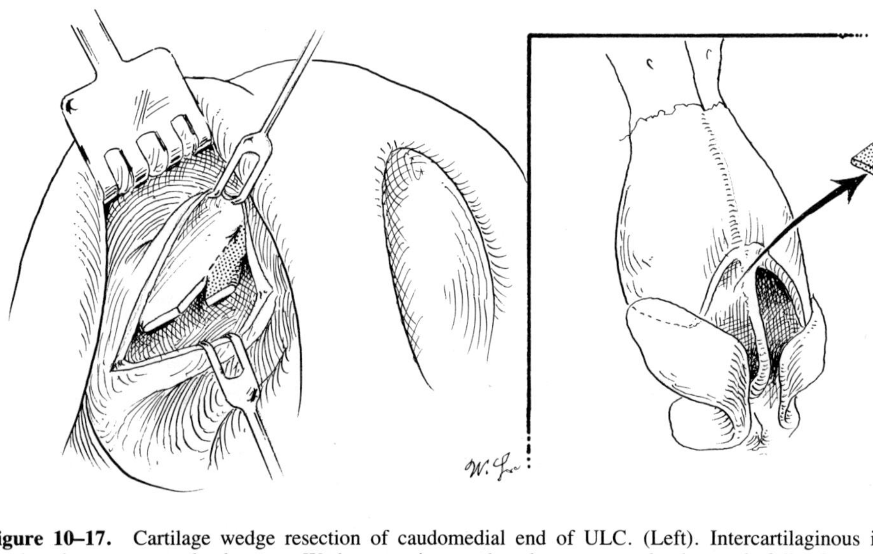

Figure 10–17. Cartilage wedge resection of caudomedial end of ULC. (Left). Intercartilaginous incision employed to access nasal valve area. Wedge resection employed to open nasal valve angle following submucoperichondral dissection.

The use of composite spreader grafts, interposed between the dorsal nasoseptum and medial edge of the ULC, has recently been described by Goode[105] for the management of valvular insufficiency secondary to loss of vestibular skin and cartilage. In his description, a composite graft measuring 10 to 12 mm × 6 to 8 mm is harvested from the upper concha, just below the inferior crus, and introduced parallel to the plane of the nasal sidewall through a closed approach. By controlling the width of the graft, lateral displacement of the ULC is achieved with increased transverse diameters of the entire nasal valve area. Similarly, if vestibular lining is adequate, but loss of medial cartilaginous support if present, placement of a narrower cartilage spreader graft (septal or conchal) only can be employed and oriented in a somewhat more transverse direction. In this configuration, the angular relationship between the nasoseptum and ULC at the valve angle is converted into a trapezoidal relationship providing intrinsic support and decreased likelihood of premature collapse (Fig. 10–18). Successful use of this technique alone is predicated upon the existence of sufficient supraalar support. An obvious tradeoff exists between the functional gain obtained from expansion of the valve angle and asesthetic compromise secondary to broadening of the cartilaginous dorsum.

In those cases where lateral support of the nasal valve area has been lost, conchal or septal cartilage batten grafts may be cantilevered off the middorsal septum, extending to the medial maxilla just above the alar crease. By placing the graft over the ULC remnant, resistance against inspiratory flaccid collapse is afforded. To prevent undesired medial displacement of the remaining ULC segment by the overlay graft, and to provide a more stable graft interface for support and revascularization, several tie-over sutures can be used from the septal/conchal onlay to the ULC to draw it outward (Fig. 10–19). A recent refinement introduced by Younger[106] employs a camber- inducing suture placed between

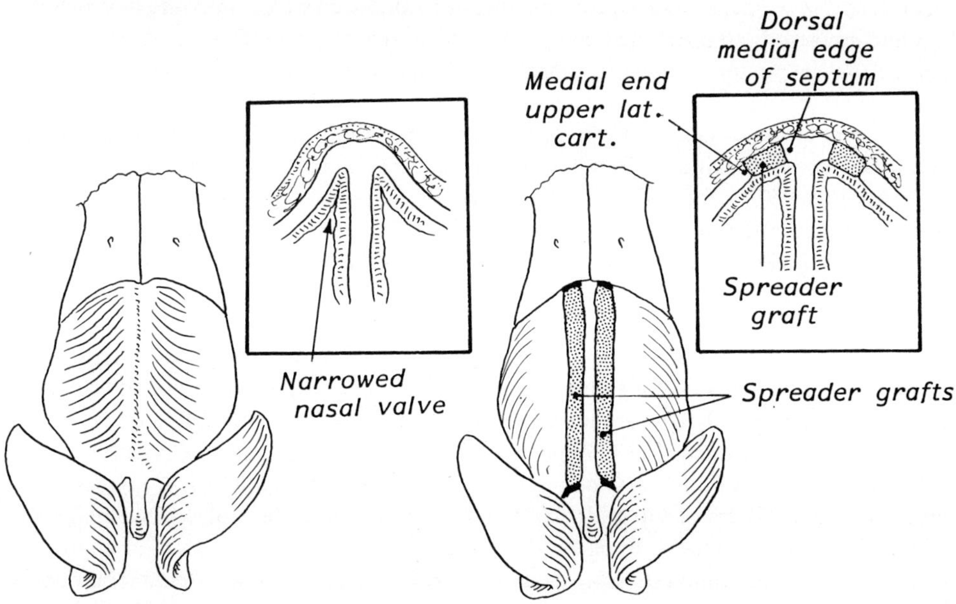

Figure 10–18. Spreader graft technique used to widen nasal valve angle. (Left). Preoperative valve relationship showing narrowing of valve angle. (Right). Postoperative effect on valve angle following intercalation of spreader grafts.

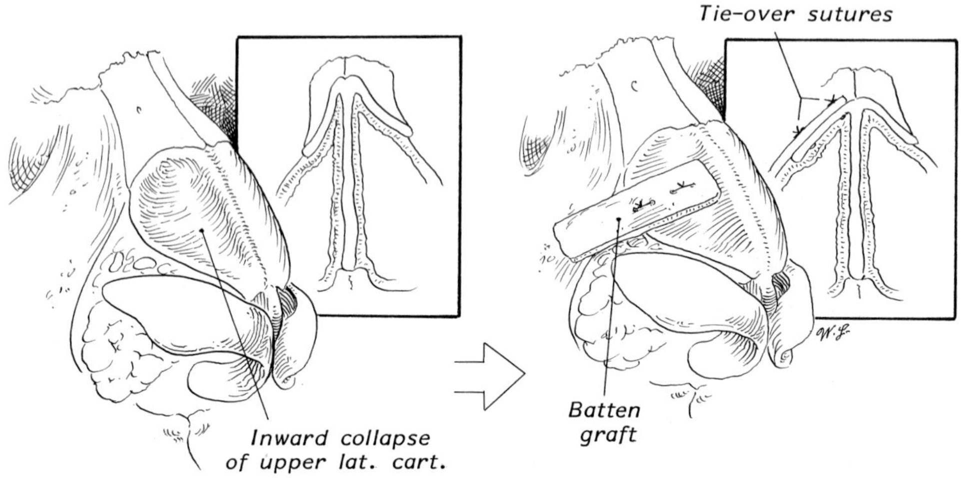

Figure 10–19. External support to collapsing nasal valve area afforded by cartilaginous batten grafts. (Left). Narrowed right nasal valve angle secondary to weakened ULC. (Right). Illustrated with stabilization obtained by fulcrumed graft.

the medial ends of two conchal battern grafts (3 to 8 mm lateral to the medial stabilization suture affixing the graft to the dorsal septum). By adjustments in the tension and mediolateral placement of the camber-inducing suture, a medial convexity can be created in the autograft, which resists flattening associated with healing forces.

The formation of intranasal adhesions (synechiae), webs, or areas of stenosis may occur in any area where there is proximity between abraded or lacerated mucosal surfaces. Left uncorrected, both functional and aesthetic disturbances may develop as scar contraction narrows inspiratory regulators (nasal or turbinal valves) or displaces mobile structure (cartilage vault components). Intranasal adhesions are easily managed by lysis immediately tangent to its surface of origin (to maximize gap width) followed by 1 to 2 weeks of intranasal stenting (bacitracin-impregnated Nugauze/Telfa or Silastic sheeting) depending on the severity. Whatever method is chosen, gentle tissue manipulation is imperative so as to avoid further mucosal injury.

Intranasal webs, by definition, involve greater surface areas of mucosal scarring and should be managed by excision and tissue replacement. Beekhuis[96] described a method of utilizing the web for intranasal closure by incising it vertically to create anterior and posterior flaps. Using a V-wedge key and lock design, the two flaps are interdigitated, thereby obviating the need for free tissue grafting. Goode[105] prefers to use full-thickness upper eyelid skin (sized 20% larger than defect to allow for shrinkage) placed via alotomy incision to enhance exposure. Although mucosal grafts represent viable alternatives to split or full-thickness skin grafts, several authors have commented on their less favorable take rates and thicker nature of the graft. Although Z-plasties have been described as a useful adjunct in the treatment of webs elsewhere (eg, epicanthal/commissural), their application intranasally is more limited (base of nasal valve rather than apex), the tissue requirements often exceed what is available, and technical execution can be difficult. For these reasons, the authors recommend direct excision of enough scar tissue to reestablish normal anatomic relationships after soft tissue undermining, followed by overlay skin grafting (upper eyelid/postauricular), and a 2-week period of stenting. Areas of stenosis associated with cartilaginous deficiencies are managed in a similar fashion but replaced with composite grafts harvested from the concha.

REFERENCES

1. Illum P. Long-term results after treatment of nasal fractures. *J Laryngol Otol*. 1986;100:273–277.
2. Courtiss EH, Goldwyn RM. The effects of nasal surgery on airflow. *Plast Reconstr Surg*. 1983;72:9–19.
3. Vaino-Mattila J. Correlations of nasal symptoms and signs in random sampling study. *Acta Otolaryngol*. 1974;318(Suppl):1–48.
4. McCaffrey TV, Kern EB. Clinical evaluation of nasal obstruction: A study of 1000 patients. *Arch Otolaryngol*. 1979;105:542–545.
5. Bachmann W. The present status of rhinomanometry. *Rhinology*. 1976;14:5–9.
6. Parkes ML. Functional sequelae of rhinoplasty. *Ann Plast Surg*. 1980;4:116–120.
7. Holt GR, Garner ET, McLarey D. Post-operative sequelae and complications of rhinoplasty. *Otolaryngol Clin North Am*. 1987;20:853–875.
8. Sherman AH. A study of nasal airway function in the post-operative period of nasal surgery. *Laryngoscope*. 1977;3:299–303.
9. Beekhuis GJ. Nasal obstruction after rhinoplasty: etiology and techniques for correction. *Laryngoscope*. 1976;86:540–548.
10. Roos R. L'obstruction nasale et les rhinites aperiodiques en Alsace. *J Med Strasbourg*. 1973;4:135–140.
11. Baker DC, Strauss RB. Intranasal injections of long acting corticosteroids. *Ann Otolaryngol*. 1962;71:525–531.
12. Allen GW. Vasomotor rhinitis: answer to a question. *JAMA*. 1982;248:988.
13. Johns KJ, Chandra AR. Visual loss following corticosteroid injection. *JAMA*. 1989;261:2413.
14. Nalebuff DJ. Allergic rhinitis. In: Cummings CW, ed. *Otolaryngology - Head and Neck Surgery*. St Louis, Mo: CV Mosby Co; 1993: chap 44.
15. Baker DC, Rees RD: Complications of rhinoplasty. In: Lewis JR, ed. *The Art of Aesthetic Plastic Surgery*. Boston, Mass: Little, Brown; 1989: chap 64.
16. Hinderer KH. Nasal problems in children. *Pediatr Ann*. 1976;5:499–509.
17. East CA, O'Donaghue G. Acute nasal trauma in children. *J Pediatr Surg*. 1987;22:308–310.
18. Holt GR. Immediate open reduction of nasal septal injuries. *Ear Nose Throat J*. 1978;57:345–354.
19. Maceri DR. Epistaxis and nasal trauma. In: Cummings CW, ed. *Otolaryngology - Head and Neck Surgery*. St Louis, Mo: CV Mosby Co, 1993: chap 41.
20. Olsen KD, Carpenter RJ, Kern EB. Nasal septum injury in children. *Arch Otolaryngol*. 1980;106:317–320.
21. Kern EB. Acute nasal trauma. In: Rees TD, ed. *Rhinoplasty Problems and Controversies: A Discussion with the Experts*. St Louis, Mo: CV Mosby Co, 1988: chap 44.
22. Fry JHJ. The pathology and treatment of haematoma of the nasal septum. *Br J Plast Surg*. 1969;22:331–335.
23. Meyer R. Secondary and functional rhinoplasty: the difficult nose. Orlando, Fla: Grune and Stratton: 1988;38.
24. Causabon JN, Dion MA, Larbrisseau A. Septic cavernous sinus thrombosis after rhinoplasty. *Plast Reconstr Surg*. 1977;59:119–123.
25. Coursey DL. Staphyloccal endocarditis following septorhinoplasty. *Arch Otolaryngol*. 1974;99:454, 455.
26. Gilden MH, Miller EM, Johnson WG. Central nervous system histoplasmosis after rhinoplasty. *Neurology* (Minneap). 1974;24:874–877.
27. Kubik CS, Adams RD. Subdural empyema. *Brain*. 1943;66:18–42.
28. Lacy GM, Conway H. Recovery after meningitis with convulsions and paralysis following rhinoplasty: cause for pause. *Plast Reconstr Surg*. 1965;36:254–256.
29. Lewin ML, Argamaso RV, Friedman S. Localized cerebritis following an esthetic rhinoplasty. *Plast Reconstr Surg*. 1979;64:720–723.
30. Thomas SM, Baird IM, Frazier RD. Toxic shock syndrome following submucous resection and rhinoplasty. *JAMA*. 1982;247:2402–2404.
31. Jacobson JA, Kasworm EM. Toxic shock syndrome after nasal surgery. *Arch Otolaryngol Head Neck Surg*. 1986;112:329–332.
32. Kemble JVH. The importance of the nasal septum in facial development. *J Laryngol Otol*. 1973;87:379–386.
33. Huizing EH. Implantations and transplantation in reconstructive facial surgery. *Rhinology*. 1974;12:93–106.

34. Pirsig W. Historical notes and actual observations on the nasal septal abscess especially in children. *Int J Pediatr Otorhinolaryngol*. 1984;8:43–54.
35. Maran AGD, Lund VJ. *Clinical Rhinology*. New York, NY: Thieme Medical Publishers; 1990: chap 2.
36. Haight JSJ, Cole P. The site and function of the nasal valve. *Laryngoscope*. 1983;93:49–55.
37. Wight RG, Jones AS, Beckingham E. Radical trimming of the inferior turbinate and its effect on nasal resistance to airflow. *J Laryngol Otol*. 1988;102:694–696.
38. Wight RG, Jones AS, Clegg RT. A comparison of anterior and radical trimming of the inferior nasal turbinates and the effect on nasal resistance to airflow. *Clin Otolaryngol*. 1988;13:223–226.
39. Courtiss EH, Goldwyn RM, O'Brien JJ. Resection of obstructing inferior nasal turbinates. *Plast Reconstr Surg*. 1978;62:249–257.
40. Thompson AC, Surgical reduction of the inferior turbinate in children: extended follow-up. *J Laryngol Otol*. 1989;103:577–579.
41. Mayell MF. Nasal fractures: their occurrence, management and some late results. *J R Coll Surg Edinb*. 1973;18:31–36.
42. Harrison DH. Nasal injuries: their pathogenesis and treatment. *Br J Plast Surg*. 1979;32:57–64.
43. Murray JAM, Maran AGD. The treatment of nasal injuries by manipulation. *J Laryngol Otol*. 1980;94: 1405–1410.
44. Murray JAM, Maran AGD, Mackenzie IJ, Raab G. Open v closed reduction of the fractured nose. *Arch Otolaryngol*. 1984;110:797–802.
45. Murray JAM, Maran AGD. A pathologic classification of nasal fractures. *Injury* 1986;17:338–344.
46. Fry HJH. Interlocked stresses in human septal cartilage. *Br J Plast Surg*. 1966;19:276–278.
47. Fry HJH. Nasal skeleton trauma and interlocked stresses on the nasal septal cartilage. *Br J Plast Surg*. 1967;20:146–158.
48. Facer GW. A blow to the nose. *Postgrad Med*. 1981;70:83–92.
49. Farrior R. Management of late sequelae of nasal fractures. In: Mathog RH, ed. *Maxillofacial Trauma*. Baltimore, Md: Williams & Wilkins; 1984: chap 20.
50. Goldman IB. When is rhinoplasty indicated for correction of recent nasal fractures? *Laryngoscope*. 1964;74:689–700.
51. Schultz RC, DeVillers YT. Nasal fractures. *J Trauma*. 1975;15:319–327.
52. Mathog RH. *Atlas of Craniofacial Trauma*. Philadelphia, Pa: WB Saunders Co; 1992: chap 49.
53. Goode RL, Spooner TR. Management of nasal fractures in children: a review of current practices. *Clin Pediatr*. 1972;11:526–529.
54. Gorney M. The septum in rhinoplasty. In: Rees TD, Baker DC, Tabbal N (eds). *Rhinoplasty Problems and Controversies: a Discussion with the Experts*. St Louis, Mo: CV Mosby Co, 1988; chap 31.
55. Rubin F. Permanent change in shape in cartilage by morselization. *Arch Otolaryngol*. 1969;89:602–608.
56. Wright W. Principles of nasal septal reconstruction. *Trans Am Acad Ophthalmol Otolaryngol*. 1969;78: 252–255.
57. Stucker FJ. Management of the scoliotic nose. *Laryngoscope*. 1982;92:128–134.
58. Thomas JR, Griner NR, Remmler DJ. Steps for a safer method of osteotomies in rhinoplasty. *Laryngoscope*. 1987;97:746, 747.
59. Webster RC, Davidson TM, Smith RC. Curved lateral osteotomy for airway protection in rhinoplasty. *Arch Otolaryngol*. 1977;103:454–458.
60. Rozner L. Nasal obstruction due to restriction of the bony nasal inlet. *Br J Plast Surg*. 1964;17:287–296.
61. Ismail HK. Closure of septal perforations. A new technique. *J Laryngol Otol*. 1964;78:620–623.
62. Frey HH, Weinang P. Zur Haufigkeit und Aitologie der Nasenseptum Perforation. *HNO*. 1968;16:33–35.
63. Fairbanks DNF, Fairbanks GR. Surgical management of large nasal septum perforations. *Br J Plast Surg*. 1971;24:382–387.
64. Fairbanks DNF. Closure of nasal septal perforations. *Arch Otolaryngol*. 1980;106:509–513.
65. Belmont JR. An approach to large nasoseptal perforations and attendant deformity. *Arch Otolaryngol*. 1985;111:450–455.
66. Facer GW, Kern EB. Nonsurgical closure of nasal septal perforations. *Arch Otolaryngol*. 1979;105:6–8.
67. Brain DJ. Septo-rhinoplasty: the closure of septal perforations. *J Laryngol Otol*. 1980;94:495–505.
68. Fairbanks DNF, Fairbanks GR. Nasal septal perforation: prevention and management: *Ann Plast Surg*. 1980;5:452–459.
69. Pallanch JF, Facer GW, Kern EB, Westwood WB. Prosthetic closure of nasal septal perforations. *Otolaryngol Head Neck Surg*. 1982;90:448–452.
70. Meyer R, Berghaus A. Closure of perforations of the septum including a single-session method for large defects. *Head Neck Surg*. 1983;5:390–400.
71. Kuriloff DB. Nasal perforations and nasal obstruction. *Otolaryngol Clin North Am*. 1989;22:333–350.
72. Gollom J. Perforation of the nasal septum. *Arch Otolaryngol*. 1968;88:84–88.
73. Bridger GP. Surgical closure of septal perforations. *Arch Otolaryngol Head Neck Surg*. 1986;112:1283–1285.

74. Goodman WS, Strelzow VV. The surgical closure of nasoseptal perforations. *Laryngoscope*. 1982;92: 121–124.
75. Strelzow VV, Goodman WS. Nasoseptal perforation - closure by external septorhinoplasty. *J Otolaryngol*. 1978;7:43–48.
76. Kridel RWH, Appling D, Wright WK. Septal perforation closure utilizing the external septorhinoplasty approach. *Arch Otolaryngol Head Neck Surg*. 1986;112:168–172.
77. Karlan MS, Ossoff R, Christu P. Reconstruction for large septal perforations. *Arch Otolaryngol*. 1982;108: 433–436.
78. Romo T, Foster CA, Korovin GS, Sachs ME. Repair of nasal septal perforation utilizing the midface degloving technique. *Arch Otolaryngol Head Neck Surg*. 1988;114:739–742.
79. Younger R, Blokmanis A. Nasal septal perforations. *J Otolaryngol*. 1985;14:125–131.
80. Kridel RWH, Appling WD, Wright WK. Closure of septal perforations: a simplified method via the external septorhinoplasty approach. In: Ward PH, Berman WE, eds. *Plastic and Reconstructive Surgery of the Head and Neck: Proceedings of the Fourth International Symposium. American Academy of facial plastic and reconstructive surgery*. Vol. 1. St Louis, Mo: CV Mosby Co; 1984:183–188.
81. Tipton JB. Closure of large septal perforations with a labial-buccal flap. *Plast Reconstr Surg*. 1970;46:514, 515.
82. Tardy ME. Sublabial mucosal flap: repair of septal perforations. *Laryngoscope*. 1977;87:275–278.
83. Fairbanks DNF, Chen SCA. Closure of large nasal septum perforations. *Arch Otolaryngol*. 1970;91:403–406.
84. Wright WK. Letter to the editor. *Arch Otolaryngol*. 1970;91:492, 493.
85. Kern EB. Surgical approaches to abnormalities of the nasal valve. *Rhinology*. 1978;16:165–189.
86. Parkes ML, Kanodia RJ. Avulsion of the upper lateral cartilage: etiology, diagnosis, surgical anatomy and management. *Laryngoscope*. 1981;91:758–764.
87. Robinson JK, Burget GC. Nasal valve malfunction resulting from resection of cancer. *Arch Otolaryngol Head Neck Surg*. 1990;116:1419–1424.
88. Mink PJ. Le nez comme voie respiratoire. *Presse Otolaryngol* (Belg). 1903;2:481–496.
89. Dishoeck van HAE. The part of the valve and turbinates in total nasal resistance. *Int Rhinol*. 1965;3:19–26.
90. Bridger GP. Physiology of the nasal valve. *Arch Otolaryngol*. 1970;92:543–553.
91. Bridger GP, Proctor DF. Maximum nasal inspiratory flow and nasal resistance. *Ann Otol Rhinol Laryngol*. 1970;79:481–488.
92. Dishoeck van HAE. Electrogram of the alar muscles and the nasal resistance curve. *Acta Otolaryngol*. 1937;25:285–295.
93. Kasperbauer JL, Kern EB. Nasal valve physiology. Implications in nasal surgery. *Otoalaryngol Clin North Am*. 1987;20:699–719.
94. Fanous N. Anterior nasal collapse: flaccid or rigid? An approach to clinical diagnosis. *J Otolaryngol*. 1990;19:110–113.
95. Stucker FJ, Smith TE. The nasal bony dorsum and cartilaginous vault. *Arch Otolaryngol*. 1976;102:695–698.
96. Beekhuis GJ. Nasal obstruction after rhinoplasty: etiology and techniques for correction. *Laryngoscope*. 1976;86:540–548.
97. Parkes ML, Borowiecki B, Binder W. Functional sequelae of rhinoplasty. *Ann Plast Surg*. 1980;4:116–120.
98. Adamson JE. Constriction of the internal nasal valve in rhinoplasty: treatment and prevention. *Ann Plast Surg*. 1987;18:114–121.
99. Bonilla JSD, McCaffrey TV, Kern EB. The nasal valve: a rhinomanometric evaluation of maximum nasal inspiratory flow and pressure curves. *Ann Otol Rhinol Laryngol*. 1986;95:229–232.
100. Proctor DF. State of the art. 1. Nasal physiology and defense of the lungs. *Am Rev Respir Dis*. 1977;115: 97–129.
101. Williams RI. The nasal index: anthropological and clinical. *Ann Otol Rhinol Laryngol*. 1956;65:171–189.
102. Kern EB. Evaluation of nasal breathing: an objective method. In: Rees RD, ed. *Rhinoplasty-Problems and Controversies*. St. Louis, Mo: CV Mosby Co; 1988: chap 23.
103. Heinberg CE, Kern EB. The Cottle sign: an aid in the physical diagnosis of nasal airflow disturbances. *Rhinology*. 1973;11:89–94.
104. Bridger GP. Split rib graft for alar collapse. *Arch Otolaryngol*. 1981;107:110–113.
105. Goode RL. Surgery of the incompetent nasal valve. *Laryngoscope*. 1985;95:546–555.
106. Younger RAL. Alar valvular collapse. *Operat Tech Otolaryngol. Head Neck Surg*. 1990;1:260–263.

Index